Health Communication Theory

Foundations of Communication Theory

The Foundations of Communication Theory series publishes innovative textbooks that summarize and integrate theory and research for advanced undergraduate and beginning graduate courses. In addition to offering state-of-the-art overviews in a broad array of subfields, authors are encouraged to make original contributions to advance the conversation within the discipline. Written by senior scholars and theorists, these books will provide unique insight and new perspectives on the core subdisciplinary fields in communication scholarship and teaching today.

Published
Health Communication Theory by Teresa L. Thompson and Peter J. Schulz
Organizational Change: Creating Change Through Strategic Communication, Second Edition by Laurie K. Lewis
Theorizing Crisis Communication, by Timothy L. Sellnow, Matthew W. Seeger

Forthcoming
The Work and Workings of Human Communication by Robert E. Sanders
Theorizing Crisis Communication, Second Edition by Timothy L. Sellnow and Matthew W. Seeger

Health Communication Theory

EDITED BY

Teresa L. Thompson

Peter J. Schulz

WILEY Blackwell

This edition first published 2021
© 2021 John Wiley & Sons, Inc.

The right of Teresa L. Thompson and Peter J. Schulz to be identified as the authors of the editorial material in this work has been asserted in accordance with law.

Registered Office
John Wiley & Sons, Inc., 111 River Street, Hoboken, NJ 07030, USA

Editorial Office
111 River Street, Hoboken, NJ 07030, USA

For details of our global editorial offices, customer services, and more information about Wiley products visit us at www.wiley.com.

Wiley also publishes its books in a variety of electronic formats and by print-on-demand. Some content that appears in standard print versions of this book may not be available in other formats.

Library of Congress Cataloging-in-Publication Data

Names: Thompson, Teresa L., editor. | Schulz, Peter J., 1958- editor.
Title: Health communication theory / edited by Teresa L. Thompson,
    University of Dayton, Professor Emerita Dayton, USA, University of
    Kansas, Edwards Campus Overland Park, USA, Peter J. Schulz, University
    of Lugano, Lugano, Switzerland.
Description: Hoboken, NJ : Wiley/Blackwell, 2021. | Series: Foundations of
    communication theory series | Includes bibliographical references and
    index.
Identifiers: LCCN 2020030502 (print) | LCCN 2020030503 (ebook) | ISBN
    9781119574439 (paperback) | ISBN 9781119574460 (adobe pdf) | ISBN
    9781119574507 (epub)
Subjects: LCSH: Communication in medicine.
Classification: LCC R118 .H4357 2021 (print) | LCC R118 (ebook) | DDC
    610.1/4–dc23
LC record available at https://lccn.loc.gov/2020030502
LC ebook record available at https://lccn.loc.gov/2020030503

Cover Design: Wiley
Cover Image: © didesign021/Getty Images

Set in 10/12.5pt CenturyStd by SPi Global, Pondicherry, India
Printed and bound by CPI Group (UK) Ltd, Croydon, CR0 4YY

10 9 8 7 6 5 4 3 2 1

To Steve and Connor....
Love, Teri/Mimi

To Magda and my sons Thomas E., Lukas P. and Markus J.
In gratitude, Peter

With warm thanks to Scott Poole
TT and PS

Contents

Contributors

Salah H. Al-Ghaithi, Department of Communication, University of Illinois at Urbana-Champaign

Austin S. Babrow, School of Communication, Ohio University

Maria Brann, Department of Communication, IUPUI

Jennifer J. Bute, Department of Communication, IUPUI

Andrea Martinez Gonzalez, School of Communication Studies, James Madison University

Evelyn Y. Ho, Department of Communication, University of San Francisco

Youjin Jang, Department of Communication, Michigan State University

Shaohai Jiang, Department of Communications and New Media, National University of Singapore

Hannah Jones, Department of Communication, Rutgers University

Maureen Keeley, Department of Communication Studies, Texas State University

Dannielle E. Kelley, National Cancer Institute

Arunima Krishna, Department of Mass Communication, Advertising, and Public Relations, Boston University

Yanqin Liu, Clinical Studies Unit, Mayo Clinic Arizona

Michael Mackert, Center for Health Communication, Stan Richards School of Advertising & Public Relations, Moody College of Communication

Marianne S. Matthias, Department of Medicine, Indiana University

Maria D. Molina, Department of Advertising and Public Relations, Michigan State University

Robin L. Nabi, Department of Communication, University of California, Santa Barbara

Rebekah H. Nagler, Hubbard School of Journalism and Mass Communication, University of Minnesota

Sarah M. Parsloe, Department of Communication, Rollins College

Sandra Petronio, Department of Communication, IUPUI

Rachyl Pines, Research Administration Department, Santa Barbara Cottage Hospital

Brian L. Quick, Department of Communication, University of Illinois at Urbana-Champaign

Tobias Reynolds-Tylus, School of Communication Studies, James Madison University

Anthony J. Roberto, Hugh Downs School of Human Communication, Arizona State University

James D. Robinson, Department of Communication, University of Dayton

Peter J. Schulz, Institute of Communication & Health, School of Communication, Culture and Society University of Lugano (Università della Svizzera italiana)

Barbara F. Sharf, Independent Scholar and Professor Emerita, Dept. of Communication, Texas A & M University

Brian G. Southwell, RTI International, Duke University, University of North Carolina at Chapel Hill

Anne M. Stone, Department of Communication, Rollins College

S. Shyam Sundar, Donald P. Bellisario College of Communications, Pennsylvania State University

Teresa L. Thompson, Professor Emerita, Department of Communication, University of Dayton

Yan Tian, Department of Communication and Media, University of Missouri-St. Louis

Jeanine W. Turner, Communication, Culture and Technology Program, Georgetown University

Monique Mitchell Turner, Department of Communication, Michigan State University

Shawn Turner, Department of Communication, Michigan State University

Bernadette Watson, Director, International Research Centre for the Advancement of Health Communication (IRCAHC), Department of English, The Hong Kong Polytechnic University

Jill Yamasaki, Jack J. Valenti School of Communication, University of Houston

Marco Yzer, Hubbard School of Journalism and Mass Communication, University of Minnesota

PART I

Perspectives on the Field of Health Communication

1

The Basics of Health Communication Theory

Teresa L. Thompson and James D. Robinson

Health problems are prevalent all over the world, and communication processes play essential roles in addressing these health problems. From Ebola, MERS, Zika, and COVID-19 to vaping and the opioid epidemic, various health crises must be confronted across the world on a constant basis. The area of study that has come to be called "health communication" is crucial as practitioners and scholars attempt to alleviate and minimize a multitude of health problems and improve health care delivery. Effective and useful health communication is foundational as we attempt to control the spread of disease and health problems.

Do *message strategies* that encourage people to manage their diet to control diabetes also inspire them to look more closely at vaccination decisions? In other words, can we generalize what we learn about health communication regarding one health problem to other health issues? Does the study of patient-centered communication have implications for mental health as well as physical health and illness? Does message targeting or tailoring allow the effective adaptation of anti-vaping messages to different audiences? These and other questions are conceptual and theoretical concerns that underlie health promotion and a broader

Health Communication Theory, First Edition. Edited by Teresa L. Thompson and Peter J. Schulz.
© 2021 John Wiley & Sons, Inc. Published 2021 by John Wiley & Sons, Inc.

understanding of health communication processes. Through health communication research one may understand not only how communication operates in relation to a particular health issue, but how health communication functions more broadly. Indeed, the ultimate hope is an increased understanding of communication processes across contexts and a healthier world.

As is evident in the title of this volume, the focus of this book is on the theories that we use to study health-related processes. Our goal is to help students, scholars, and practitioners more adequately examine health communication concerns by grounding their work in solid theory. We thus begin the volume by briefly defining health communication, health, health care delivery, and theory. We then talk about why theory is important in the study of health communication. We follow this with brief discussions of the traditions of health communication theory and generative tensions in health communication scholarship. This chapter concludes with a preview of the remainder of the book and a discussion of ethical concerns.

What is Health Communication?

It is frequently noted that the area of study that has become known as health communication began to emerge from research in the 1940s that looked at the persuasive impact of health information and promotion, although Salmon and Poorisat (2019) point to even earlier traditions from the field of public health. This work goes back to the development of germ theory and can be traced to the beginning of the twentieth century. Starting with newspapers and then moving to film, radio, and television, media campaigns about health issues began to appear. The emergence and refinement of social science research methods, including the development of Thurstone and Likert-type scales and sampling techniques à la George Gallup, was another central factor in the progress that was made during earlier decades of the twentieth century. Salmon and Poorisat (p. 1) identify four key factors that influenced and characterized this growth:

1. the early use of mass communication for public health campaigns (1900–1910s);
2. the search for effects (1920–1930s);
3. the search for explanation from interdisciplinary perspectives (1940–1950s); and
4. the formal recognition of health communication as a distinct and valuable field of practice and research (1960s).

The reader will see these influences reflected in the theories and chapters that follow.

The Stanford Heart Disease Prevention Program, which began in 1971, was also an important development in the history of health communication. During the early 1970s scholars such as Barbara Korsch and her colleagues (e.g. Korsch and Negrete, 1972) conducted work that served as the foundation of research on physician–patient communication. This work, published in such prestigious outlets as *Scientific American*, created interest within the broader field of communication. Some of this work was labeled "medical communication." Simultaneously, scholars building on the interactional view articulated in Watzlawick, Beavin, and Jackson's (1967) *Pragmatics of Human Communication* and further developing the conceptualization of communication processes offered by Gregory Bateson (1972) focused on what was called "therapeutic communication." These traditions came together beginning in the early-1970s to prompt the development of the new area of study called "health communication." The inception of the Health Communication Division of the International Communication Association in 1975 (following the founding of the Health Communication Interest Group in 1972) most clearly demarcated this new area of study. The movement within medicine, public health, and the social sciences from a biomedical approach to a biopsychosocial view was simultaneously occurring (see Ho and Sharf, Chapter 14 in this volume, for more discussion of this).

The area of health communication did not take long to develop. Books on the topic, most notably Kreps and Thornton's (1982) *Health Communication: Theory and Practice*, began to emerge in the early 1980s. By 1986, enough work was being conducted in the area that the publisher Lawrence Erlbaum Associates expressed interest in a journal on health communication. The first author of the present chapter, who is also the editor of the journal *Health Communication*, began soliciting submissions in 1987, and the first issue of the journal came out in January of 1989. The journal originally published four issues a year, but at the time of the writing of this chapter is publishing 14 lengthy issues a year. During 2019, the journal processed 776 submissions. Two hundred and nine issues of the journal have now been published. *Health Communication* was shortly followed by *The Journal of Health Communication: International Perspectives, Patient Education and Counseling, Journal of Communication in Healthcare, Communication and Medicine*, and several other outlets. The *Journal of Health Communication* began publishing in 1996. The first edition of the *Handbook of Health Communication* (chapters of which were translated into Korean) was published in 2003, and the second edition, *The Routledge*

Handbook of Health Communication was published in 2011. The third edition of the handbook is in press at the time of the writing and will be published in 2021. *The Sage Encyclopedia of Health Communication* came out in 2014. All of these publications are evidence of the rapid growth of this area of study.

International interest in health communication has also increased notably over the last three decades. This is reflected in the subtitle of the *Journal of Health Communication: International Perspectives*, but is really reflected in the work published in all the health communication outlets. The journals all receive and publish submissions from a variety of countries. As continents, Europe, Oceania (Australia and New Zealand), and Asia are particularly active in health communication scholarship, as is North America. Within Europe, scholars in the Netherlands, Switzerland, and the UK are highly involved in health communication research. The Asian countries of Korea, China, Taiwan, and Singapore are also replete with active health communication researchers. In North America, health communication research is conducted in both the US and Canada.

The initial issue of *Health Communication* included many invited pieces by such important scholars as Barbara Korsch, Gary Kreps, David Smith, and Jon Nussbaum. These pieces attempted to set the agenda for the field – and they did, continuing to be cited during subsequent decades. Several articles in the 100th issue of the journal referred back to these articles and identified the progress that had been made over the last 100 issues. Much advancement was, indeed, apparent. Many of the directions suggested by these scholars have now been actualized.

Early submissions to and publications in *Health Communication* tended to be atheoretical and offered relatively simplistic views on communicative processes, although not as simplistic as those that are still apparent in the research conducted today by submitters without a background in the social sciences. The quality and focus of most of the work that is now submitted to the journal has changed substantially in the 30-some years in which the journal has been publishing, and work is rarely accepted for publication without a guiding theoretical foundation.

As is the case with any area of study or phenomenon, varying definitions of health communication have been offered. The process of communication focuses on simultaneous, transactional message co-creation of meaning through interaction. Health communication focuses on such processes as they relate to and impact health and health care delivery. The primary areas of study that are the foci of health communication work include provider–patient communication, health campaigns and other types of health promotion, health information in the media, eHealth and mHealth, health risk communication, communicative processes within health organizations, and everyday health communication (see Kreps 2020, for more detailed discussion of many of these areas). Everyday health communication focuses on communication *about* health and as it *impacts* health among family members and friends, as opposed to that communication which takes place with formal health care providers and through mediated channels of communication (Cline 2011; Head and Bute 2018).

What are Health and Health Care Delivery?

Although most of us probably have an ordinary conception of health as a state of being disease-free, more precise conceptualizations of it have been offered. The World Health Organization defines health as "a state of complete physical, mental and social well-being and not merely the absence of disease or infirmity" (The World Health Organization 2020, n.p.). Please note the focus on mental and social issues as well as physical health.

Building on this, the US National Institutes of Health (NIH) defines health care delivery as "The concept concerned with all aspects of providing and distributing health services to a patient population" (NIH 2020, n.p.). Although this definition appears to focus on formal health care delivery, health communication scholarship goes well beyond this traditional emphasis. The best health communication work is that which is grounded in theory.

What is Theory? What is Health Communication Theory?

The term "theory" is used rather loosely in ordinary conversation ("I have a theory about why my brother is so messed up") but has a more precise meaning in scholarship. Once again, many different definitions are offered of theory. Put fairly simply, a theory is an attempt to explain a phenomenon or set of phenomena in a testable manner. It provides guidance for research and can serve as a lens or a map. It is a supposition that is based on past research. This makes it an educated guess.

It should not be tautological or based on circular reasoning. The theory should be independent of the phenomenon to be explained. Theories make predictions which are then testable.

Theory plays a different role in qualitative/interpretive research than it does in positivist/quantitative research. Whereas good quantitative research is typically grounded in and tests theory, qualitative research is more likely to generate theory. The goal of interpretive work is to reform society and generate understanding more than to test predictions and hypotheses. Jill Yamasaki (Chapter 3 in this volume) articulates this difference in more detail and makes clearer the role of theory in interpretive work.

Babrow and Mattson (2011) offered a useful definition of health communication theory in the 2nd edition of the *Routledge Handbook of Health Communication*. They define health communication theory "as consciously elaborated, justified, and uncertain understanding developed for the purpose of influencing practice related to health and illness" (p. 19). This will be our working definition of health communication theory in this volume.

Why Do We Need Health Communication Theory?

As is the case with any area of scholarly study, health communication work that is guided by a theoretical framework is stronger than work that is atheoretical. Some work that falls within the general category of health communication is problem-focused but not theoretically framed. Work that is based in theory is more systematic than is work that is problem-oriented but atheoretical. Work that is grounded in theory is generalizable beyond the particular context or health condition that was the focus of the original study. Good theories are not content- or health-problem-specific. They apply to broader communicative processes, not just to a particular health problem or in a particular setting. Good theory is, most importantly, practical and applicable to social concerns.

If a study on diabetes management is grounded in a perspective such as the theory of reasoned action, findings from that study will provide insights that scholars may apply to other health problems and contexts. Although generalizability is partially based on sampling, design issues, and ecological validity concerns, it is also based on theoretical framing.

Through the theoretical grounding of a study the broader base of knowledge is extended. This is the goal of scholarship. This is how a body of knowledge is built.

One of the more interesting examples of theory being extended into new areas of study is cybersecurity. If imitation is the sincerest form of flattery, theories of health and health communication should at least blush occasionally. Several theories discussed within this volume have gained theoretical traction in research on computer security.

Scholars studying how to motivate end users to engage in safe computer practices use the health belief model (Rosenstock 1974), the protection motivation theory (Rogers 1975), and the transtheoretical model (Prochaska and DiClemente 1983) to guide their research.

For example, Ng et al. (2009) found that perceptions of susceptibility, benefits, and feelings of self-efficacy were the best predictors of opening email attachments. The analogue of "don't click on links or open unexpected email attachments" in the realm of health is "maintain social distance and wash your hands." Viruses move through contact and malware moves through virtual contact or email.

Recently researchers from Carnegie Mellon (Faklaris, Dabbish, and Hong 2018) recognized the value of the transtheoretical model for designing security interventions. Their recommendations acknowledge that, just like the public in a general health information campaign, end users are not equally accepting or ready for making changes to their behavior. By targeting messages based on users' current readiness or stage of change, cybersecurity professionals may increase the effectiveness of their campaigns and training materials. Also important, developing targeted messages may help reduce the feelings of cyber-fatigue that are now recognized as the bane of security training efforts.

Training programs for avoiding phishing attacks and ransomware attacks require different lists of rules. It is no wonder that end users receiving information not targeted to their readiness produce fatalistic attitudes about cybersecurity training.

Fortunately, health communication theory has come to the rescue here, too. Recent research by Zhang and Borden (2019) employed the extended parallel processing model (Witte 1994) and found fear and anxiety mediated end-user behavior. Specifically, negative emotions were shown to influence the impact of threat on end-user intentions to comply and seek additional information. Efforts to motivate end-user cybersecurity behavior need to consider the role self-efficacy plays in the process. It remains to be seen how effective these theories will be, but it is clear scholars from other disciplines are looking to health and health communication for theoretical models. The next section of this chapter focuses on the different types of theories. The breadth and depth of these theoretical traditions have certainly helped us grow the discipline.

Traditions of Health Communication Theory

Much has been written about communication theory as an area of study over the last several decades. Perhaps the most frequently cited and well-known work on communication theory was published by Robert Craig (1999) in the journal *Communication Theory*. Among the many important points made by Craig is an insightful discussion of the multiple disciplines from which communication theory has developed. These varying disciplinary roots have led to rather different conceptualizations of the nature of theory and its application in the broad field of communication. Craig notes that acknowledging these differing roots is more fruitful than arguing about the validity of varying theoretical approaches. Craig identifies seven traditions of communication theory. His discussion has become foundational to our understanding of theory in the field of communication.

Building on this work, Babrow and Mattson (2003, 2011) identify how these traditions apply to health communication scholarship. They trace the following lines of research and knowledge in this discussion: (i) rhetorical ("the practical art of persuasive discourse", Babrow and Mattson 2011, p. 25); (ii) semiotic ("intersubjective mediation by signs and sign systems", p. 26); (iii) phenomenological ("communication as dialogue or experience of otherness", p. 26); (iv) cybernetic ("information processing by which systems are able to function", p. 27); (v) sociopsychological (a focus on behavior expressing psychological systems, states, and traits producing a variety of effects); (vi) sociocultural (symbolic processes producing and reproducing sociocultural patterns that are shared within a group); and (vii) critical traditions (which focus on "material practices and hegemonic ideologies that distort communication" p. 29). More of the theories to be discussed in the remainder of this volume focus upon sociopsychological and sociocultural traditions than on the other traditions (for exceptions see Ho and Sharf, Chapter 14 in this volume).

Understanding the conceptualization of communication and theory on which a particular theory is based is important in order to adequately assess the value of that theory and research.

Generative Tensions in Health Communication

Understanding theory in health communication is also directly related to comprehension of the "generative tensions" underlying the study of health communication (Babrow and Mattson 2011, p. 19). One of these tensions focuses upon the interplay of the body and communication that is inherent in the biopsychosocial turn that has been key to changes in views of medicine in the last few decades. The guiding principles after the turn are: Disease shapes communication. Communication shapes disease and other aspects of health. Social and cultural factors influence all aspects of health communication. How disease is defined and the manner in which we communicate about it determine how it is treated.

A second generative tension is related to this – the opposition between science and humanism. Contrasts between the potentialities of science vs the actualization of being human epitomize this. Babrow and Mattson (2011) exemplify this tension through a discussion of death and dying. The contemporary fear of mortality is but one factor that captures and typifies this tension.

The strain between idiosyncrasy and communality characterizes the third generative tension that they identify. The contrast between ontological and holistic views of medicine makes this apparent. Finally, the experience of uncertainty and values are central to the fourth generative tension described by Babrow and Mattson (2011). This tension will be most apparent in the chapter written by Babrow, Matthias, Parsloe, and Stone (Chapter 13 in this volume), which focuses on uncertainty management theories.

Preview of the Book

Many of the theories that are commonly used in health communication scholarship are applied across contexts and areas of health communication study. Dividing these theories into chapters is somewhat arbitrary, but it was necessary to do so in some manner in order to make the presentation of the theories manageable. We looked in part at the origins of various theories to shape the various chapters. All theories in the book are applied to the field of health communication but might originate elsewhere. Four origins can be distinguished: (i) theories developed in the field of *health communication* proper, (ii) theories developed in the context of *health* in general (and then specified or made useful in the more narrow area of health communication), (iii) theories developed in *communication* (and then also specified to health communication), and (iv) theories of provenance from fields *beyond health or communication*, but which are nevertheless applied in health communication. The book begins with an overview in Part I and then moves to narrower interpersonal contexts. We broaden the context from there.

Some of the conceptual constructs that frame health communication scholarship are not proper theories, per se, but function in ways similar to that which is found in theoretical scholarship. We elected to include them in Chapter 2 by Brian L. Quick et al. that follows this introduction and occasionally throughout the other chapters. These variables/processes are frequently used to segment audiences and allow the adaptation of messages. They include notions such as tailoring and targeting health messages based on demographic, geographic, psychographic, and behavioral considerations. Other individual difference variables are also used and discussed in the chapter by Quick et al. Important amongst these are involvement, reactance proneness, locus of control, self-monitoring, and sensation-seeking. Health literacy is a key concept in much health communication research, although it is not specifically theoretical, so we have also added this notion into Chapter 2. This first section culminates with Jill Yamasaki's chapter (Chapter 3) on interpretive health communication scholarship. This chapter is appropriately called "When Theory and Methods Intertwine" because interpretive scholarship does not typically begin with a particular theory that is then tested, as is the case with the other theories discussed throughout the book. Yamasaki introduces several interpretive approaches to research that frame health communication theory.

As is common in books focusing on communication, we then move in Part II to dyadic contexts and a discussion of the theories most commonly used in that area of health communication research. These dyadic contexts tend to be interpersonal in focus. Three theories are the focus of discussion in the following chapter (Chapter 4) – communication accommodation theory, communication privacy management theory, and the theory of negotiated morality. Although these theories have different origins, they all illuminate interpersonal interaction as it relates to health and health care delivery. It should be noted that none of the theories are used exclusively in health and illness contexts, but they all have been applied extensively and fruitfully in health communication scholarship. This chapter is presented in an unusual manner, in that we had experts on the different theories write separate sections, with authorship of each section noted within the chapter. The authors of this chapter are Maria Brann, Jennifer J. Bute, Maureen Keeley, Sandra Petronio, Rachyl Pines, and Bernadette Watson.

Broadening the context a bit to the family, we move to four important theories that illuminate our understanding of how health processes operate within familial settings. Maureen Keeley and Hannah Jones's chapter (Chapter 5) discusses inconsistent nurturing as control theory, Olson's circumplex model of marital and family systems, affection exchange theory, and the double ABCX model of family stress and coping. These theories have important implications for mental health concerns as well as physical health.

Still focusing on the interpersonal context is Peter J. Schulz and Shaohai Jiang's discussion in Chapter 6 of several theories that are important in the study of provider–patient interaction. We selected the following theories for this chapter: narrative medicine, politeness theory, dialectical tensions, the relational health communication competence model, the care model/productive interaction change approaches, and argumentation theory. Narrowing this chapter to the theories we selected was challenging because provider–patient communication is one of the dominant areas of study within health communication. This area of study, however, is the least theoretically based. Schulz and Jiang speculate on reasons for this limitation within the chapter.

Part III of the book broadens to a focus on persuasive communication, although this label should not be interpreted to imply that there is communication that does not have persuasive elements. Certainly, the theories prior to this section also pertain to persuasion in some ways. This section of the volume begins with Monique Mitchell Turner, Youjin Jang, and Shawn Turner's discussion of information processing and cognitive theories (Chapter 7), and includes a focus on the following theories: the risk information seeking and processing model; the risk perception attitude framework; PRISM (planned risk information seeking model); the health belief model and the reconceptualized health belief model; dual-processing models; and attribution theory and attribution error. Moving to theories of affective impact, Robin Nabi outlines for us in Chapter 8 the concept of psychological reactance; work on fear appeals and the extended parallel process model; and action tendency emotions.

A focus on behavior is then found in the chapter by Marco Yzer and Rebekah Nagler in Chapter 9 of the book. This discussion is extensive and includes the following important theories: theory of normative social behavior; theory of planned behavior; theory of reasoned action; the integrative model; the transtheoretical/stages of change model; social cognitive theory; and the societal risk reduction motivation model. We conclude Part III with a focus on message effects by James Robinson, Yan Tian, and Jeanine W. Turner (Chapter 10). Their discussion emphasizes agenda setting; cultivation theory; inoculation effects; use and gratifications theory; narrative engagement theory; media complementarity theory; and framing theories (regulatory focus, construal level theory).

Part IV turns our focus to theories of organizations and society. We begin with Yanquin Liu and Anthony J. Roberto's thorough discussion of sociopsychological theories in Chapter 11, which includes: the diffusion of innovations model; social judgment theory; self-determination theory; and social comparison theory. None of these theories were originally developed to apply to health communication contexts, but all of them have come to play important roles in our understanding of such processes. Also taking a comprehensive focus is Chapter 12 on public relations by Arunima Krishna. This chapter focuses on situational theory and organizational-public relations theory. The reader will notice the broadening contexts of the chapters as the book moves toward its culmination.

Chapter 13, by Austin S. Babrow, Marianne S. Matthias, Sarah M. Parsloe, and Anne M. Stone, provides an insightful discussion of uncertainty management theories and health. These include the theory of motivated information management; uncertainty management theory; problematic integration theory, and harm reduction theory. As uncertainty management processes are fundamental to all health and illness contexts, these theories operate on the same broad level as do the other theories in this section. Also discussing theories at a broad, cultural level is Chapter 14, written by Evelyn Y. Ho and Barbara F. Scharf. This focus on cultural perspectives provides insightful analysis of the evolution of the study of health communication and the notion of culture as well as in-depth discussion of social construction perspectives; ecological perspectives; culture-centered approaches; the rhetoric of health and medicine; the cultural variance model; the communication theory of identity; critical approaches; and globalization theory.

The world in which we live requires an understanding of communication technology as it currently operates and will continue to change.

To address this, Shyam Sundar and Maria D. Molina (Chapter 15) discuss some key theories that frame research on digital information technologies in health communication. These important theories include the motivational technologies model; network influence; and gamification.

Danielle E. Kelley and Brian G. Southwell (Chapter 16) conclude the volume for us with a focus on underdeveloped directions in health communication research. This chapter provides insight that will guide the work of health communication scholars and practitioners in the decades to come. As is implicit in this chapter and others throughout the book, ethical concerns are fundamental to all health communication research.

Ethics

As any area of scholarship or practice develops, it takes a bit of time for those within the field to begin to develop awareness of ethical issues that are especially relevant to their work. Bioethics are, of course, relevant to almost all health communication research. The first explicit mention of ethics in the title of a *Health Communication* article appeared in 1995 in work by Thomas Addington and Jeanne Wegescheide-Harris. This work focused upon ethics in communication with the terminally ill. Subsequent work on end-of-life communication has continued to provide a strong focus on ethical concerns, as has much other work related to provider–patient and family–patient communication.

The work on health promotion and campaigns has important ethical implications, as well. This work is most notably articulated by Nurit Guttman, beginning with her 1997 article describing 13 ethical dilemmas in health campaigns. Guttman extended this argument in her 2000 book on ethical dilemmas, and continues to be a primary source on the ethical concerns of which health communication scholars and practitioners should be aware (see also Guttman and Thompson, 2010).

Conclusion

The goal of this volume is to facilitate the process of understanding and applying health communication theory in future scholarship. It is hoped that this presentation of the theories we have selected for inclusion accomplishes this goal. Health communication research has made and will continue to make important contributions on both scholarly and practical levels. The grounding of future research in a theoretical foundation will undoubtedly serve to further these contributions.

At some point we have to decide if we believe what Kurt Lewin (1935) said. Everyone knows that he said "There is nothing so practical as a good theory" (p. 169) but he also said "If you want truly to understand something, try to change it" (in Tolman 1996, p. 31). The development of theory depends on research identified and tested by what Lewin called "basic social scientists" and evaluated by applied behavioral scientists. These tests provide critical information that enables basic scientists to revise, refine, or reject their initial principles.

Toward that goal, strident theoretically based tests such as structural equation modeling are useful because they allow the researcher to better understand both the relationships between observed and unobserved variables and their influence on some outcome. Because there is no standard model, the researcher must carefully specify the relationships between variables based on the theory. Unexpected relationships are consequently more difficult to ignore and point out the relative value of measured variables compared to unmeasured variables. As a multivariate test, structural equation modeling identifies boundary conditions and demands explanations for relationships that fit or do not fit the theory.

The use of experimental design as a test of the theory is also critical because as, Lewin points out, if you understand something about human behavior you should be able to change it. The use of experiments – both laboratory and field – allow those behavioral scientists charged with testing the models to demonstrate that the theory works as advertised.

It is also hoped that in the experimentation phase of theory development the researchers will focus on health behaviors. Attitudes and intentions are important but ultimately we want to see how communication behavior influences health. So at some point our research programs need to move in that direction. With the advent of new measurement technologies, we should begin looking at physiological responses to communication right along with our examination of overt behavior. We need not become neuroscientists or physicians but we do need to consider how such expertise can be incorporated within our research. Demonstrating that A1C scores, which indicate blood sugar levels, change along with the way people communicate with a health care professional is a start but ultimately we would like to demonstrate the direction of causality and we would like to see if changes in communication produce changes in health. This may best be done with longitudinal research studies. More stringent testing of our theories should help ensure that we progress as a discipline and increase our understanding the role of communication and health.

References

Addington T., & Wegescheide-Harris, J. (1995). Ethics and communication with the terminally ill. *Health Communication, 7*, 267–281.

Babrow, A., & Mattson, M. (2003). Theorizing about health communication. In T.L. Thompson, A.M. Dorsey, K.I. Miller, and R. Parrott (Eds.), *The handbook of health communication* (pp. 35–61). Mahwah, NJ: Lawrence Erlbaum Associates.

Babrow, A., & Mattson, M. (2011). Building health communication theories in the 21st century. In T.L. Thompson, R. Parrott, and J.F. Nussbaum (Eds.), *The Routledge handbook of health communication* (2nd ed). New York, NY: Routledge.

Bateson, G. (1972) *Steps to an ecology of mind.* Chicago, IL: University of Chicago Press.

Cline, R.W.C. (2011). Everyday interpersonal communication and health. In T.L. Thompson, R. Parrott, and J.F. Nussbaum (Eds.) *The Routledge handbook of health communication* (2nd ed; pp. 377–396). New York, NY: Routledge.

Craig, R. (1999). Communication theory as a field. *Communication Theory, 9*, 119–161.

Faklaris, C., Dabbish, L., & Hong, J. (August 13, 2018). Adapting the transtheoretical model for the design of security interventions. A paper presented at the Symposium on Usable Privacy and Security Conference, Baltimore, MD.

Guttman, N. (1997). Ethical dilemmas in health campaigns. *Health Communication, 9*, 155–190.

Guttman, N. (2000). *Public health communication interventions: Values and ethical dilemmas.* Thousand Oaks, CA: Sage.

Guttman, N., & Thompson, T.L. (2010). Health communication ethics. In C. Cheney, S. May, & D. Munshi (Eds.), *ICA handbook of communication ethics* (pp. 293–308). Mahwah, NJ: Lawrence Erlbaum Associates.

Head, K., & Bute, J. (2018). The influence of everyday interpersonal communication on the medical encounter: An extension of Street's ecological model. *Health Communication, 33*, 786–792.

Korsch, B.M., & Negrete, V.F. (1972). Doctor–patient communication. *Scientific American, 227*(2), 66–74.

Kreps, G. (2020). The value of health communication scholarship: New directions for health communication inquiry. *International Journal of Nursing Sciences, 7*(2s).

Kreps, G., & Thornton, B.C. (1982*). Health communication: Theory and practice.* Prospect Heights, IL: Waveland.

Lewin, K. (1935). *A dynamic theory of personality.* New York, NY: McGraw Hill.

National Institutes of Health. (2020). The delivery of health care. https://www.semanticscholar.org/topic/Delivery-of-Health-Care/16054

Ng, B-Y, Kankanhalli, A., & Xu, C. (2009). Studying users' computer security behavior: A health belief perspective. *Decision Support System, 46,* 815–825.

Prochaska, J.O., & DiClemente, C.O. (1983). Stages and processes of self-change of smoking: Toward an integrative model of change. *Journal of Consulting & Clinical Psychology, 51,* 390–395. doi:10.1037/0022-006X.51.3.390

Rogers, R.W. (1975). A protection motivation theory of fear appeals and attitude change. *Journal of Psychology, 91,* 93–114.

Rosenstock, I.M. (1974). Historical origins of the health belief model. *Health Education Monographs, 2,* 328–335.

Salmon, C., & Poorisat, T. (2019) The rise and development of public health communication. *Health Communication,* online first.

Tolman, C. (1996*). Problems in theoretical psychology.* International Society for Theoretical Psychology.

Watzlawick, P. Beavin, J. and Jackson, D. (1967). *The pragmatics of human communication.* New York, NY: W.W. Norton.

Witte, K. (1994). Fear control and danger control: A test of the extended parallel process model. *Communication Monographs, 61,* 113–134.

World Health Organization: 2020. Definition of Health. https://8fit.com/lifestyle/the-world-health-organization-definition-of-health/ n.p.

Zhang, X. A., & Borden, A. (2019). How to communicate cyber-risk? An examination of behavioral recommendations in cybersecurity crises. *Journal of Risk Research.* doi: 10.1080/13669877.2019.1646315

2

Segmenting Priority Audiences Employing Individual Difference Variables to Improve Health Promotion Efforts

Brian L. Quick, Tobias Reynolds-Tylus, Andrea Martinez Gonzalez, Salah H. Al-Ghaithi, and Michael Mackert

Promotional efforts aimed at a priority audience are an important feature of effective health communication efforts (Lee and Kotler 2020). Tailoring and directing messages to a specific audience segment based on demographic, geographic, psychographic, and behavioral variables, as opposed to disseminating promotional messages to the general public, is a much more efficient and effective strategy (McKenzie and Smeltzer 2001). For this reason, during the early stages of a campaign, social marketers and health communication practitioners devote considerable resources to formative research efforts to identify the appropriate psychographics (e.g. barriers, benefits, competition) associated with the specific behavior of interest (Andreasen 1995). Traditionally, social marketers reject the notion of experts designing, implementing, and evaluating promotional efforts without an adequate understanding of the priority audience's perceptions and self-efficacy with respect to performing the behavior (Finnell and John 2017).

Health Communication Theory, First Edition. Edited by Teresa L. Thompson and Peter J. Schulz.
© 2021 John Wiley & Sons, Inc. Published 2021 by John Wiley & Sons, Inc.

Audience segmentation has long been considered a necessary practice for the success of communication campaigns (Atkin and Salmon 2013; Donahew 1990; Grunig 1989; Trump 2016). To segment the audience, one divides the population into subpopulations with meaningful shared qualities (Slater 1995), seeking similar audience responses (Atkin and Salmon 2013). This practice is key to designing systematically tailored messages to fulfill the communication needs of the priority audience (Slater 1995), and it provides the basis for selecting channels to reach the intended audience (e.g. radio, word-of-mouth, etc; Moriarty et al. 2014). Identifying and understanding the idiosyncrasies of the priority audience enables social marketers and health communication practitioners the opportunity to create messages that resonate with the priority audience's needs (Andreasen 1995; Lee 2016; Slater 1995). Specifically, tailored messages provide social marketers with benefits such as (i) disseminating messages more effectively to potential adopters, (ii) effectively meeting the needs of potential adopters, (iii) providing greater satisfaction to adopters, and subsequently (iv) increasing the likelihood of sustained adoption (Kotler and Roberto 1989). Slater (1995) suggests meticulous campaign planners rarely overlook careful targeting and audience segmentation strategies, noting that it is important to adapt the style and content of our promotional messages to adequately fit the needs of the priority audience. By carefully tailoring a message to a particular audience segment, Andreasen (1995) suggests campaigners can more effectively meet the priority audience's needs, thus resulting in desired outcomes. In general, the more health communicators know about their intended audience, the better they can describe them, and as a result, practitioners can tailor messages and utilize appropriate channels with greater specificity and precision (McKenzie and Smeltzer 2001).

Segmentation strategies rely on an educated selection of variables (e.g. demographic, geographic, psychographic, and behavioral) known or assumed to influence attitudes and behaviors (Slater 1996). Among the many available determinants of audience responses, an extensive amount of communication research has identified a handful of individual difference variables to utilize when segmenting audiences. Individual difference variables including involvement (Petty and Cacioppo 1979), health literacy (Aldoory 2017), locus of control (Rotter 1966), reactance proneness (Hong and Faedda 1996), self-monitoring (Briñol and Petty 2015; Snyder 1979), and sensation seeking (Zuckerman 1979), stand to offer health communication professionals with important psychographics to consider when designing their next social influence initiative. The aforementioned individual difference variables serve as potential audience segmentation variables as extant research demonstrates how each affects individuals' response to promotional messages (O'Keefe 2013; Shen and Dillard 2009; Shen, Mercer, and Kollar 2015). In this chapter, each of these individual difference variables are discussed with an emphasis on their application as audience segmentation variables for use in future health communication campaigns.

Involvement

Involvement is a commonly invoked concept to better understand the situations under which individuals are more or less likely to be persuaded (Johnson and Eagly 1989). Though conceptual definitions of involvement are varied (cf. Allport 1943; Eagly and Chaiken 1993; Johnson and Eagly 1989; Petty and Cacioppo 1986), the term involvement has broadly been defined as the extent to which a topic or issue is considered personally relevant or significant to an individual (Perloff 2003). Several theories of persuasion – including social judgment theory (Sherif and Hovland 1961; Sherif, Sherif, and Nebergall 1965), the elaboration likelihood model (Petty and Cacioppo 1986), and the heuristic-systematic model (Chaiken 1980) – posit that involvement is a fundamental variable affecting how individuals process and respond to persuasive messages. Despite widespread agreement that involvement affects message processing, the directionality of its influence is variable. For instance, according to social judgment theory (Sherif and Hovland 1961; Sherif et al. 1965), involvement is hypothesized to have a direct, albeit negative, effect on attitude change. In contrast, the elaboration likelihood model (Petty and Cacioppo 1986) posits that involvement is positively associated with an individual's elaboration motivation, or desire to engage in issue-relevant thinking about a topic (see O'Keefe 2013). These mixed findings propelled researchers to develop more nuanced conceptualizations for the involvement construct.

In their meta-analysis of the effects of involvement on persuasion, Johnson and Eagly (1989) argued that involvement is a multidimensional construct comprising three distinct types of involvement: value-relevant involvement, impression-relevant involvement, and outcome-relevant involvement. Johnson and Eagly (1989) contend that these different types of involvement activate different "aspect[s] of the message recipients' self-concept" (p. 290). Accordingly, the persuasive effects of each type of involvement are dependent on the aspect of the self that is activated by the persuasive message. Cho and Boster (2005) validated a measure for assessing Johnson and Eagly's (1989) three involvement types. Cho and Boster's (2005) involvement measures have received support across various topics and populations (Lapinski, Zhuang, Koh, and Shi 2017; Marshall, Reinhart, Feeley, Tutzauer, and Anker 2008; Pfau et al. 2010; Quick and Heiss 2009).

The first type of involvement identified by Johnson and Eagly (1989) is value-relevant involvement. Value-relevant involvement represents the relationship between an attitude object and an individual's enduring values. In Johnson and Eagly's (1989) words, value-relevant involvement is "the psychological state that is created by the activation of attitudes that are linked to important values" (p. 290). These values refer to the traits and ideals that are particularly salient to individuals and correspondingly are used by individuals in defining their self-concept. Value-relevant involvement is analogous to ego-involvement as originally studied by Sherif and his colleagues (Sherif and Cantril 1947; Sherif and Hovland 1961; Sherif et al. 1965). In their meta-analysis, Johnson and Eagly (1989) concluded that the effects of value-relevant involvement on persuasion are quite straightforward. Individuals who are highly value-involved are harder to persuade than those who have low value-involvement, although this can be overcome with strong arguments. In line with Johnson and Eagly's (1989) finding, subsequent research has demonstrated that individuals who have high value-relevant involvement in an issue are in fact more difficult to persuade (Cho and Boster 2005; Pfau et al. 2010).

The second type of involvement identified by Johnson and Eagly (1989) is impression-relevant involvement. Impression-relevant involvement refers to concerns about self-presentation, social desirability, and identity management. High impression-relevant involved individuals are concerned with "holding an opinion that is socially acceptable" (Johnson and Eagly 1989, p. 291), and often have more flexible or less extreme positions on topics. In contrast to value-relevant involvement, individuals high in impression-relevant involvement are motivated to behave in a manner that is considered acceptable by others (Cho and Boster 2005), whereas high value-relevant involved individuals tend to behave in a way that is consistent with their own beliefs (Lapinski et al. 2017). Correspondingly, high levels of impression-relevant involvement have been found to be associated with other-directedness (Cho and Boster 2005), the level to which individuals have concerns for "pleasing others, conforming to the social situation, and masking one's true feelings" (Briggs, Cheek, and Buss 1980, p. 681). Of the three involvement types, impression-relevant involvement has received the least amount of academic investigation. Furthermore, research examining impression-relevant involvement (Lapinski et al. 2017; Marshall et al. 2008; Pfau et al. 2010; Quick and Heiss 2009) has often failed to find support for impression-relevant involvement's persuasive function as specified by Johnson and Eagly (1989).

The final type of involvement identified by Johnson and Eagly (1989) is outcome-relevant involvement. Outcome-relevant involvement refers to the relevance of the issue to an individual's important goals or outcomes. In short, if an issue or topic potentially will help an individual achieve some goal, she or he is said to have high outcome-relevant involvement (Johnson and Eagly 1989). Outcome-relevant involvement is conceptually similar to Petty and Cacioppo's (1979) concept of issue involvement, defined as "the extent to which the attitudinal issue under consideration is of personal importance" (p. 1915). Research on the role of outcome-relevant involvement on persuasion has been somewhat inconsistent, with findings suggesting that outcome-relevant involvement can both enhance and inhibit attitude change (Cho and Boster 2005; Maio and Olson 1995). These inconsistent findings can be best explained by the elaboration likelihood model (Petty and Cacioppo 1986), which proposes that as outcome-relevant involvement prompts greater message processing, attitude change should be expected only when strong persuasive messages are presented. In support of this reasoning, research has found that individuals with high outcome-relevant involvement engage in more information seeking (Cho and Boster 2005; Quick and Heiss 2009) and more objective cognitive processing (Hubbell, Mitchell, and Gee 2001; Levin, Nichols, and Johnson 2000).

Health communicators can benefit by considering audience members' involvement in an issue, given the central role involvement plays in message processing and attitude change. Formative research into a target audience's type and level of involvement in an issue allows for subsequent audience segmentation and message tailoring. One illustrating example of this comes from Marshall and colleagues (2008) who examined college students' impression-, outcome-, and value-relevant involvement for alcohol use (as well as several other health behaviors). Though participants had similar (and relatively high) levels of involvement for alcohol use, Marshall and colleagues (2008) found that outcome-relevant involvement was positively associated with alcohol use, whereas value-relevant involvement was negatively associated with alcohol use, and impression-relevant involvement was unrelated with alcohol use. From a message design standpoint, this negative relationship between value-relevant involvement and drinking suggests that anti-drinking messages that resonate with college students' existing values (e.g. healthy lifestyle) represent a potentially fruitful avenue for health communication efforts. Furthermore, given the positive association between outcome-relevant involvement and drinking, these results suggest that social marketing efforts will likely benefit from finding new and innovative ways to convey the negative effects of alcohol use, given the existence of perceived positive benefits of alcohol use (e.g. socialization, stress management; Marshall et al. 2008). With an overview of involvement provided, we next move to the concept of health literacy.

Health Literacy

Another concept that merits attention in the development of social marketing campaigns and health promotion programs is health literacy, a set of characteristics that allow for the understanding and use of health information to make health decisions (Aldoory 2017). Berkman and colleagues (Berkman, Davis, and McCormack 2010) conducted a review of 13 definitions of health literacy and then proposed a new definition: the degree to which individuals can obtain, process, understand, and communicate about health-related information needed to make informed health decisions. Given this definition, it is no surprise that lower health literacy is linked to poorer health outcomes and substantial increased costs to the overall health care system (Nielsen-Bohlman, Panzer, and Kindig 2004; Paasche-Orlow and Wolf 2007). Paasche-Orlow and Wolf (2007) developed a framework to demonstrate the causal pathways between limited health literacy and patients' health outcomes. It is estimated that between one third to one half of US adults have limited health literacy (Nielsen-Bohlman et al. 2004).

Given the evolution of the concept of health literacy, which was initially strongly tied to math and reading capabilities in the health context, one of the most frequent areas of health communication research focused on health literacy has been around the readability of various kinds of health promotion materials. Weiss (2015) noted that in a search of medical literature from 2000 to 2013 there were at least 160 studies investigating readability of patient education materials, and argued that the consistent finding – the reading demand of patient materials is too high – is well-established and research should focus on more productive avenues. Other studies have considered everything from informed consent documents (Donovan-Kicken, Mackert, Guinn, et al. 2012) to patient–provider communication (Hironaka and Paasche-Orlow 2008) to approaches for improving medication instructions (Katz, Kripalani, and Weiss 2006) to how advertising and journalism professionals understand health literacy (Hinnant and Len-Rios 2009; Mackert 2011). Finally, in a thoughtful study, Meppelink and colleagues (2015) make the important point that all individuals regardless of their health literacy level benefit from simpler, clearer messages – a universal precautions approach. There is both a solid foundation on which to build regarding the role of health literacy in health communication and social marketing efforts, as well as substantial room for improving the field's understanding the mechanisms of health literacy on eventual outcomes.

Those interested in health literacy as an individual-level variable that can affect the potential impact of social marketing efforts and contribute to overall health face several challenges. As already noted, there is a variety of definitions of health literacy, and the different definitions can create confusion and a lack of consensus within the field (Mackert, Champlin, Su, and Guadagno 2015); a recent proposal by the US Department of Health and Human Services to adopt a new definition of health literacy which would emphasize the role of society in providing accessible and comprehensible health information has some potential benefits (e.g. increasing the focus on those delivering health information) but could also exacerbate some of the challenges of a lack of consensus around the definition of health literacy (e.g. the indexing of academic literature focused on health literacy; Ancker, Grossman, and Benda 2019). It is perhaps a natural consequence of lack of consensus around definitions which leads to a host of measures around health literacy, as well as accompanying calls for consensus and better measures of health literacy that reflect newer perspectives on health literacy as an avenue for health promotion (Pleasant, Cabe, Patel, et al. 2015; Pleasant, McKinney, and Rikard 2011). Perhaps the most pressing issue is that there is limited, quality evidence about what kind of interventions can change the negative outcomes associated with limited health literacy (Berkman, Sheridan, Donahue, et al. 2011; Weiss 2015). Focused research on the different steps of building health promotion efforts – from the message design process to audience reception to health outcomes – with health literacy as a consideration throughout the process will contribute to a growing evidence based of how best to build health literacy and improve the health of those with limited health literacy. Aldoory (2017) lays out a number of existing research gaps and opportunities for future research related to health literacy and health communication. With a discussion of health literacy behind us, we next turn to locus of control by defining the concept and dimensions, as well as discussing how it provides opportunities and challenges to health practitioners.

Locus of Control

Another individual difference variable to consider when segmenting an audience is locus of control, which refers to individuals' acknowledgement of accountability for their life outcomes (Latimer, Katulak, Mowad, and Salovey 2005). The term locus of control was coined by Rotter (1966) more than five decades ago and refers to the degree individuals feel their life circumstances result from their actions and characteristics or are due to external forces considered to be out of their control such as chance, luck, or powerful others. Said differently, locus of control captures the extent to which people believe events in their life are caused by their actions or circumstances outside of their control (Kim and Baek 2019). The former is referred to as internal control whereas the latter reflects external control. Within the context of health outcomes, Wallston, Wallston, and DeVellis (1978) developed the multidimensional health locus of control scale. Health locus of controls reflects the degree to which people feel their health outcomes are contingent on their behavior or the behavior of others or the environment (Kannan and and Veazie 2015). The scale consists of three dimensions including internality (i.e. health outcomes are internally based and our individual responsibility) and externality, which features both chance (i.e. health outcomes are due to fate and out of our control) and powerful others (i.e. health outcomes are determined by powerful others such as a physician and thereby out of our control).

Locus of control is important to health practitioners considering its relation to a myriad of important behavior change variables. For instance, Brehm and Brehm (1981) identified locus of control as an individual difference variable closely linked to psychological reactance. Reactance is conceptualized as an aversive motivational state emanating from a threatened or eliminated freedom (Brehm 1966). Despite a cogent theoretical connection between locus of control and reactance, we are aware of only one study to examine the association between these theoretical constructs (Xu 2017). Xu demonstrated a stronger association between controlling language and reactance among individuals with an internal, as opposed to an external, locus of control. Delivering messages congruent with one's locus of control beliefs stands as a fruitful approach to mitigating reactance following experimental work by Latimer and colleagues (2005). For example, it is reasonable to expect delivering a personal responsibility message to people with an internal locus of control while at the same time disseminating a health care provider responsibility message to those favoring an external locus of control would mitigate the reactance experienced. Although matching messages to one's controllability beliefs is intuitively appealing, a fear persists that people with an external locus of control mindset may lack confidence in their ability to avoid aversive health complications (Booth-Butterfield, Anderson, and Booth-Butterfield 2000).

The relationship between an internal locus of control and self-efficacy continues to emerge within the literature. Specifically, research has found the controllability of health outcomes beliefs is positively linked to increased self-efficacy among individuals (Armitage 2003). For example, within the context of parental alcoholism effects on their adult children, Richards and Nelson (2012) discovered a positive association between self-efficacy and an internal locus of control whereas a negative association emerged for individuals with an external locus of control. Health practitioners must remain aware of the positive association between control beliefs and one's confidence in performing an advocated behavior. Moreover, maintaining an internal locus of control is positively correlated with conscientiousness and overall life satisfaction (Morrison 1997). Interestingly, recent research has connected heavy television viewers to maintaining an external locus of control (Kim and Baek 2019). Health promotion messages delivered to people with an external locus of control should emphasize self- and response efficacy through modeling as well as identifiable narratives in order to increase adoption rates. However, a heightened internal locus of control can have a downside. There remains speculation that an elevated internal locus of control could be positively associated with increased anxiety and unreasonable self-blame (Richards and Nelson 2012). Future research should continue to investigate the benefits and costs with both a heightened internal or external locus of control. Taking the range of locus of control into consideration is important for health practitioners. Equally important is to consider one's resistance to influential attempts as is discussed with the next individual difference variable, reactance proneness.

Reactance proneness

Although generally considered a psychological state (Brehm 1966), reactance can also be conceived as a variable that differentiates individuals on their likelihood to experience reactance, a motivational state operationalized as anger and negative cognitions following exposure to a freedom threat (Dillard and Shen 2005) in response to restrictions in autonomy and threats to behavioral freedom (Brehm and Brehm 1981; Chartrand, Dalton, and Fitzsimons 2007; Lienemann and Siegel 2016; Steindl et al. 2015). Reactance proneness is defined as an individual's proclivity to feel reactance when one's freedom is threatened or eliminated (Brehm and Brehm 1981; Lienemann and Siegel 2016; Steindl et al. 2015; Van Petegem, Soenens, Vansteenkiste, and Beyers 2015). Among several measures of reactance proneness (Dowd, Milne, and Wise 1991; Hong 1992; Hong and Faedda 1996; Hong and Page 1989; Merz 1983), Hong and Faedda's (1996) reactance proneness scale is one of the most commonly utilized by researchers to capture individuals' innate proclivity to experience reactance. Hong and Faedda's (1996) scale measures one's agreement with statements such as, "Regulations trigger a sense of resistance in me," "I become frustrated when I am unable to make free and independent decisions," and "When someone forces me to do something, I feel like doing the opposite." Measuring reactance proneness is useful for targeting at-risk and consistently resistant audiences (e.g. adolescents, substance-dependent individuals, mental health patients; De las Cuevas, et al. 2014; Grandpre et al. 2003; LaVoie, Quick, Riles, and Lambert 2017; Miller et al. 2006; Miller and Quick 2010; Missotten et al. 2017; Quick, Bates, and Quinlan 2009; Quick, Shen, and Dillard 2013), as individuals high in reactance proneness are more likely to engage in risky behaviors (e.g. Miller and Quick 2010; Quick et al. 2013).

Audience segmentation based on reactance proneness is logical because reactance-prone individuals respond similarly to messages (Quick et al. 2013; Trump 2016). For example, highly reactance-prone individuals process and respond similarly to language perceived to threaten their autonomy (Dillard and Shen 2005), giving health communication professionals the possibility to anticipate responses to autonomy-supporting versus autonomy-restricting language. Highly reactance prone individuals are self-driven, self-reliant, resistant to external influences, and confrontational (Quick et al. 2013; Seibel and Dowd 2001). These individuals will defend their freedom at all costs (Wicklund 1974) and feel particularly attacked by persuasive messages and intentional influence attempts (LaVoie et al. 2017; Quick and Stephenson 2008). As a result, reactance proneness might often lead to message rejection (for a review, see Quick et al. 2013). For example, reactance proneness is associated with boomerang effects in response to smoking cessation messages (Grandpre et al. 2003; Henriksen et al. 2006; LaVoie et al. 2017; Miller et al. 2006), risky sex (Miller and Quick 2010), and with effective parent–child communication (Missotten et al. 2017). Given the increased likelihood of maladaptive responses, it is recommended that promotional messages be tailored to reactance-prone individuals in a way that bolsters their autonomy. Segmenting an audience with reactance proneness in mind can help practitioners plan for less autonomy-suppressing appeals and prevent maladaptive freedom restoration outcomes (Trump 2016). Related to autonomy preservation and maintaining a favorable impression, the next section introduces self-monitoring and how this individual difference variable can be used as an audience segmentation psychographic variable.

Self-monitoring

Self-monitoring is defined as individuals' tendency to "exercise control over their expressive behavior, self-presentation, and nonverbal displays of affect" (Snyder 1979, p. 86). This tendency is shaped by one's individual perspective, as well as by personal and social experiences. Snyder's (1974, 1979) original 25-item self-monitoring scale was composed to capture individuals' (i) concern for social appropriateness (e.g. "It's important for me to fit into the group I'm with"); (ii) attention to social comparison (e.g. "I try to pay attention to the reactions of others to my behavior in order to avoid being out of place"); (iii) ability to control and modify one's behavior and image (e.g. "In social situations, I have the ability to alter my behavior if I feel that something else is called for"); (iv) ability to adapt oneself to fit particular situations (e.g. "I may deceive people by being friendly when I really dislike them"); and (v) ability to tailor one's behavior and image to fit in (e.g. "In different situations and with different people, I often act like very different persons"). Since the conception of Snyder's (1979) original scale, a revised shortened version of the self-monitoring scale has been validated (e.g. 12-items, Lennox and Wolfe 1984, O'Cass 2000), but there has been little recent measurement work on the scale.

As an audience segmentation variable, self-monitoring allows for functional message matching (Briñol and Petty 2015; Carpenter, Boster, and Andrews 2013; Teeny, Briñol, and Petty 2016; Petty et al. 2017). Self-monitoring is especially useful to promote health behaviors which may vary at the public versus private level (e.g. nutrition, exercise) as it has been successfully used to differentiate individuals in key compatible contexts (e.g. relationships, emotional displays, purchasing and brand selection, social media use; Graeff 1996; Kim, Seely, and Jung 2017; Oh et al. 2013; Snyder 1987). Compared to low self-monitors, high self-monitors tend to (a) identify socially-appropriate expectations and adapt to them, and (b) seek to fit in with others, which results in them behaving differently in public versus private environments (DeBono 2006a, 2006b). High self-monitors are easily influenced by advertising tactics that help them fit in (DeBono and Packer 1991; Shavitt, Lowrey, and Han 1992; Snyder and DeBono 1985), and they are more willing to try and maintain favorable attitudes toward products that help them look socially appropriate (DeBono and Packer 1991; Snyder and DeBono 1985). They need to look good in others' eyes (Smith, Lair, and O'Brien 2019), they are notorious status seekers (Fuglestad and Snyder 2010), and impression managers (Kudret, Erdogan, and Bauer 2019), extrinsically motivated buyers (Shao, Grace, and Ross 2019), and more easily persuaded by attractive sources over expert sources (Evans and Clark 2012). In many respects, high self-monitors are similar to individuals with high impression-relevant involvement (Johnson and Eagly 1989). Conversely, low self-monitors are less driven by social expectations or belonging, and their public and private behaviors are quite consistent with each other (DeBono 2006a, 2006b). Given these contrasts, health messages tailored to high self-monitors ought to emphasize public gratification for the individual, improved social image, status, and need for belonging, and should be delivered by attractive sources. Such messages may involve a public pledge or affiliation with a visible cause, such as Susan G. Komen's breast cancer awareness' pink merchandize and fundraising runs (Susan G. Komen Foundation, n.d.), as well as organ donation logos and blood donation stickers for recognition. When addressing low self-monitors, health communication campaigns may focus on intrinsically derived values, satisfaction, and using an expert source. Individuals with a range of self-monitoring tendencies can create a host of challenges and opportunities for our priority audience. The final individual difference variable discussed in this chapter is sensation seeking.

Sensation Seeking

Sensation seeking refers to people's need to satisfy their desire for stimulating, exciting, and novel experiences (Zuckerman 1994). Individuals high in sensation seeking enjoy such experiences as riding extreme thrill rides (e.g. sky diving), and as a result, experience what they describe as a "rush" (Bardo, Donohew, and Harrington 1996). Since sensation seekers enjoy novel and intense experiences, they seek gratification in taking financial, legal, physical, and social risks (Zuckerman 1979, 1994). With relation to health behaviors, sensation seekers engage in risky behaviors such as drug use (Donohew 1990) and unsafe sexual activity (Donohew et al. 2000). Given their need and desire to perform risky behaviors, not surprisingly, sensation seeking has been recognized by health communication researchers and practitioners as an effective audience segmentation variable (e.g. Palmgreen et al. 2001).

The activation model of information exposure provides the theoretical framework for much of sensation seeking research (Donohew, Lorch, and Palmgreen 1998; Donohew, Palmgreen, and Duncan 1980), which stipulates that an individual has an ideal level of arousal at which they feel optimal comfort and that individuals seek to achieve and maintain this level of arousal when they are in situations of information exposure. Stephenson (2002) argued that individuals will continue paying attention to a stimulus that meets their arousal threshold. Otherwise, they look for another source of excitement to fulfill such a need. Therefore, the activation model of information exposure provides an explanation of how low and high sensation seekers react differently to health campaign messages, such that messages with structural and content features that are adequately arousing will appeal more to sensation seekers, whereas non-sensation seekers may attend more to messages that cater more to their optimal level of arousal. Donohew, Lorch, and Palmgreen (1991) assert that "only when the message satisfies a desired level of arousal that individuals are likely to stay with it" (p. 207). It follows that a marketing message that appeals to non-sensation seekers may not be adequately stimulating for sensation seekers to maintain attention to it. Conversely, messages that sensation seekers find stimulating may be perceived as too arousing by non-sensation seekers. Hence, perceived message sensation is a determinant of the attention to and processing of messages.

Sensation seeking has also been studied in the contexts of HIV/AIDS prevention messages (Hull and Hong 2016), risky driving behaviors (Lemarié, Bellavance, and Chebat 2019; Zhang, Qu, Tao, and Xue 2019), student procrastination (Chen 2019), food supplement use (Hatch et al. 2019), and body piercing (Hong and Lee 2017). Among these studies, previous research investigated the role of sensation seeking on message processing with some finding no difference between low and high sensation seekers (Stephenson and Palmgreen 2001) and others reporting an interaction between sensation seeking and message processing and attitude (Stephenson 2002). An explanation for the mixed findings lies in topic differences. Stephenson (2002) argued that message topics which normally have more severe consequences tend to be of a higher sensation value. Messages considered high in sensation value are characterized as being dramatic, emotional, and novel (Palmgreen et al. 2001). On the other hand, messages with less severe consequences may be of a moderate sensation value, which makes it harder to detect message processing differences between low and high sensation seekers. Much like the previous individual difference variables introduced in this chapter, we see sensation seeking as an important segmentation variable to consider when advocating the health consequences associated with performing a risky behaviors.

Conclusion

Carefully disseminating promotional messages to the priority audience can be improved by considering the role of the individual difference variables. For decades, social marketing professionals have recognized the value of targeting specific audience segments in the greatest need of a behavioral change (Lee 2016; Lee and Kotler 2020). The impetus behind the current chapter is not to do away with or discourage tailoring messages to a specific audience segment based on demographic, geographic, psychographic, and behavioral variables. Rather, we are advocating for a handful of individual difference variables to be considered as additional audience segmentation variables, with a history of moderating how an audience processes promotional messages. Specifically, future health campaigns should consider segmenting priority audiences along the dimensions of involvement (Petty and Cacioppo 1979), health literacy (Aldoory 2017), locus of control (Rotter 1966), reactance proneness (Hong and Faedda 1996), self-monitoring (Briñol and Petty 2015; Snyder 1979), and sensation seeking (Zuckerman 1979). Inclusion of these factors will likely shed light into a more nuanced understanding of the priority audiences' perceived barriers, benefits, and competition as each relate to the desired behavior (Andreasen 1995). With a greater understanding of these factors, social marketers and health campaign professionals' ability to design, implement, and evaluate campaigns will only improve (Finnell and John 2017).

References

Aldoory, L. (2017). The status of health literacy research in health communication and opportunities for future scholarship. *Health Communication, 32,* 211–218. doi:10.1080/10410236.2015.1114065

Allport, G. W. (1943). The ego in contemporary psychology. *Psychological Review, 50,* 451– 478. doi:10.1037/h0055375

Ancker, J. S., Grossman, L. V., & Benda, N. C. (2019). Health literacy 2030: Is it time to redefine the term?" *Journal of General Internal Medicine.* doi:10.1007/s11606-019-05472-y

Andreasen, A. R. (1995). *Marketing social change: Changing behavior to promote health, social development, and the environment.* San Francisco, CA: Jossey-Bass.

Armitage, C. J. (2003). The relationship between multidimensional health locus of control and perceived behavioural control: How are distal perceptions of control related to proximal perceptions of control? *Psychology & Health, 18*(6), 723–738. doi:10.1080/0887044031000141216

Atkin, C. K., & Salmon, C. (2013). Persuasive strategies in health campaigns. In J. P. Dillard & L. Shen (Eds.), *The Sage handbook of persuasion: Developments in theory and practice* (pp. 278–295). Thousand Oaks, CA: Sage.

Bardo, M., Donohew, L., & Harrington, N. G. (1996). Psychobiology of novelty-seeking and drugseeking behaviour. *Brain and Behaviour, 77,* 23–43. doi:1 0.1016/0166-4328(95)00203-0

Berkman, N. D., Davis, T. C., & McCormack, L. (2010). Health literacy: What is it? *Journal of Health Communication, 15*(supp. 2), 9–19.

Berkman, N. D., Sheridan, S. L., Donahue, K. E., Halpern, D. J., Viera, A., Crotty, K., . . . Viswanathan. M. (2011). Health literacy interventions and outcomes: An updated systematic review. Evidence Report/Technology Assessment, No. 99. Rockville, MD: Agency for Healthcare Research and Quality.

Booth-Butterfield, M., Anderson, R. H., & Booth-Butterfield, S. (2000). Adolescents' use of tobacco, health locus of control, and self-monitoring. *Health Communication, 12,* 137–148.

Brehm, J. W. (1966). *A theory of psychological reactance.* New York, NY: Academic Press.

Brehm, J. W., & Brehm, S. S. (1981). *Psychological reactance: A theory of freedom and control.* San Diego, CA: Academic Press.

Briggs, S. R., Cheek, J. M., & Buss, A. H. (1980). An analysis of The Self-Monitoring Scale. *Journal of Personality and Social Psychology, 38,* 679–686. doi:10.1037/0022-3514.38.4.679

Briñol, P., & Petty, R. E. (2015). Elaboration and validation processes: Implications for media attitude change. *Media Psychology, 18*, 267–291. doi:10.1080/152 13269.2015.1008103

Carpenter, C., Boster, F. J., & Andrews, K. R. (2013). Reactance theory and persuasion. In J. P. Dillard & L. Shen (Eds.), *The Sage handbook of persuasion: Developments in theory and practice* (pp. 104–119). Thousand Oaks, CA: Sage.

Chaiken, S. (1980). Heuristic versus systematic information processing and the use of source versus message cues in persuasion. *Journal of Personality and Social Psychology, 39*, 752–756. doi:10.1037/0022-3514.39.5.752

Chartrand, T. L., Dalton, A. N., & Fitzsimons, G. J. (2007). Nonconscious relationship reactance: When significant others prime opposing goals. *Journal of Experimental Social Psychology, 43*, 719–726. doi:10.1016/j.jesp.2006.08.003

Chen, B.B. (2019). Academic procrastination and bedtime among Chinese undergraduates: The indirect and moderating effects of sensation seeking and goal disengagement. *Current Psychology, 38*, 187–193. doi:10.1007/s12144-017-9605-9

Cho, H., & Boster, F. J. (2005). Development and validation of value-, outcome-, and impression-relevant involvement scales. *Communication Research, 32*, 235–264. doi:10.1177/0093650204273764

DeBono, K. G. (2006a). Attitude functions and consumer psychology: Understanding perceptions of product quality. In G. R. Maio & J. M. Olson (Eds.), *Why we evaluate: Functions of attitudes* (pp. 195–221). Mahwah, NJ: Erlbaum.

DeBono, K. G. (2006b). Self-monitoring and consumer psychology. *Journal of Personality, 74*, 715–738. doi:10.1111/j.1467-6494.2006.00390.x

DeBono, K. G., & Packer, M. (1991). The effects of advertising appeal on perceptions of product quality. *Personality and Social Psychology Bulletin, 17*, 194–200. doi:10.1177/014616729101700212

De las Cuevas, C., Peñate, W., Betancort, M., & de Rivera, L. (2014). Psychological reactance in psychiatric patients: Examining the dimensionality and correlates of the Hong Psychological Reactance Scale in a large clinical sample. *Personality and Individual Differences, 70*, 85–91. doi:10.1016/j.paid.2014.06.027

Dillard, J. P., & Shen, L. (2005). On the nature of reactance and its role in persuasive health communication. *Communication Monographs, 72*, 144–168. doi:10.1080/03637750500111815

Donohew, L. (1990). Public health campaigns: Individual message strategy. In E. B. Ray & L. Donohew (Eds.), *Communication and health* (pp. 136–152). Hillsdale, NJ: Erlbaum.

Donohew, L., Lorch, E. P., & Palmgreen, P. (1991). Sensation seeking and targeting of televised antidrug PSAs. In L. Donohew, H. E. Sypher, & W. J. Bukoski (Eds.), *Persuasive communication and drug abuse prevention* (pp. 209–226). Hillsdale, NJ: Erlbaum.

Donohew, L., Lorch, E. P., & Palmgreen, P. (1998). Applications of a theoretic model of information exposure to health interventions. *Human Communication Research, 24*, 454–468. doi:10.1111/j.1468-2958.1998.tb00425.x

Donohew, L., Palmgreen, P., & Duncan, J. (1980). An activation model of information exposure. *Communication Monographs, 47*, 295–303. doi:10.1080/03637758009376038

Donohew, L., Zimmerman, R., Cupp, P. S., Novak, S., Colon, S., & Abell, R. (2000). Sensation seeking, impulsive decision-making, and risky sex: Implications for risk-taking and design of interventions. *Personality and Individual Differences, 28*, 1079–1091. doi:10.1016/S0191-8869(99)00158-0

Donovan-Kicken, E., Mackert, M., Guinn, T., Tollison, A., Breckinridge, B., & Pont, S. (2012). Health literacy, self-efficacy, and patients' assessment of medical disclosure and consent documentation. *Health Communication, 27*, 581–590.

Dowd, E. T., Milne, C. R., & Wise, S. L. (1991). The Therapeutic Reactance Scale: A measure of psychological reactance. *Journal of Counseling & Development, 69*, 541–545. doi:10.1002/j.1556-6676.1991.tb02638.x

Eagly, A. H., & Chaiken, S. (1993). *The psychology of attitudes*. New York, NY: Harcourt Brace Jovanovich.

Evans, A. T., & Clark, J. K. (2012). Source characteristics and persuasion: The role of self-monitoring in self-validation. *Journal of Experimental Social Psychology, 48*, 383–386. doi:10.1016/j.jesp.2011.07.002

Finnell, K. J., & John, R. (2017). Formative research to understand the psychographics of 1% milk consumption in a low-income audience. *Social Marketing Quarterly, 23*, 169–184. doi:10.1177/1524500417697205

Fuglestad, P. T., & Snyder, M. (2010). Status and the motivational foundations of self-monitoring. *Social and Personality Psychology Compass, 4*, 1031–1041. doi:10.1111/j.1751-9004.2010.00311.x

Graeff, T. R. (1996). Image congruence effects on product evaluations: The role of self-monitoring and public/private consumption. *Psychology & Marketing, 13*, 481–499.

Grandpre, J., Alvaro, E. M., Burgoon, M., Miller, C. H., & Hall, J. R. (2003). Adolescent reactance and anti-smoking campaigns: A theoretical approach. *Health Communication, 15*, 349–366. doi:10.1207/s15327027hc1503_6

Grunig, J. (1989). Publics, audiences, and market segments: Segmentation principles for campaigns. In C. Salmon (Ed.), *Information campaigns: Balancing social values and social change* (pp. 199–228). Newbury Park, CA: Sage.

Hatch, A. M., Cole, R. E., DiChiara, A. J., McGraw, S. M., Merrill, E. P., Wright, A. O., . . . Bukhari, A. S. (2019). Personality traits and occupational demands are linked to dietary supplement use in soldiers: A cross-sectional study of sensation seeking behaviors. *Military Medicine, 184*, e253–e262. doi:10.1093/milmed/usy201

Henriksen, L., Dauphinee, A. L., Wang, Y., & Fortmann, S. P. (2006). Industry sponsored anti-smoking ads and adolescent reactance: Test of a boomerang effect. *Tobacco Control, 15*, 13–18. doi:10.1136/tc.2003.006361

Hinnant, A., & Len-Rios, M. E. (2009). Tacit understandings of health literacy: Interview and survey research with health journalists. *Science Communication, 31*, 84–115.

Hironaka, L. K., & Paasche-Orlow, M. K. (2008). The implications of health literacy on patient–provider communication. *Archives of Disease in Childhood, 93*, 428–32. doi.org/10.1136/adc.2007.131516

Hong, B. K., & Lee. H. Y. (2017). Self-esteem, propensity for sensation seeking, and risk behavior among adults with tattoos and piercings. *Journal of Public Health Research, 6*, 158–163. doi:10.4081/jphr.2017.1107

Hong, S. M. (1992). Hong's Psychological Reactance Scale: A further factor analytic validation. *Psychological Reports, 70*, 512–514. doi:10.2466/pr0.1992.70.2.512

Hong, S.-M., & Faedda, S. (1996). Refinement of the Hong Psychological Reactance Scale. *Educational and Psychological Measurement, 56*, 173–182. doi:10.1177/0013164496056001014

Hong, S.-M., & Page, S. (1989). A psychological reactance scale: Development, factor structure and reliability. *Psychological Reports, 64*, 1323–1326. doi:10.2466/pr0.1989.64.3c.1323

Hubbell, A. P., Mitchell, M. M., & Gee, J. C. (2001). The relative effects of timing of suspicion and outcome involvement on biased message processing. *Communication Monographs, 68*, 115–132. doi:10.1080/03637750128056

Hull, S. J., & Hong, Y. (2016). Sensation seeking as a moderator of gain- and loss-framed HIV-test promotion message effects. *Journal of Health Communication, 21*, 46–55. doi:10.1080/10810730.2015.1033113

Johnson, B. T., & Eagly, A. H. (1989). Effects of involvement on persuasion: A meta-analysis. *Psychological Bulletin, 106*, 290–314. doi:10.1037/0033-2909.106.2.290

Kannan, V. D., & Veazie, P. J. (2015). Who avoids going to the doctor and why? Audience segmentation analysis for application of message development. *Health Communication, 30*, 635–645. doi:10.1080/10410236.2013.878967

Katz, M. G., Kripalani, S., & Weiss, B. D. (2006). Use of pictorial aids in medication instructions: A review of the literature. *American Journal of Health-System Pharmacy: AJHP: Official Journal of the American Society of Health-System Pharmacists, 63*, 2391–97. doi.org/10.2146/ajhp060162

Kim, S., & Baek, Y. M. (2019). Medical drama viewing and healthy lifestyle behaviors: Understanding the role of health locus of control beliefs and education level. *Health Communication, 34*, 392–401. doi:10.1080/10410236.2017.1405483

Kim, D. H., Seely, N. K., & Jung, J.-H. (2017). Do you prefer, Pinterest or Instagram? The role of image-sharing SNSs and self-monitoring in enhancing ad effectiveness. *Computers in Human Behavior, 70*, 535–543. doi:10.1016/j.chb.2017.01.022

Kotler, P., & Roberto, E. (1989). *Social marketing: Strategies for changing public behavior*. New York, NY: The Free Press.

Kudret, S., Erdogan, B., & Bauer, T. N. (2019). Self-monitoring personality trait at work: An integrative narrative review and future research directions. *Journal of Organizational Behavior, 40*, 193–208. doi:10.1002/job.2346

LaVoie, N. R., Quick, B. L., Riles, J. M., & Lambert, N. J. (2017). Are graphic cigarette warning labels an effective message strategy? A test of psychological reactance theory and source appraisal. *Communication Research, 44*, 416–436. doi:10.1177/0093650215609669

Lapinski, M. K., Zhuang, J., Koh, H., & Shi, J. (2017). Descriptive norms and involvement in health and environmental behaviors. *Communication Research, 44*, 367–387. doi:10.1177/0093650215605153

Latimer, A. E., Katulak, N. A., Mowad, L., & Salovey, P. (2005). Motivating cancer prevention and early detection behaviors using psychologically tailored messages. *Journal of Health Communication, 10*, 137–155. doi:10.1080/10810730500263364

Lee, N. R. (2016). Corporate social marketing: Five key principles for success. *Social Marketing Quarterly, 22*, 340–344. doi:10.1177/1524500416672550

Lee, N. R., & Kotler, P. (2020). *Social marketing: Behavior change for good* (6th ed.). Thousand Oaks, CA: Sage.

Lemarié, L., Bellavance, F., & Chebat, J. C. (2019). Regulatory focus, time perspective, locus of control and sensation seeking as predictors of risky driving behaviors. *Accident Analysis & Prevention, 127*, 19–27. doi:10.1016/j.aap.2019.02.025

Lennox, R. D., & Wolfe, R. N. (1984). Revision of the Self-Monitoring Scale. *Journal of Personality and Social Psychology, 4*, 1349–1364. doi:10.1037/0022-3514.46.6.1349

Levin, K. D., Nichols, D. R., & Johnson, B. T. (2000). Involvement and persuasion: Attitude functions for the motivated processor. In G. R. Maio & J. M. Olson (Eds.), *Why we evaluate: Functions of attitude* (pp. 163–194). Mahwah, NJ: Erlbaum.

Lienemann, B. A., & Siegel, J. T. (2016). State psychological reactance to depression public service announcements among people with varying levels of depressive symptomatology. *Health Communication, 31*, 102–116. doi:10.1080/10410236.2014.940668

Mackert, M. (2011). Health literacy knowledge among direct-to-consumer pharmaceutical advertising professionals. *Health Communication, 26*, 525–33. doi:10.1080/10410236.2011.556084

Mackert, M., S. Champlin, Z. Su, & Guadagno, M. (2015). The many health literacies: Advancing the field or fragmentation?" *Health Communication, 30*, 1161–1165.

Maio, G., & Olson, J. (1995). Involvement and persuasion: Evidence for different types of involvement. *Canadian Journal of Behavioural Science, 27*, 64–78. doi:10.1037/008-400X.27.1.64

Marshall, H. M., Reinhart, A. M., Feeley, T. H., Tutzauer, F., & Anker, A. (2008). Comparing college students' value-, outcome-, and impression-relevant involvement in health-related issues. *Health Communication, 23*, 171–183. doi:10.1080/10410230801968252

McKenzie, J., & Smeltzer (2001). *Planning, implementing, and evaluating health promotion programs: A primer* (3rd ed.). Boston, MA: Allyn and Bacon.

Meppelink, C. S., Smit, E. G., Buurman, B. M., & van Weert, J. C. M. (2015). Should we be afraid of simple messages? The effects of text difficulty and illustrations in people with low or high health literacy. *Health Communication, 30*, 1181–1189.

Merz, J. (1983). A questionnaire for the measurement of psychological reactance. *Diagnostics, 29*, 75–72.

Miller, C. H., Burgoon, M., Grandpre, J. R., & Alvaro, E. M. (2006). Identifying principal risk factors for the initiation of adolescent smoking behaviors: The significance of psychological reactance. *Health Communication, 19*, 241–252. doi:10.1207/s15327027hc1903_6

Miller, C. H., & Quick, B. L. (2010). Sensation seeking and psychological reactance as health risk predictors for an emerging adult population. *Health Communication, 25*, 266–275. doi:10.1080/10410231003698945

Missotten, L. C., Luyckx, K., Branje, S., & Van Petegem, S. (2017). Adolescents' conflict management styles with mothers: Longitudinal associations with parenting and reactance. *Journal of Youth and Adolescence, 47*, 260–274. doi:10.1007/s10964-017-0634-3

Moriarty, S., Mitchell, N. D., Wells, W. D., Crawford, R., Brenan, L., & Spence-Stone, R. (2014). *Advertising: Principles and practice* (3rd ed.). Melbourne, VIC, Australia: Pearson.

Morrison, K. A. (1997). Personality correlates of the five-factor model for a sample of business owners/managers: Associations with scores on self-monitoring, type a behavior, locus of control, and subjective well-being. *Psychological Reports, 80* (1), 255–272. doi:10.2466/pr0.1997.80.1.255

Nielsen-Bohlman, L., Panzer, A., & Kindig, D. (2004). *Health literacy: A prescription to end confusion*. Washington, DC: National Academy of Sciences.

O'Cass, A. (2000). A psychometric evaluation of a revised version of the Lennox and Wolfe revised self-monitoring scale. *Psychology & Marketing, 17*, 397–419.

Oh, I.-S., Charlier, S. D., Mount, M. K., & Berry, C. M. (2013). The two faces of high self-monitors: Chameleonic moderating effects of self-monitoring on the relationships between personality traits and counterproductive work behaviors. *Journal of Organizational Behavior, 35*, 92–111. doi.org/10.1002/job.1856

O'Keefe, D. (2013). The elaboration likelihood model. In J. P. Dillard & L. Shen (Eds.), *The Sage handbook of persuasion: Developments in theory and practice* (pp. 137–149). Thousand Oaks, CA: Sage.

Paasche-Orlow, M. K., & Wolf, M. S. (2007). The causal pathways linking health literacy to health outcomes. *American Journal of Health Behavior, 31*, S19–26.

Palmgreen, P., Donohew, L., Lorch, E. P., Hoyle, R., & Stephenson, M. T. (2001). Television campaigns and adolescent marijuana use: Tests of sensation-seeking targeting. *American Journal of Public Health, 91*, 292–296.

Perloff, R. M. (2003). *The dynamics of persuasion: Communication and attitudes in the 21st century* (2nd ed.). Mahwah, NJ: Erlbaum.

Petty, R. E., Briñol, P., Teeny, J., & Horcajo, J. (2017). The elaboration likelihood model. In B. Jackson, J. Dimmock, & J. Compton (Eds.) *Persuasion and communication in sport, exercise, and physical activity* (pp. 22–37). New York, NY: Routledge.

Petty, R. E., & Cacioppo, J. T. (1979). Issue involvement can increase or decrease persuasion byenhancing message-relevant cognitive responses. *Journal of Personality and SocialPsychology, 37*, 1915–1926. doi:10.1037/0022-3514.37.10.1915

Petty, R. E., & Cacioppo, J. T. (1986). *Communication and persuasion: Central and peripheral routes to attitude change.* New York: Springer-Verlag.

Pfau, M., Banas, J., Semmler, S. M., Deatrick, L., Lane, L., Mason, A., . . . Underhill, J. (2010). Role and impact of involvement and enhanced threat in resistance. *Communication Quarterly, 58*, 1–18. doi:10.1080/01463370903520307

Pleasant, A., Cabe, J., Patel, K., Cosenza, J., & Carmona. R. (2015). Health literacy research and practice: A needed paradigm shift. *Health Communication, 30*(12), 1176–1180.

Pleasant, A., McKinney, J., & R. V. Rikard. (2011). Health literacy measurement: A proposed research agenda. *Journal of Health Communication, 16*, 11–21.

Quick, B. L., Bates, B. R., & Quinlan, M. R. (2009). The utility of anger in promoting clean indoor air policies. *Health Communication, 24*, 548–561. doi:10.1080/10410230903104939

Quick, B. L., & Heiss, S. N. (2009). An investigation of value-, impression-, and outcome-relevant involvement on attitudes, purchase intentions, and information seeking. *Communication Studies, 60*, 253–267. doi:10.1080/10510970902956008

Quick, B. L., Shen, L., & Dillard, J. P. (2013). Reactance theory and persuasion. In J. P. Dillard & L. Shen (Eds.), *The Sage handbook of persuasion: Developments in theory and practice* (pp. 167–183). Thousand Oaks, CA: Sage.

Quick, B. L., & Stephenson, M. T. (2008). Examining the role of trait reactance and sensation seeking on perceived threat, state reactance, and reactance restoration. *Human Communication Research, 34*, 448–476. doi:10.1111/j.1468-2958.2008.00328.x

Richards, S., & Nelson, C. (2012). Problematic parental drinking and health: Investigating differences in adult children of alcoholic status, health locus of control, and health self-efficacy. *Journal of Communication in Healthcare: Strategies, Media and Engagement in Global Health, 5*, 84–90. doi:10.1179/1753807612Y.0000000006

Rotter, J. B. (1966). Generalized expectancies for internal versus external control of reinforcement. *Psychological Monographs: General and Applied, 80*, 1–28.

Seibel, C. A., & Dowd, E. T. (2001). Personality characteristics associated with psychological reactance. *Journal of Clinical Psychology, 57*, 963–969. doi:10.1002/jclp.1062

Shao, W., Grace, D., & Ross, M. (2019). Consumer motivation and luxury consumption: Testing moderating effects. *Journal of Retailing and Consumer Services, 46*, 33–44. doi:10.1016/j.jretconser.2018.10.003

Shavitt, S., Lowrey, T. M., & Han, S.-P. (1992). Attitude functions in advertising: The interactive role of products and self-monitoring. *Journal of Consumer Psychology, 1*, 337–364. doi:10.1016/s1057-7408(08)80059-9

Shen, L., & Dillard, J. P. (2009). Message frames interact with motivational systems to determine depth of message processing. *Health Communication*, *24*, 504–514. doi:10.1080/10410230903104897

Shen, L., & Mercer Kollar, L. M. (2015). Testing moderators of message framing effect: A motivational approach. *Communication Research*, *42*, 626–648. doi:10.1177/0093650213493924

Sherif, M., & Cantril, H. (1947). *The psychology of ego-involvements: Social attitudes and identifications*. New York, NY: Wiley.

Sherif, M., & Hovland, C. I. (1961). *Social judgment: Assimilation and contrast effects in communication and attitude change*. New Haven, CN: Yale University Press.

Sherif, C. W., Sherif, M., & Nebergall, R. E. (1965). *Attitude and attitude change: The social judgment-involvement approach*. Philadelphia, PA: Saunders.

Slater, M. D. (1995). Choosing audience segmentation strategies and methods for communication. In E. W. Maibach & R. Parrott (Eds.), *Designing health messages: Approaches from communication theory and public health practice* (pp. 186–198). Thousand Oaks, CA: Sage.

Slater, M. D. (1996). Theory and method in health audience segmentation. *Journal of Health Communication, 1,* 267–284. doi:10.1080/108107396128059

Smith, C. V., Lair, E. C., & O'Brien, S. M. (2019). Purposely stoic, accidentally alone? Self-monitoring moderates the relationship between emotion suppression and loneliness. *Personality and Individual Differences, 149*, 286–290. doi:10.1016/j.paid.2019.06.012

Snyder, M. (1974). Self-monitoring of expressive behavior. *Journal of Personality and Social Psychology*, *30*, 526–537. doi:10.1037/h0037039

Snyder, M. (1979). Self-monitoring processes. *Advances in Experimental Social Psychology*, *12*, 85–128. doi:10.1016/S0065-2601(08)60260-9

Snyder, M. (1987). *Public appearances, private realities: The psychology of self-monitoring*. New York, NY, W. H. Freeman.

Snyder, M., & DeBono, K. G. (1985). Appeals to image and claims about quality: Understanding the psychology of advertising. *Journal of Personality and Social Psychology, 49*, 586–597. doi:10.1037/0022-3514.49.3.586

Steindl, C., Jonas, E., Sittenthaler, S., Traut-Mattausch, E., & Greenberg, J. (2015). Understanding psychological reactance. *Zeitschrift für Psychologie, 223*, 205–214. doi:10.1027/2151-2604/a000222

Stephenson, M. T. (2002). Sensation seeking as a moderator of the processing of anti-heroin PSAs. *Communication Studies*, *53*, 358–380. doi:10.1080/10510970209388598

Stephenson, M. T., & Palmgreen, P. (2001). Sensation seeking, perceived message sensation value, personal involvement, and processing of anti-marijuana PSAs. *Communication Monographs, 68,* 49–71. doi:10.1080/03637750128051

Susan G. Komen Foundation. (n.d.) Get involved. Retrieved from https://ww5.komen.org/unacceptable/?utm_source=Komen.org&utm_medium=GlobalHeaderCTA&utm_campaign=Unacceptable

Teeny, J., Briñol, P., & Petty, R. E. (2016). The elaboration likelihood model: Understanding consumer attitude change. In C. V. Jansson-Boyd & M. J.

Zawisza (Eds.), *Routledge international handbook of consumer psychology* (pp. 390–410). New York, NY: Routledge.

Trump, R. K. (2016). Harm in price promotions: When coupons elicit reactance. *Journal of Consumer Marketing, 33,* 302–310. doi:10.1108/jcm-02-2015-1319

Van Petegem, S., Soenens, B., Vansteenkiste, M., & Beyers, W. (2015). Rebels with a cause? Adolescent defiance from the perspective of reactance theory and self-determination theory. *Child Development, 86,* 903–918. doi:10.1111/cdev.12355

Wallston, K. A., Wallston, B. S., & DeVellis, R. (1978). Development of the Multidimensional Health Locus of Control (MHLC) Scales. *Health Education Monographs, 6,* 160–170.

Weiss, B. D. (2015). Health literacy research: Isn't there something better we could be doing? *Health Communication, 30,* 1173–1175.

Wicklund, R. A. (1974). *Freedom and reactance.* Potomac, MD: Erlbaum.

Xu, J. (2017). The impact of locus of control and controlling language on psychological reactance and ad effectiveness in health communication. *Health Communication, 32,* 1463–1471. doi:10.1080/10410236.2016.1230807

Zhang, X., Qu, X., Tao, D., & Xue, H. (2019). The association between sensation seeking and driving outcomes: A systematic review and meta-analysis. *Accident Analysis & Prevention, 123,* 222–234. doi:10.1016/j.aap.2018.11.023

Zuckerman, M. (1979). *Sensation seeking: Beyond the optimal level of arousal.* Hillsdale, NJ: Erlbaum.

Zuckerman, M. (1994). *Behavioral expressions and biosocial bases of sensation seeking.* Cambridge, UK: Cambridge University Press.

3

When Theory and Method Intertwine

Jill Yamasaki

Given the nature of interpretive/critical approaches to health communication research, it is not always possible, practical, or desirable to consider theory as distinct from methodology and representation. Theories exist in this context as explanatory concepts that are related but not unified and generated rather than extended, challenged, or confirmed. To that end, contemporary interpretive/critical scholarship often intertwines theory with method and combines findings with discussion in carefully crafted expressions (i.e. written, oral, and/or visual) that emphasize local knowledge, in-depth understandings, and intersubjectivity. Despite these differences from theory-driven (often post-positivist) work, however, rigor, validity, and ethical considerations throughout the research process remain paramount.

In this chapter, I offer a brief introduction to four common theoretical frameworks that incorporate these tenets and help guide interpretive/critical health communication research. First, I present shared philosophical foundations underlying interpretive scholarship, followed by explanations of grounded theory, narrative theorizing, autoethnography, and rhetoric of health and medicine. None of these theoretical

Health Communication Theory, First Edition. Edited by Teresa L. Thompson and Peter J. Schulz.
© 2021 John Wiley & Sons, Inc. Published 2021 by John Wiley & Sons, Inc.

approaches or methods originated in health communication; however, they have been employed extensively in health contexts and by health communication scholars, many of whom have expanded, shaped, and/or strengthened them through health communication research.

Philosophical Foundations

Interpretive/critical scholars approach knowledge and the world in very different ways from post-positivist theorists. Rather than engaging in a scientific search for universal explanations and causal relationships, interpretive/critical theorists instead seek in-depth understandings of social life and lived experiences. For them, reality is subjective, multiple, and socially constructed, with participants creating, interpreting, and challenging shared meanings through communicative behavior. People build their own understandings from cultural norms, values, and beliefs, and these understandings then evolve and develop through interaction. Because we come to agreement about what is real intersubjectively, interpretive/critical scholarship does not measure the (in) accuracies of messages against an objective reality; instead, researchers embrace their own subjectivity and acknowledge that they are "interpreting others' interpretations" (Zoller and Kline 2008, p. 93). In this double hermeneutic (Giddens 1984), interpretive/critical scholars seek to understand socially constructed realities and, in doing so, contribute to them, as well. While interpretive scholars strive for thick description of a particular context, critical scholars examine how communication in health contexts creates, reproduces, or challenges dominant power relations and ideologies (Zoller and Kline 2008).

Miller (2005) distinguished between theories that (i) examine general processes of meaning construction for consideration across situational boundaries and (ii) seek to understand local and emergent communication phenomena in specific situations and contexts (see also Dutta and Zoller 2008). Some of these theories are discussed elsewhere in this book (see, for example, Chapters 4, 5, 13, and 14). Regardless, interpretive/critical research is often viewed as "an ongoing process in which there is a continual intertwining – even a blurring – of data collection, analysis, and theorizing" (Miller 2005, p. 63). Just as meaning arises in interaction, concepts and issues of study emerge through the research process itself. Thus, like the social reality being theorized about, interpretive/critical theory is created inductively through observation and interaction. Rejecting the desirability or possibility of separating the knower from the known, researchers immerse themselves in local contexts, combine qualitative methods with their own perspectives and experiences, and seek inside understandings in research conducted jointly with participants. Accordingly, a single study often represents several theoretical commitments (e.g. grounded theory, ethnography, and narrative analysis) in what is usually a back-and-forth, rather than linear, process (Zoller and Kline 2008).

The following theoretical frameworks serve as popular, robust examples of the continual intertwining of data collection, analysis, and theorizing in interpretive/critical health communication research. As Zoller and Kline (2008) note, they overlap and may be employed alone as combined theory and method or used as theory, method, or both with other approaches. I offer exemplary scholarship throughout the chapter – with a focus on theory rather than method – to illustrate their growing and influential contributions to heath communication research.

Grounded Theory

Grounded theory – in various guises – is an especially popular and fruitful approach to research in health contexts and by health communication scholars. Originally developed in the 1960s by medical sociologists Barnie Glaser and Anselm Strauss studying the experiences of hospitalized dying patients, the first conceptualization of grounded theory has been recast by other scholars from different paradigms over the years. The basic steps have remained similar across these formulations; however, significant variability continues to exist in the understanding and application of grounded theory principles and practices within and beyond health communication.

Theory as Process

Research methods and theory development are intimately connected in the grounded theory approach with researchers placing particular emphasis on the *comparative process*. Indeed, Glaser and Strauss (1967) originally claimed that the "strategy of comparative analysis for generating theory puts a high emphasis on theory as process; that is, theory as an ever-developing entity, not as a perfected product" (p. 32). As researchers gather data, they compare new data to existing data, sort those data into meaningful and related categories, and then expand or alter existing categories as needed for theoretical sampling. This process of constant comparison occurs at every step of the research process as scholars compare and refine data and emerging findings. Researchers also consult extant research throughout data gathering and analysis, using it to make sense of emic (participant) categories and drawing relationships to etic (researcher and theoretical) ideas that may be used as sensitizing concepts for further analysis. These comparisons occur within an evolving study design in which research questions are shifted, added, or deleted as initial findings prompt new forms of data or additional data from new participants. Ideally, the goal is to abstract categories into a single statement of theory; however, most health communication research stops short of new theory generation, offering useful typologies, extensions to current theory, or pragmatic implications for improving communication instead (Ellingson and Borofka 2014).

Glaser and Strauss (1967) introduced grounded theory as a way to develop theories from research rather than deduce testable hypotheses from existing theories. This traditional systematic formulation was steeped in the tenants of positivism pervading social sciences at the time and focused on discovering themes that emerged naturally and dispassionately from the data. They originally believed that (i) theory is embedded in and emerges from the data; (ii) researchers should remain objective during data collection and analysis (and even save the literature review until after analysis to ensure a blank slate); and (iii) even without one truth, research can capture a semblance of reality in the data and present that reality as a set of theoretical findings (Corbin 2009). Later, Strauss broke from Glaser and, with his colleague Juliet Corbin, recast grounded theory in a postpositivist vein. Their evolved conceptualization (Strauss and Corbin, 1990) acknowledged the researcher's more active role in generating themes while still emphasizing validity checks and systematic procedures for doing so.

More recently, medical sociologist Kathy Charmaz (2006) situated grounded theory within social constructionism, contending that researchers create both data and analysis from shared experiences and relationships with participants and other sources of data, including the researcher's own perspectives, positions, and privileges. Unlike earlier conceptualizations of grounded theory, she claimed that theories do not emerge from the data but are instead constructed through the researcher's past and present participation in the social world. Constructivist grounded theorists take a reflexive stance toward the research process and products to consider *how* theories evolve from shared meanings and situated practices. From this perspective:

> Theorizing means stopping, pondering, and thinking afresh. We stop the flow of studied experience and take it apart. To gain theoretical sensitivity, we look at studied life from multiple vantage points, make comparisons, follow leads, and build on ideas. . . The acts involved in theorizing foster *seeing* possibilities, *establishing* connections, and *asking* questions. (Charmaz 2006, p. 244; emphasis in original)

This approach explicitly assumes that any theoretical rendering offers an interpretive portrayal – rather than an exact picture – of the studied world (Charmaz 2006, p. 17). While all approaches to grounded theory can be found in health communication literature, the post-positivist and social constructionist types are far more common than the original conceptualization, paralleling larger trends in qualitative methodology (Ellingson and Borofka 2014).

Theory as Product

With roots in medical sociology and nursing, grounded theory has had meaningful impacts on health-related research. Within health communication, Ellingson and Borofka (2014) cited three specific strengths of this approach. First, they claimed that grounded theory highlights participant voices and experiences through categories grounded in participant perspectives. For example, Donovan-Kicken et al. (2012) grounded their analysis in 40 cancer survivors' descriptions of the demands, obligations, and preparatory activities involved in discussing their illness. From these results, they then theorized the construct of communication work, which focuses on the labor and resources devoted to managing talk while living with illness. In another study, Peterson (2010) grounded her analysis in descriptions of the challenges that 45 women living with HIV or AIDS face while seeking and receiving social support. The research served as an initial step toward the development of a normative model of social support for women living with HIV.

Second, Ellingson and Borofka (2014) noted that grounded theory "often generates pragmatic, heuristic implications for improving communication within a variety of health contexts that, while not generalizable, are widely applicable and useful" (p. 538). For example, Martin's

(2016) study of the experience and communicative management of identity threats among 47 people with Parkinson's disease offered insights that could be utilized in healthcare and interventions for combating identity loss and responding to identity challenges in adaptive ways. In another study, Ellingson (2007)'s ethnography of a dialysis unit yielded implications for several areas of health communication research, including improved staff training and delivery of care, further articulation of the relationship between communication and technology in contemporary healthcare, and the development of models of nursing leadership.

Finally, Ellingson and Borofka (2014) claimed grounded theory in health communication research "produces findings rich in contextual and interactional details that complement and contextualize other qualitative, critical, and quantitative analyses" (p. 538). To illustrate, critical health communication scholars have paired grounded theory with (i) the culture-centered approach (see Chapter 14) to reveal enrollment disparities among African Americans and hospice care (Dillon and Basu 2016); (ii) media framing to elaborate tensions that emerge within the discursive space of HIV/AIDS in Indian newspapers (de Souza 2007); and (iii) functional theories of stigma to acknowledge the role of medical power, discrimination, and authority in healthcare encounters with transgender patients (Poteat, German, and Kerrigan 2013). Further, as a well-known health communication scholar specializing in feminist and grounded theory methodologies, Laura Ellingson has advocated for studies that embrace a continuum approach across social science methodologies. From this approach – which Ellingson (2009) deemed crystallization – grounded theory, which is typically represented in traditional research report genres, can be creatively paired with more artistic representation, including photovoice techniques (e.g. Evans-Agnew, Boutain, and Rosemberg 2017) and poetic transcription (e.g. Ellingson 2011).

Narrative Theorizing

The communication discipline boasts a rich history of narrative theory (see Bochner 2014; Fisher, 1987), and communication scholars have contributed meaningfully to the narrative turn in health contexts (see Harter et al. 2020; Harter, Japp, and Beck 2005; Sharf et al. 2011; Sharf and Vanderford 2003). At the heart of his narrative paradigm, rhetorician Walter Fisher (1984) claimed that people are *homo narrans* – or natural storytellers who think in stories: "Narratives enable us to understand the actions of others 'because we all live out narratives in our lives and because we understand our own lives in terms of narratives'" (p. 8). These ideas both incorporated and extended literary theorist Kenneth Burke's (1935/1984) arguments that narratives represent "equipment for living" – or the symbolic resources that allow individuals to size up circumstances and chart future action. According to Sharf et al. (2011), the robustness of narrative theorizing in current health communication scholarship rests in part in its focus on webs of interwoven social (and material) forces. "No story is solely personal, organizational, or public," they explained. "Personal stories cannot escape the constraints of institutional interests, nor are they separate from cultural values, beliefs, and expectations. Meanwhile, institutional structures and scripts intertwine to form the social milieu in which performances unfold" (p. 38).

Although narrative is a broad term that encompasses a multidisciplinary collection of theories and methods, the maturation of health narrative theorizing speaks to enduring and emerging issues of concern for health communication scholars (Harter et al. 2020). To illustrate, Lynn Harter, one of the premiere narrative theorists in health communication, launched Defining Moments, a forum in *Health Communication* and a complementary podcast dedicated to showcasing the social and material power of storytelling. In the first 10 years, authors of the collective essays narrated "myriad maladies, infirmities, and oddities of the human condition" and storied a vast number of topics with particular import for fostering well-being, humanizing healthcare, and advocating for change (Harter et al. 2020, p. 262).

Illness as a Call for Stories

In foundational work based on his own and others' experiences, sociologist Arthur Frank (1995) positioned illness as a call for stories. His popular typology presents three common plotlines that "wounded storytellers" use to first understand and then to explain their illnesses. The most familiar and socially condoned is the restitution plot, which posits that health problems can be remedied and the body restored to its pre-illness state. In contrast, the chaos plotline stories illness as incoherent and disordered, with no hope for control and no promise of getting better. Frank (1995) argued wounded storytellers learn to tell the quest narrative – the third plotline, in which illness is deemed a source of insight to be shared with others – when they "meet suffering head on. They accept illness and seek to *use* it" (p. 115). Scholars have employed this typology as a theoretical framework in research especially focused on life with chronic illness, impairment, or loss (e.g. Titus and de Souza 2011); however, it may not be applicable for all illness situations, including ailments that are chronic but managed, and successful recoveries/remissions that provoke new emotional, cognitive, and physical challenges, like long-term cancer survivors' late effects from treatment (e.g. Ellingson 2017).

Illness narratives are generated in response to a rupture or turning point in a person's life (Bruner 1990) and are told in and through the body (Frank 1995), meaning "the body is simultaneously cause, topic, and instrument of whatever story is told" (Sparkes and Smith 2008, p. 302). Inherently, narratives of health and illness are embodied and dialogic, calling upon listeners (or readers, viewers, touchers) to join with tellers (or writers, filmmakers, artists) in the creation and re-creation of meaning (Harter et al. 2020). Narrative theorists (Frank, 1995; Kleinman, 1988) underscore the importance of reciprocity for bearing witness to individual or community suffering and trauma. Storytellers have the moral responsibility to guide others who may follow, just as storylisteners have the moral – and often uncomfortable – obligation to listen and respond to that suffering.

Core dimensions of narrative theorizing from health communication scholars encompass the functions (e.g. identity construction and community building), grammars (e.g. emplotment and temporality), and types (e.g. institutional and societal stories) of narrative activity (Harter et al. 2005). Narratives endow experience with meaning by organizing events across space and time, identifying characters and their relationships, and determining causes and effects (Harter 2013). Personal narratives provide a way of sensemaking in uncertain or chaotic circumstances and enable a sense of control in the face of threat or disorder. They help transform personal identities regarding how individuals view themselves and are perceived by others, and they help create identification among people experiencing similar problems, thereby building a sense of community in place of social isolation (Sharf and Vanderford 2003; Sharf et al. 2011). Finally, narratives increase public awareness, challenge master narratives (i.e. stories that underlie, reflect, and perpetuate predominant cultural values), and propel health advocacy and social activism (Sharf 2001; Zoller 2005). Sharf et al. (2011) envision the latter contributing to new directions in health communication scholarship, namely "a parallel continuum of stories of illness to stories of prevention, healing, and mobilizing resources" (p. 42).

Narrative Problematics

In their seminal collection of health and illness narratives, Harter et al. (2005) advanced a typology of what they consider core dimensions – or vital problematics (i.e. assumptions) – of narrative theorizing that are pervasive but often unarticulated in the way scholars do narrative work. First, the problematic of knowing and being foregrounds how individuals narratively co-construct and understand personal and social life. As one example, Yamasaki and Hovick (2015) revealed how African American older adults characterize their understandings of health-related conditions from storied family histories and then rationalize their motivations and constraints for sharing that information with current family members. Second, the problematic of continuity and disruption, which "concerns disorder and the human desire for coherence" (Harter et al. 2005, p. 14), describes how storytellers construct and weigh "the past/present/future flow of continuity and disruption to give force to some understanding of the distinction between 'now' and 'then'" (pp. 15–16). To illustrate, Pangborn (2019) poignantly demonstrated how teenagers at a family bereavement camp rely upon aesthetic and embodied narrative experiences to reject confining scripts for "appropriate" grief, acknowledge the value of their perspectives, and reengage in life in affirming ways.

Next, the problematic of creativity and constraint "foregrounds the human struggle to be individuated (i.e. assert creativity) and still identify with a group (i.e. respond to social and institutional constraints)," emphasizing connections between the personal and cultural (Harter et al. 2005, p. 19). Health communication scholars have engaged this problematic in studies that explore how "narratives emerge as contested terrains, open to challenge by those who seek to reshape perceptions of health issues and construct alternate narratives" (Harter et al. 2005, p. 23), including embodied, aesthetic stories that transform meanings of age (e.g. Sharf 2017; Yamasaki 2014), disability (e.g. Harter et al. 2006; Quinlan and Harter 2010), and baby loss (e.g. Willer 2016; Willer et al. 2019), among others. Finally, the problematic of the partial and indeterminate recognizes that the nature of narrative knowledge is always situated and shifting: "People live stories, and in the living of these stories, reaffirm them, modify them, and create new ones" (Harter et al. 2005, p. 27).

Narrative Medicine

Storytelling in healthcare reflects the narrative impulse and is a powerful form of experiencing and expressing suffering, loss, and healing (Sharf 1990; Sharf et al. 2011; Vanderford, Jenks, and Sharf 1997).

Indeed, healthcare would be impossible if not for the capacities of participants (i.e. patients and providers) to order and represent experience in narrative form (Harter 2013). These clinical encounters involve both patient and provider in the creation and negotiation of a plot structure within clinical time, which Mattingly (1994) termed *therapeutic emplotment*. Patients story pared-down autobiographical accounts of illness that reveal lay beliefs about cause and effect, while healthcare providers rely on narrative activity to gather information, keep records, make therapeutic decisions, build relationships with patients, and respond to their concerns in the contexts of their unfolding lives.

The narrative medicine movement signifies growing acknowledgment that clinical judgment is an interpretive act of coupling narrative logics with the scientific reasoning of biomedicine (Harter 2013; Sharf et al. 2011). Widely recognized as the authority in the practice of narrative medicine, Dr. Rita Charon (2006, 2009) – who is both a general internist (with an MD from Harvard University) and a literary scholar (with a PhD from Columbia University) – claims that narrative sensibilities humanize healthcare by enabling providers to join with patients who are suffering and to be responsive to their plight. Narrative medicine (see also Chapter 6) calls for providers to study literary texts to deepen their abilities – what Charon (2006) deems *narrative competence* – to absorb, interpret, and respond to the stories of others. Because narrative provides an important "road toward empathy and reflection" (Charon 2006, p. 131) by orienting individuals aesthetically and imaginatively to the way they live, literary ways of thinking can help providers adopt contradictory points of view, embrace the metaphorical as well as the factual, and be moved by what they hear (Charon 2006).

Physicians who practice narrative medicine make sense of their patients' experiences through a mutual dialogue of storytelling and story-listening. First, they attend to what their patients are saying and how they are saying it; then, they represent what they have witnessed by creating something new, by writing their experiences to perceive and display their thoughts, feelings, and perceptions of the situation (Charon 2006). From this perspective, narratives invite providers to stretch their imaginations to empathically grasp events befalling their patients: "The boldness of the imagination is the courage to relinquish one's own coherent experience of the world for another's unplumbed, potentially volatile viewpoint" (Charon 2006, p. 122). Ultimately, narrative medicine is a relational accomplishment: providers must be attentive without becoming overwhelmed, and patients must be willing and empowered to story their experiences (Harter 2013).

Autoethnography

Autoethnography has become increasingly popular in the social sciences, especially in health-related research (Chang 2016). By definition, autoethnography "operates as a bridge, connecting autobiography and ethnography in order to study the intersection of self and others, self and culture" (Ellingson and Ellis 2008, p. 446). Autoethnographers incorporate the "I" into research but analyze the self as if an "other" (Ellingson and Ellis 2008, p. 448), describing and systematically analyzing their personal experiences to understand cultural, social, and political meanings. Autoethnographic research is socially just and often critically reflective of taken-for-granted aspects of the social world (Ellis et al. 2011). Indeed, autoethnographers "seek the good" for society and themselves, sharing "the hope (and determination) that the moral, political, and practical work of autoethnography can give meaning to our lives and the lives of other people touched by this work" (Bochner and Ellis 2016a, p. 213).

As with other approaches described in this chapter, autoethnography intertwines theory and method from a social constructionist perspective, rendering it both process and product. Forms of autoethnography differ in a variety of ways, including how much emphasis is placed on the study of others and on the researcher's self in interaction with others (Ellis et al. 2011). Indeed, scholars view autoethnography as a "broad and wonderfully ambiguous category that encompasses a wide array of practices" (Ellingson and Ellis 2008, pp. 449–450) – with analysis and representation once again falling across a continuum. Still, autoethnographers have begun to recently distinguish their work as either evocative or analytic (Anderson 2006), with the former focused on narrative presentations that evoke emotions and inspire conversations (i.e. storyteller) and the latter concerned with developing theoretical explanations of broader social phenomena (i.e. story-analyst; Bochner and Ellis 2016b; Ellingson and Ellis 2008). Although autoethnographies often incorporate elements of both at varying points on a paradigmatic continuum (Allen-Collinson 2013; Wall 2016), I present them here as dichotomous to better explain how theorizing is understood and engaged in each. In doing so, I recognize that I have inserted scholarly examples somewhat artificially, based on my own subjective understandings rather than the authors' implicit intentions.

Evocative Autoethnography

Communication scholars Carolyn Ellis and Art Bochner are widely recognized for conceptualizing, curating, and promoting autoethnography, in general, and *evocative autoethnography*, in particular.

To them, autoethnographies are personal "stories with raw and naked emotion that investigate life's messiness, including twists of fates and chance" (Bochner and Ellis 2016b, p. 10). Researchers craft these intimate, vulnerable stories with evocation as a goal, wanting to move audiences "to care, to feel, to empathize, and to do something, to act" (Ellis and Bochner 2006, p. 433). From this perspective, stories can and do theorize (Ellis and Bochner 2006). Rather than privileging analysis over story (i.e. treating stories as data to be analyzed), scholars instead write or perform stories that frame their lived experiences in hindsight and invite others into conversation about what those experiences mean for themselves and others (Bochner and Ellis 2016b). In other words, evocative autoethnographers place themselves and their experiences under a "narrative analytic microscope," thereby applying the same theoretical scrutiny to themselves that they readily apply to the lives of others (Goodall 2004, p. 189).

To that end, evocative autoethnography embodies emotionality and subjectivity, blurs the boundaries between the social sciences and humanities, and claims conventions of literary writing (i.e. dialogue, scenes, unfolding action, characterization) in first-person accounts of lived experiences. As Bochner and Ellis (2016b) explain in their writings and yearly workshops:

> We encouraged researchers to think of themselves as writers and to tell stories the way novelists do; we promoted emotional, vulnerable, and heartful writing; we discouraged jargon and celebrated erotic and close to the bone prose in which knowledge is delivered through emotional arousal, identification, and self-examination rather than abstraction and explanation. "Let the story do the work," we insisted. "Be evocative. Make your readers feel stuff; activate their subjectivity; compel them to respond viscerally." What mattered most to us was intimate detail, not abstracted facts. (pp. 59–60)

As a small illustrative sample, evocative accounts of health and illness have offered important insights into negotiating the social effects of life with chronic pain (Birk 2013); navigating patriarchal healthcare while living with invisible illness (Edley and Battaglia 2016) or giving birth (Ohs 2020); managing emotions outside of an eating disorder (Tillmann 2009); adjusting to new normals after a difficult diagnosis (Baglia 2019) or permanent disability (Kellett 2017; Smith 2019); and raising cultural and political consciousness of pregnancy loss (Silverman and Baglia 2014).

Analytic Autoethnography

The term *analytic autoethnography* refers to ethnographic research in which the researcher combines self-narrative with dialogic engagement and is committed to developing theoretical understandings of broader social phenomena (Anderson 2006). The latter is what especially defines and distinguishes analytic autoethnography from Ellis and Bochner's evocative autoethnography. Indeed, "the definitive feature of analytic autoethnography is this value-added quality of not only truthfully rendering the social world under investigation but also transcending that world through broader generalization" (Anderson 2006, p. 388). This is a more conservative position that incorporates the researcher's perspective within traditional elements of scholarly inquiry, leading some critics to claim analytic autoethnography is really no different than realist ethnography (see Ellis and Bochner 2006).

Anderson (2006) outlined five key features characterizing analytic autoethnography. First, the researcher is a complete member of the studied social world. Second, as a complete member conducting research, the researcher is also aware of her reciprocal influence on the social world under study (i.e. analytic reflexivity) and, third, is visible in the narrative representation of her work to demonstrate her personal engagement in that world. Fourth, the researcher grounds her autoethnography in her subjective experience but reaches beyond it as well in dialogue with other participants. Finally, to that end, the researcher is committed to analysis directed toward theoretical elaboration, refinement, and extension that transcends beyond the local data for broader understandings of social processes.

To illustrate, consider Laura Ellingson's (2005) innovative ethnography of an interdisciplinary geriatric oncology team at a regional cancer center. A cancer survivor herself, she combined autoethnography with narrative ethnography, grounded theory, and feminist analyses to theorize backstage communication processes (e.g. formal reporting, informal information sharing, and relationship building) for improved frontstage patient care. While her layered account shared many of the characteristics of analytic autoethnography, Ellingson also embraced crystallization, embodied ways of knowing, and her talents as a narrative writer to evoke emotional responses that traditional analysis and representation usually eschew.

Like Ellingson (2009; Ellingson and Ellis 2008), some scholars call for a moderate approach to autoethnography that is both self-focused and analytical:

> What I wish to do in this article is draw attention to the middle ground, to encourage would-be autoethnographers to consider a balanced perspective that lies between the warring factions of evocative and analytic approaches to this method, one that captures the meanings and events of one life in an ethical way but also in a way that moves collective thinking forward – a moderate autoethnography. (Wall 2016, p. 7)

Erin Willer's (2020) compelling autoethnography of running as an embodied practice under the load of infertility, baby loss, and motherhood provides an apt example. Willer drew from her detailed running log, which consisted of "the successes and challenges of my runs themselves, but also my memories, experiences, and sense-making surrounding my infertility, losses, motherhood, and transitioning into being 40 years old that running conjures up" (Willer 2020, p. 3), to explore meanings born from this running-in-process state and to expose the sociocultural challenges that women similarly experience. Willer writes with striking sensory detail, literary artfulness, and soulful heart (i.e. evocative) while also theorizing feminist embodiments of health and unsteady spaces of freedom (i.e. analytic). In other studies, autoethnographers in health communication have combined singular personal stories with theoretical understandings of – for example – disenfranchised grief when an ex-spouse dies (Tullis 2017), feminist perspectives on patient consent during illness (Cole 2020), revealing and concealing invisible illness (Defenbaugh 2013), and the moral process of bearing witness to suffering in the intensive care unit (Sharf 2019). Moderate autoethnographies like these "tap into legitimate and unique sources of knowledge and insight that come from a particular view of one's place in the world" in evocative tellings that are supported by theory and connected to relevant literature (Wall 2016, p. 7).

Rhetoric of Health and Medicine

Within a university communication department, shared theoretical constructs (e.g. narrative, metaphor, ideology, hegemony) can unite methodological differences – namely, the critical-interpretive health communication and the rhetoric of health and medicine – as scholars investigate meaning-making in a variety of health-related contexts (see Keranën 2015; Lynch and Zoller 2015). Rhetoric can be defined in various ways, but it generally refers to the study of persuasive discourses in any number of forms, including spoken, written, mediated, or face-to-face. In health communication, rhetorical criticism has been "invaluable in answering important questions about how best to communicate health information, the consequences of those messages, and how cultures come to understand and address particular health concerns" (Stokes 2014, p. 279).

Beyond and within health communication (see Lynch and Zoller 2015), rhetoric of health and medicine is a burgeoning, robust area of scholarship, spanning rhetorical studies and the medical humanities, as well as multiple communicative contexts and a wide swath of discourse domains. Indeed, "health and medical rhetoric infuses every aspect of healthcare" (Keranën 2014, p. 1173) from insurance forms, patient intake histories, and clinical notes through online support groups, digital health information, pharmaceutical advertisements, email exchanges between patients and providers, and mass-mediated representations of illness. Scholarship in the rhetoric of health and medicine offers a humanistic perspective on the exigencies, functions, and impacts of health-related discourse.

Stokes (2014) outlined four theoretical assumptions that – echoing the other frameworks in this chapter – demonstrate the commitment of rhetoricians as critics to keep close relationship with the discourses they critique. First, rhetoricians assume reality is constructed through language and culture is perpetuated through discourse. To that end, they are interested in both the measurable outcomes of a campaign and in the ways that campaign could shift cultural views, as demonstrated, for example, in campaign analyses of the use of humor in combating stigma about mental health in men (Mocarski and Butler 2016) and in the endorsement of personal responsibility for managing risks of infection (Brown 2019). Second, rhetoricians acknowledge that a neutral stance is both impossible and unethical, given that they bring their own ideologies and biases to bear when studying a particular phenomenon. Third, rhetoricians recognize that their perspective is selective. As such, any rhetorical act can be read in numerous ways, and audiences may take away different meanings from a particular health message. Finally, rhetoricians debate what constitutes an object of critique, noting that it could be one particular persuasive discourse or an assembly of texts and artifacts. As Lisa Keranën, an influential rhetorician of health and medicine, noted:

> Rhetorical studies of health and medicine have increasingly embraced theoretical frameworks and methods that can account for the complexities of language as social action, shifting our focus from texts to the networks, ecologies, and activity systems that shape health-related discourse and its effects. Many rhetoricians of health and medicine are looking beyond traditional rhetorical theory and methods – with their emphases on the persuasive moves of authors in texts – to explore other means of rhetorical inquiry. . . that foreground interconnectedness, materiality, and movement in health and medicine. (Scott, Segal, and Keranën 2013, p. 3)

Indeed, Jensen (2015) positioned the articulation and tracing of health-related arguments in and through time as a major objective of scholarship in rhetoric of health and medicine, and she offered two different but related orientations for engaging this approach. In the first, research focuses on the interaction of different kinds of rhetoric across a largely chronological timeline to constitute broader health landscapes. As an example, Jensen (2016) drew from doctor–patient correspondence, oral histories, and contemporary popular and scientific news coverage to trace the transformation of language surrounding infertility and the implications of those rhetorical constructions on individuals and the societies in which they live.

In the second approach, research demonstrates how historical arguments about health percolate up at distinct, chronologically disjointed moments: "The exploration of health as it was conceptualized in even the distant past can be understood. . . as a valuable contribution to delineating conceptualizations of health today that may not follow a linear or rational logic" (Jensen 2015, p. 524). To illustrate, consider the notable study on mothering, media, and medical expertise conducted by historian Bethany Johnson and health communication scholar Maggie Quinlan (2019). They engaged historical texts (e.g. doctors' notes and family papers) and present-day social media texts (e.g. comments and hashtags) to discover how such discourses have challenged and continue to challenge and create expertise and power relations in defining the good mother. Other studies have examined the rhetorical work of genres, such as Cole and Carmon's (2019) analysis of addiction-related obituaries, and the rhetoric of a particular area or topic, like Miller's (2019) analysis of fat stigma as rhetorical disability or Alderton's (2018) analysis of the aesthetics of self-harm (i.e. visual rhetoric) in online communities.

Conclusion

Zoller and Kline (2008) defined the goal of interpretive, critical, and rhetorical health communication research as seeking "to better understand interpretation and the process of meaning making . . . [and] to provide in-depth understanding of lived experience or a unique, well-argued and defended interpretation of a discourse to impart some insight into the multiple ways in which communication fosters particular meanings" (p. 93). From these paradigms, grounded theory, narrative theorizing, autoethnography, and rhetoric of health and medicine intertwine theory and method to contribute a rich body of interdisciplinary scholarship in health-related contexts.

Acknowledgment

Special thanks to Barbara Sharf for the insightful comments that prompted the creation of this chapter and the generous feedback provided as I wrote it.

References

Alderton, Z. (2018). *The aesthetics of self-harm: The visual rhetoric of online self-harm communities*. Abingdon, UK: Routledge.

Allen-Collinson, J. (2013). Autoethnography as the engagement of self/other, self/culture, self/politics, and selves/futures. In S. Holman Jones, T. E. Adams, & C. Ellis (Eds.), *Handbook of autoethnography* (pp. 281–299). Walnut Creek: CA: Left Coast Press.

Anderson, L. (2006). Analytic autoethnography. *Journal of Contemporary Ethnography, 35*(4), 373–395. doi:10.1177/0891241605280449

Baglia, J. (2019). Beginning again: Diagnosis as breach, survival as a new normal. In L. W. Peterson & C. E. Kiesinger (Eds.), *Narrating midlife: Crisis, transition, and transformation* (pp. 107–130). Lanham, MD: Lexington Books.

Birk, L. B. (2013). Erasure of the credible subject: An autoethnographic account of chronic pain. *Cultural Studies – Critical Methodologies, 13*(5), 390–399. doi:10.1177/1532708613495799

Bochner, A. P. (2014). *Coming to narrative: A personal history of paradigm change in the human sciences*. New York, NY: Routledge.

Bochner, A. P., & Ellis, C. (2016a). The ICQI and the rise of autoethnography: Solidarity through community. *International Review of Qualitative Research, 9*(2), 208–217. doi:10.1525/irqr.2016.9.2.208

Bochner, A. P., & Ellis, C. (2016b). *Evocative ethnography: Writing lives and telling stories.* New York, NY: Routledge.

Brown, M. M. (2019). Don't be the "fifth guy": Risk, responsibility, and the rhetoric of handwashing campaigns. *Journal of Medical Humanities, 40,* 211–224. doi:10.1007/s10912-017-9470-4

Bruner, J. (1990). *Acts of meaning.* Cambridge, MA: Harvard University Press.

Burke, K. (1984 [1935]). *Permanence and change* (3rd ed.). Berkeley, CA: University of California Press. (Original work published 1935).

Chang, H. (2016). Autoethnography in health research: Growing pains? *Qualitative Health Research, 26*(4), 443–451. doi:10.1177/1049732315627432

Charmaz, K. (2006). *Constructing grounded theory: A practical guide through qualitative analysis.* London: Sage.

Charon, R. (2006). *Narrative medicine: Honoring the stories of illness.* Oxford: Oxford University Press.

Charon, R. (2009). Narrative medicine as witness for the self-telling body. *Journal of Applied Communication Research, 37*(2), 118–131. doi:10.1080/00909880902792248

Cole, K. L. (2020). The paradox of patient consent: A feminist account of illness and healthcare. *Health Communication,* 1–10. doi:10.1080/10410236.2020.1724645

Cole, K. L., & Carmon, A. F. (2019). Changing the face of the opioid epidemic: A generic rhetorical analysis of addiction obituaries. *Rhetoric of Health & Medicine, 2*(3), 291–320. doi:10.5744/rhm.2019.1014

Corbin, J. (2009). Taking an analytic journey. In J. M. Morse, P. N. Stern, J. Corbin, B. Bowers, K. Charmaz, & A. E. Clarke (Eds.), *Developing grounded theory: The second generation* (pp. 35–54). Walnut Creek, CA: Left Coast Press.

de Souza, R. (2007). The construction of HIV/AIDS in Indian newspapers: A frame analysis. *Health Communication, 21*(3), 257–266. doi:10.1080/10410230701307733

Defenbaugh, N. L. (2013). Revealing and concealing ill identity: A performance narrative of IBD disclosure. *Health Communication, 28*(2), 159–169. doi:10.1080/10410236.2012.666712

Dillon, P. J., & Basu, A. (2016). African Americans and hospice care: A culture-centered exploration of enrollment disparities. *Health Communication, 31*(11), 1385–1394. doi:10.1080/10410236.2015.1072886

Donovan-Kicken, E., Tollison, A. C., & Goins, E. S. (2012). The nature of communication work during cancer: Advancing the theory of illness trajectories. *Health Communication, 27*(7), 641–652. doi:10.1080/10410236.2011.629405

Dutta, M. J., & Zoller, H. M. (2008). Theoretical foundations: Interpretive, critical, and cultural approaches to health communication. In H. M. Zoller & M. J. Dutta (Eds.), *Emerging perspectives in health communication: Meaning, culture, and power* (pp. 1–27). New York, NY: Routledge.

Edley, P., & Battaglia, J. (2016). Dying of dismissal: An autoethnographic journey of chronic illness. *Women & Language, 39*(1), 33–48.

Ellingson, L. L. (2005). *Communicating in the clinic.* Creskill, NJ: Hampton Press.

Ellingson, L. L. (2007). The performance of dialysis care: Routinization and adaptation on the floor. *Health Communication, 22*(2), 103–114. doi:10.1080/10410230701453926

Ellingson, L. L. (2009). *Engaging crystallization in qualitative research: An introduction.* Thousand Oaks, CA: Sage.

Ellingson, L. L. (2011). The poetics of professionalism among dialysis technicians. *Health Communication, 26*(1), 1–12. doi:10.1080/10410236.2011.527617

Ellingson, L. L. (2017). Realistically ever after: Disrupting dominant narratives of long-term cancer survivorship. *Management Communication Quarterly, 31*(2), 321–327. doi:10.1177/0893318917689894

Ellingson, L. L., & Borofka, K. G. E. (2014). Grounded theory. In T. L. Thompson (Ed.), *Encyclopedia of health communication* (pp. 537–538). Thousand Oaks, CA: Sage.

Ellingson, L. L., & Ellis, C. (2008). Autoethnography as constructionist project. In J. A. Holstein & J. F. Gubrium (Eds.), *Handbook of constructionist research* (pp. 445–465). New York, NY: The Guilford Press.

Ellis, C., Adams, T. E., & Bochner, A. P. (2011). Autoethnography: An overview. *Historical Social Research, 36*(4), 273–290.

Ellis, C., & Bochner, A. P. (2006). Analyzing analytic autoethnography: An autopsy. *Journal of Contemporary Ethnography, 35*(4), 429–449. doi:10.1177/0891241606286979

Evans-Agnew, R. A., Boutain, D. M., & Rosemberg, M.-A. S. (2017). Advancing nursing research in the visual era: Reenvisioning the photovoice process across phenomenological, grounded theory, and critical theory methodologies. *Advances in Nursing Science, 40*(1), E1–E15. doi:10.1097/ANS.0000000000000159

Fisher, W. R. (1984). Narration as a human communication paradigm: The case of public moral argument. *Communication Monographs, 51*(1), 1–22. doi:10.1080/03637758409390180

Fisher, W. R. (1987). *Human communication as narration: Toward a philosophy of reason, value, and action.* Columbia, SC: University of South Carolina Press.

Frank, A. W. (1995). *The wounded storyteller: Body, illness, and ethics.* Chicago, IL: University of Chicago Press.

Giddens, A. (1984). *The constitution of society: Outline of the theory of structuration.* Berkeley, CA: University of California Press.

Glaser, B., & Strauss, A. (1967). *The discovery of grounded theory: Strategies for qualitative research.* Chicago, IL: Aldine.

Goodall, H. L. (2004). Narrative ethnography as applied communication research. *Journal of Applied Communication Research, 32*(3), 185–194. doi:10.1080/0090988042000240130

Harter, L. M. (2013). The poetics and politics of storytelling in health contexts. In L. M. Harter & Associates (Eds.), *Imagining new normals. A narrative framework for health communication* (pp. 3–27). Dubuque, IA: Kendall Hunt.

Harter, L. M., Ellingson, L. E., Yamasaki, J., Hook, C., & Walker, T. (2020). Defining moments. . . Telling stories to foster well-being, humanize healthcare, and advocate for change. *Health Communication, 35*, 262–267.

Harter, L. M., Japp, P. M., & Beck, C. S. (2005). Vital problematics of narrative theorizing about health and healing. In L. M. Harter, P. M. Japp, & C. S. Beck (Eds.), *Narratives, health, and healing: Communication theory, research, and practice* (pp. 7–29). Mahwah, NJ: Erlbaum.

Harter, L. M., Scott, J. A., Novak, D. R., Leeman, M., & Morris, J. F. (2006). Freedom through flight: Performing a counter-narrative of disability. *Journal of Applied Communication Research, 34*(1), 3–29. doi:10.1080/00909880500420192

Jensen, R. E. (2015). An ecological turn in rhetoric of health scholarship: Attending to the historical flow and percolation of ideas, assumptions, and arguments. *Communication Quarterly, 63*(5), 522–526. doi:10.1080/014633 73.2015.1103600

Jensen, R. E. (2016). *Infertility: Tracing the history of a transformative term.* University Park, PA: Pennsylvania State University Press.

Johnson, B. L., & Quinlan, M. M. (2019). *You're doing it wrong! Mothering, media, and medical expertise.* New Brunswick, NJ: *Rutgers* University Press.

Kellett, P. M. (2017). *Patienthood and communication: A personal narrative of eye disease and vision loss.* New York, NY: Peter Lang.

Keränën, L. (2014). Rhetoric: Health and medicine. In T. L. Thompson (Ed.), *Encyclopedia of health communication* (pp. 1173–1175). Thousand Oaks, CA: Sage.

Keränën, L. (2015). Biopolitics, contagion, and digital health production: Pathways for the rhetoric of health and medicine. *Communication Quarterly, 63*(5), 504–509. doi:10.1080/01463373.2015.1103596

Kleinman, A. (1988). *The illness narratives: Suffering, healing, and the human condition.* New York, NY: Basic Books.

Lynch, J. A., & Zoller, H. (2015). Recognizing differences and commonalities: The rhetoric of health and medicine and critical-interpretive health communication. *Communication Quarterly, 63*(5), 498–503. doi:10.1080/01463373.201 5.1103592

Martin, S. C. (2016). The experience and communicative management of identity threats among people with Parkinson's disease: Implications for health communication theory and practice. *Communication Monographs, 83*(3), 303–325. doi:10.1080/03637751.2016.1146407

Mattingly, C. (1994). The concept of therapeutic "emplotment." *Social Science & Medicine, 38*(6), 811–822. doi:10.1016/0277-9536(94)90153-8

Miller, E. (2019). Too fat to be president? Chris Christie and fat stigma as rhetorical disability. *Rhetoric of Health & Medicine, 2*(1), 60–87. doi:10.5744/rhm.2019.1003

Miller, K. (2005). *Communication theories: Perspectives, processes, and contexts* (2nd ed.). Boston, MA: McGraw-Hill.

Mocarski, R., & Butler, S. (2016). A critical, rhetorical analysis of *Man Therapy*: The use of humor to frame mental health as masculine. *Journal of Communication Inquiry, 40*(2), 128–144. doi:10.1177/0196859915606974

Ohs, J. E. (2020). Healthy mother, healthy baby: An autoethnography to challenge the dominant cultural narrative of the birthing patient. In P. Kellett (Ed.), *Narrating patienthood: Engaging diverse voices on health, communication, and the patient experience* (pp. 227–258). Lanham, MD: Lexington Books.

Pangborn, S. M. (2019). Narrative resources and unspeakable grief: Teens foster connection and resilience in family storytelling. *Journal of Family Communication, 19*(2), 95–109.

Peterson, J. L. (2010). The challenges of seeking and receiving support for women living with HIV. *Health Communication, 25*(5), 470–479. doi:10.108 0/10410236.2010.484878

Poteat, T., German, D., & Kerrigan, D. (2013). Managing uncertainty: A grounded theory of stigma in transgender health care encounters. *Social Science & Medicine, 84*, 22–29. doi:10.1016/j.socscimed.2013.02.019

Quinlan, M. M., & Harter, L. M. (2010). Meaning in motion: The embodied poetics and politics of Dancing Wheels. *Text and Performance Quarterly, 30*(4), 374–395. doi:10.1080/10462937.2010.510911

Scott, B., Segal, J. Z., & Keranën, L. (2013). The rhetorics of health and medicine: Inventional possibilities for scholarship and engaged practice. *POROI, 9*(1), 1–6. doi:10.13008/2151-2957.1157

Sharf, B. F. (1990). Physician–patient communication as interpersonal rhetoric: A narrative approach. *Health Communication, 2*(4), 217–231. doi:10.1207/s15327027hc0204_2

Sharf, B. F. (2001). Out of the closet and into the legislature: Breast cancer stories. *Health Affairs, 20*(1), 213–218. doi:10.1377/hlthaff.20.1.213

Sharf, B. F. (2017). Communicating health through narratives. In J. Yamasaki, P. Geist-Martin, & B. F. Sharf (Eds.), *Storied health and illness: Personal, cultural, and political complexities* (pp. 29–52). Long Grove, IL: Waveland Press.

Sharf, B. F. (2019). On witnessing the precipice between life and death. *Health Communication*, 1–4. doi:10.1080/10410236.2019.1600102

Sharf, B. F., Harter, L. M., Yamasaki, J., & Haidet, P. (2011). Narrative turns epic: Continuing developments in health narrative scholarship. In T. L. Thompson, R. Parrott, & J. F. Nussbaum (Eds.), *Routledge handbook of health communication* (2nd ed., pp. 36–51). New York, NY: Routledge.

Sharf, B. F., & Vanderford, M. L. (2003). Illness narratives and the social construction of health. In T. L. Thompson, A. Dorsey, K. I. Miller, & R. Parrott (Eds.), *Handbook of health communication* (pp. 9–34). Mahwah, NJ: Erlbaum.

Silverman, R. E., & Baglia, J. (Eds.) (2014). *Communicating pregnancy loss: Narrative as a method for change.* New York, NY: Peter Lang.

Smith, C. (2019). Reflections on a midlife crisis: My chang(ed)(ing) life after severe traumatic brain injury. In L. W. Peterson & C. E. Kiesinger (Eds.), *Narrating midlife: Crisis, transition, and transformation* (pp. 177–190). Lanham, MD: Lexington Books.

Sparkes, A. C., & Smith, B. (2008). Narrative constructionist inquiry. In J. A. Holstein & J. F. Gubrium (Eds.), *Handbook of constructionist research* (pp. 295–314). New York, NY: The Guilford Press.

Stokes, A. Q. (2014). A matter of interpretation: Rhetorical criticism of health communication. In B. B. Whaley (Ed.), *Research methods in health communication* (pp. 279–297). New York, NY: Routledge.

Strauss, A., & Corbin, J. (1990). *Basics of qualitative research: Techniques and procedures for developing ground theory.* Beverly Hills, CA: Sage.

Tillmann, L. M. (2009). Body and bulimia revisited: Reflections on "A Secret Life." *Journal of Applied Communication Research, 37*(1), 98–112. doi:10.1080/00909880802592615

Titus, B., & de Souza, R. (2011). Finding meaning in the loss of a child: Journeys of chaos and quest. *Health Communication, 26*(5), 450–460. doi:10.1080/10410236.2011.554167

Tullis, J. A. (2017). Death of an ex-spouse: Lessons in family communication about disenfranchised grief. *Behavioral Sciences, 7*(2), 1–7. doi:10.3390/bs7020016

Vanderford, M. L., Jenks, E. B., & Sharf, B. F. (1997). Exploring patients' experiences as a primary source of meaning. *Health Communication, 9*(1), 13–26. doi:10.1207/s15327027hc0901_2

Wall, S. S. (2016). Toward a moderate autoethnography. *International Journal of Qualitative Methods, 15*(1), 1–9. doi:10.1177/1609406916674966

Willer, E. K. (2016). BIRTHing ARTiculations. In S. L. Faulkner (Ed.), *Inside relationships: A creative casebook in relational communication* (pp. 80–85). New York, NY: Routledge.

Willer, E. K. (2020). Running-in(to) transition: Embodied practice under the load of infertility, baby loss, and motherhood. *Health Communication.* doi:10.1080/10410236.2020.1748830

Willer, E. K., Krebs, E., Castaneda, N., Hoyt, K. D., Droser, V. A., Johnson, J. A., & Hunniecutt, J. (2019). Our babies['] count[er story]: A narrative ethnography of a baby loss remembrance walk ritual. *Communication Monographs.* doi:10.1080/03637751.2019.1666289

Yamasaki, J. (2014). Age accomplished, performed, and failed: Liz Young as old on *The Biggest Loser. Text and Performance Quarterly, 34*(4), 354–371. doi:10.1080/10462937.2014.942871

Yamasaki, J., & Hovick, S. R. (2015). "That was grown folks' business": Narrative reflection and response in older adults' family health history communication. *Health Communication, 30*(3), 221–230. doi:10.1080/10410236.2013.837569

Zoller, H. M. (2005). Health activism: Communication theory and action for social change. *Communication Theory, 15*(4), 341–364. doi:10.1111/j.1468-2885.2005.tb00339.x

Zoller, H. M., & Kline, K. N. (2008). Theoretical contributions of interpretive and critical research in health communication. In E. L. Cohen (Ed.), *Communication yearbook 38* (pp. 89–135). New York, NY: Routledge.

PART II

Perspectives on Dyads and Groups

4

Interpersonal Health Communication Theories

Maria Brann, Jennifer J. Bute, Maureen Keeley, Sandra Petronio, Rachyl Pines, and Bernadette Watson*

The process of health communication has in many ways traditionally been studied as an interpersonal context. Some of the later chapters in this volume will focus on contexts that are more likely to be mediated, but three theories are used frequently enough to study the interpersonal dimensions of health communication that the editors elected to have experts on each of them describe the theories separately. The three theories are communication accommodation theory, communication privacy management theory, and the theory of negotiated morality. All these theories are dyadic in focus. We combine them into one chapter to allow comparison and contrast, but all are equally useful and must be included in a volume such as this. None of these theories is applied exclusively in the health communication context, but all have seen productive application within it. Authorship of each section is identified below.

Health Communication Theory, First Edition. Edited by Teresa L. Thompson and Peter J. Schulz.
© 2021 John Wiley & Sons, Inc. Published 2021 by John Wiley & Sons, Inc.

Communication Accommodation Theory and Health

Rachyl Pines and Bernadette Watson

Communication accommodation theory (CAT) is an intergroup theory of interpersonal interactions in communication that has been applied to a number of diverse contexts (see Giles 2016; Harwood et al. 2019; Weatherall, Watson, and Gallois 2007). CAT provides explanatory mechanisms of interpersonal adjustment (i.e. social identity and uncertainty reduction) and is not tied to any one specific method (see Gasiorek 2016 for a review of theories of interpersonal adjustment and CAT). The theory recognizes that sometimes it is a speech partner's group identity (e.g. professional role [medical doctor] or social membership [e.g. supporter of a rival sporting team]) that can be more salient to another person than the personal attributes of that speech partner. Over the past 20 years researchers have applied CAT to explore interactions between health professionals and their patients as well as between health professionals from different disciplines and specialties who work together to negotiate patient care (Gallois et al. 2015; Watson and Gallois 1998, 1999; Watson, Jones, and Cretchley 2014). This research has highlighted the hierarchical nature of health communication and the complexity of health interactions (Watson, Hewett and Gallois 2012). In this section we will first explain the main concepts and origins of the theory. We will then discuss its focus on health and how researchers have applied the theory to actual health contexts rather than relying on laboratory experiments. We will close with an overall appraisal of the theory.

CAT: Concepts and Origins

CAT was developed in the early 1970s (see Giles and Powesland 1975). Formerly Speech Accommodation Theory (SAT; Giles et al. 1987), CAT expanded its focus (see Gallois, Ogay, and Giles 2005) to explore how an individual's affective and cognitive dispositions towards a speech partner can influence their communication behaviors with that person in a given interaction. Interactions can be both spoken and written. It takes account of the communication of both interactants and recognizes that communication is a dynamic process whereby an individual can experience a number of psychological states immediately prior to, during, and after the conversation (Coupland et al. 1988). Coupland and colleagues posited that these states are derived from an individual's biases and expectations that form from their sociohistorical background and cultural norms. CAT calls this a speaker's *initial orientation*. A person's initial orientation then shapes the goals of each interactant, which drives their communication behaviors in the interaction.

Several social psychological theories form the basis of CAT (i.e. social identity, social exchange, and uncertainty reduction theories). It uses assumptions from Tajfel and Turner's (1978) social identity theory in order to understand interactions where power between interactants is not equitable and to explain why miscommunication can occur. This emphasis on social identity is a key part of the theory and differentiates CAT from many other communication approaches where the focus is interpersonal relations rather than group membership. CAT investigates how individuals in an interpersonal encounter often focus on the group membership of their speech partner rather than on personal idiosyncrasies or characteristics. CAT's focus on group memberships makes it a valuable framework with which to explore health communication, particularly in the healthcare space. Even in a time of patient empowerment and physician–patient matching options, health professional identity (an important social grouping) is highly salient in the health setting where power differentials exist between different health professions and in the relationships between healthcare provider and patients (Baker and Watson 2015).

Another motivation proposed by Giles (e.g. 1977) for changes in communication behavior was for one speaker to gain the approval of the other interactant. This notion draws on similarity-attraction theory, which suggests we are attracted to individuals who are similar to us (Byrne 1969). Giles also invoked social exchange theory, which posits that people seek to maximize rewards and minimize costs (Homans 1961). All of the aforementioned theories are critical to understanding the dynamics of CAT and explain whether an interactant takes an accommodative or nonaccommodative stance in a given encounter. A competent accommodative communication stance is one where an interactant uses appropriate communication behaviors to facilitate effective communication and build rapport between speakers. In contrast, a nonaccommodative stance may result in miscommunication and poor levels of rapport. The choice of accommodative or nonaccommodative communication may depend on the interactant's goals and intended outcomes for that interaction.

CAT outlines three ways that a person may interact with their communicative partner. The first of these, called convergence, concerns speech production. Individuals may adapt toward their speech partner in their language (increasing similarity on speech production such as volume, pitch, accent, or speech rate). Second, individuals can diverge away from the interactant and choose to accentuate differences in their speech. Third, there is maintenance, where no speech adaptation to the partner occurs. Maintenance is often regarded as a form of divergence. Giles and Powesland (1975) proposed that motivation to converge may be explained by a reward and cost process. If an interactant perceives that speech convergence will bring about more rewards than the costs incurred by the physical and/or mental effort of doing so, then they will be motivated to converge with the other speaker. However, Giles (1977) acknowledged that costs would sometimes outweigh rewards. Thus, if the reward for speech convergence was a high approval rating from the listener, but the cost was the speaker's loss of individuality (e.g. not standing up for one's principles), then the speaker may not converge toward the speech partner. Speech divergence, on the other hand, emphasizes differences between the two speech partners and may (though not always) serve to signal dislike or differentiation from the other person.

Lower status individuals may converge to higher status ones, again to gain approval. The extent to which the interaction is important for each speaker and the likelihood of future encounters will also influence convergence levels. However, in all cases, convergence is only within the constraints of each person's speech repertoire, with some speakers more able to converge or, contrastingly, diverge (Giles 1977). In the health context social identity is important. Junior doctors seeking the approval of senior doctors may engage in linguistic convergence to gain their approval. However, senior doctors may engage in divergence if they wish to differentiate themselves from junior doctors and emphasize their high status. Such behaviors can serve to highlight differences between the two speakers as individuals, and in many cases, to accentuate their different status and health professional memberships.

There are five CAT strategies a person can use in interaction to either consciously or unconsciously engage in convergence, divergence, or maintenance. The strategies are approximation, interpretability, discourse management, interpersonal control, and emotional expression. *Approximation*, often synonymous with convergence, entails using the same speech repertoire as one's conversation partner and also matching on other linguistic variables like pitch, rate, and volume. An example would be a physician speaking at a rate that matches the pace of their patient. Communicators use accommodative *interpretability* strategies to ensure their message is comprehensible. An example is a physician not using medical jargon with a patient who is unfamiliar with such terms in order to maximize the patient's understanding. Interpretability can be used to emphasize group differences or to reduce them. Physicians may reduce the salience of their group identity with patients who they perceive as more similar to themselves. For example, a physician may use technical terms when the physician knows that the patient has medical knowledge, such as a fellow physician.

Accommodative *discourse management* strategies focus on the macro-conversation, such as ensuring that both parties are actively involved in the conversation (both have the opportunity to hold the floor and engage in the conversation). Such accommodative behavior can reduce group differentiation and signal interest in the other speech partner and what they have to say. According to the paternalistic medical model (Beisecker and Beisecker 1993), the patient is often seen as passive so the physician may not use accommodative discourse management strategies to encourage patient engagement but rather hold the floor for longer periods and not encourage patient engagement. Such nonaccommodative behavior highlights the salience of the group memberships of each interactant.

Nonaccommodative *interpersonal control* strategies refer to any communication that emphasizes the status and role of each speaker in the conversation in a way that constrains the lower status speaker. An example is a doctor introducing themselves as Dr. with the expectation that a patient will use the honorific "Doctor" when addressing them but addressing the patient by their first name. Nonaccommodative interpersonal control also includes behaviors such as the doctor not allowing the patient or junior doctor to query decisions, terminating a discussion, or abruptly changing topic. Accommodative interpersonal control results in both the patient and doctor feeling empowered during the interaction.

Emotional expression and relationship management strategies occur when a person appropriately recognizes and validates the emotions of the other speaker and in so doing demonstrates empathy in the conversation (Watson and Gallois 2004; Williams et al. 1990). For example, a patient may share with the physician that they are afraid of an upcoming procedure. In response, the physician may validate the patient's fear and reassure them before administering the treatment. Such an accommodative stance recognizes the patient as an *individual* with concerns and needs. In sum, the five strategies when used accommodatively increase effective communication and rapport. When used nonaccommodatively, messages may not be appropriately adapted to a speaker and so decrease effective communication and reduce rapport; nonaccommodative strategies may even be used deliberately, or (perceived to be used deliberately) with malice and can result in highly negative outcomes. This type of nonaccommodation is termed counter-accommodation and reflects active hostility. For example, a senior doctor may interrupt and reprimand a junior doctor (interpersonal control) to demonstrate their higher status and knowledge. Previous research has found that older adults in care who experience nonaccommodation such as patronizing speech and interpersonal control reported perceptions of reduced quality of life (Lagacé et al. 2012).

CAT takes account of different interactants' predetermined perceptions about an upcoming interaction (initial orientation) and the salience of the intergroup identities of the interactants. Understanding the initial orientation of, say, a patient or junior doctor toward a high status senior physician is important information in the healthcare setting because it can help predict the accommodative stance that may play out in the interaction. By contrast, purely interpersonal communication approaches in healthcare (i.e. interpersonal communication skills approaches; see Street 2003 for a review) often focus on each person's communication responses based on the interpersonal circumstances of the conversation. For example, in the 1990s health communication research mostly concentrated on patient satisfaction and adherence by focusing on the interpersonal communication skills of the health provider. Healthcare practitioners and researchers alike were focused on interpersonal communication skills that achieved mutually effective communication outcomes. However, the CAT studies reported below show that mutually effective communication is not always the intent of an interactant.

Applications of CAT

There are two main applications of CAT in the health domain: health provider–patient interactions, and interprofessional and interspecialty interactions. Recognizing the intergroup nature of healthcare interactions, the first seminal studies using CAT in health examined which CAT strategies patients found satisfying when they rated their health providers, and which strategies used by physicians predicted patient adherence to medical advice from their physician (Watson and Gallois 1998, 1999). Their findings showed that patients rated a blend of accommodation strategies often emphasizing emotional expression as being most appropriate. Recognizing this intricate blend of accommodation strategies and unique patient needs, Pitts and Harwood (2015) argue that CAT should focus on communication accommodation competence.

This means that patients and providers should actively strive to establish competent relationships, which may be achieved by considering interlocuters' group identities and the unique context of the interaction.

In one specific context, for example, some researchers used CAT to investigate new mothers' experiences in hospital (Jones, Woodhouse, and Rowe 2007). Previous research had found that adolescent as opposed to adult mothers with a preterm infant are more likely to experience negative intergroup communication with a nurse in the neonatal intensive care unit (NICU). The mother's young age is a salient social category, and in some circumstances increases the potential for health-care practitioners to engage in negative stereotyping of, for example, a young unmarried mother which in turn can lead to nonaccommodation by the nurses. The findings showed that the young mothers were more likely to be dissatisfied with these interactions and even be inhibited in their ability to parent as they dealt with feelings of judgement and marginalization by the nurses (Sheeran, Jones, and Rowe 2013). Another hospital maternity study focused on pain management in obese women in labor. In this study, framed by CAT, the researchers found that although the anesthesiologists generally accommodated to their patients, at times it was done reluctantly and against their own ideas of appropriate care in that situation (Eley et al. 2017). Reluctant accommodation, especially when detectible by the receiver, can foster resentment and further ingrain or worsen negative stereotypes (Soliz and Bergquist 2016).

We now turn to interprofessional and interdisciplinary communication. Setchell et al. (2015) surveyed Australian gastroenterologists about whether some of their specific procedures could be transferred to and performed by nurse practitioners; their open-ended responses demonstrated a sense of threat to their specialist identity. They displayed threat through highlighting the incompetence of nurses who they considered not capable of performing these procedures, even though in Europe these are routine procedures performed by nurses. From a CAT perspective, the language used was highly counter-accommodative (i.e. hostile) and emphasized the intergroup relations between these physicians and the outgroup "nurses." This finding demonstrates that health providers can be highly territorial and often wish to preserve their power and status either in their specialty, or with patients.

The notion of "turf war" has been observed in the hospital health context. Hewett et al. (2009) demonstrated that strong intergroup relations which are observed between different health professions are also apparent between subspecialties (e.g. between physicians from different specialties such as intensivists and surgeons). Using CAT to better understand the communication consequences of this intergroup setting, they found that communication behaviors were described as counter-accommodative and were often caused by senior physicians demanding immediate and often scarce resources for their patients. One senior consultant said that he would put pressure on the more junior doctors and continue until, in his words "they fold" (pp. 1738), meaning the more junior doctor succumbs to the demands of the senior doctor.

These health studies which focused on interspecialty interactions using CAT demonstrate that, in some cases, prejudice or dislike of a speech partner's salient group means that speakers deliberately use a nonaccommodative stance. As opposed to CAT, communication theories that emphasize that the key goal of a conversation is to achieve mutual understanding ignore the fact that the dissatisfying and ineffective behavior may have been purposeful by one or both interactants. A strength of CAT is that it recognizes a broad range of interaction goals and stances that patients and healthcare professionals may have for interacting with one another.

Research Applications of CAT

Chevalier et al. (2017) recognized that insights from CAT could be used to create better communication interventions for healthcare staff. They created a learning experience using CAT accommodation strategies for students completing pharmacy school. Their study recognized the key role that communication plays in pharmacy consultations where patients were instructed how to comply with and correctly use their medications. Pharmacists underwent several face-to-face tutorials where they learned and practiced communication skills that were taught in the form of the five CAT strategies situated in the pharmacist–patient context. The results showed that participants realized the need to have actual conversations with their patients, and that the learning experience changed the way pharmacists communicated with patients for the better.

Similarly, CAT has also recently been applied in healthcare to prevent patient violence. To address the critique that research in this arena is largely atheoretical (Johnson and Hauser 2001), Pines and colleagues developed a training program for healthcare staff of all types, framing previously known de-escalation and limit-setting skill strategies alongside CAT strategies (Pines, Giles, and Watson 2019). In this training, staff learned about the five CAT strategies as applied in this context and role-played their skills with a simulated patient. Using CAT to address patient aggression and violence is helpful as it affords attention to attitudes and organizational norms that have previously not been adequately addressed in these healthcare interactions. CAT has also been used as an intergroup approach to create a communication toolkit for carers, either lay or trained professionals, for the purpose of communicating with people with dementia (Young et al. 2011).

In sum, the scope and range of health communication research framed by CAT in the twenty-first century has expanded beyond patient and health provider interactions. While space constraints preclude in-depth discussion of all these studies, we have highlighted key findings across the diverse domains in healthcare that have been investigated. The strong hierarchical structure of the hospital setting which produces the intergroup context has been noted by many social science scholars from a range of perspectives and is not contested (Bartunek 2010; Fiol, Pratt, and O'Connor 2009). CAT scholars have been able to clearly demonstrate how this hierarchical structure is made explicit through language.

Appraisal of CAT

Previous research has found that accommodative behaviors are robustly associated with increased well-being (i.e. self-esteem, life satisfaction, and mental health), compliance (message agreement and persuasiveness), credibility and trust, quality of contact (communication satisfaction and evaluation of the conversation) and relational solidarity (relational satisfaction closeness, common ingroup identity and intimacy; for a review, see Soliz and Bergquist 2016). Healthcare providers strive to appear credible, gain patient trust, achieve patient compliance with medical direction and help develop a working relationship with their patients, especially in cases of repeated interactions for patients with chronic illness. CAT is less explicitly tied to any particular methodology or methodological tool than are many other theories, which has encouraged its use in applied healthcare research (Farzadnia and Giles 2015).

However, there are some criticisms of CAT that must be highlighted. Gallois, Watson and Giles (2018) argued that intergroup theories of communication such as CAT are highly complex. Although complexity has meant that the theory can and has been applied in many contexts, the number of variables in the CAT model, for example, make it very difficult to test all in one study. Researchers must consider the overlapping nature of an individual's goals and the changes in goals across an interaction.

They must also recognize that the communication strategies do not occur in isolation and are not orthogonal. For example, discourse management occurs across the whole interaction process while other strategies may be consciously or unconsciously pursued simultaneously. The number of resulting variables makes hypothesis testing challenging. With the introduction of new analytical techniques (Angus and Gallois 2017), the obstacles are being reduced, but raising awareness of these techniques is slow. In the health domain, CAT requires mixed methods in order to unpack the conversational dynamics. It is not a theory that can be quickly applied in order to predict and explain individuals' goals, motivations and perceptions. Instead, it requires time and healthcare organizational access to truly apply multiple components of the theory. However, over the past 20 years, it has been one of the theories to highlight existent problems in healthcare settings.

CAT: Conclusion

This discussion has briefly overviewed the strengths of using CAT in healthcare communication research, and highlighted examples of ways it has been used thus far. This has shown that CAT provides an important lens through which to study health communication and create interventions to improve healthcare. Ultimately, using CAT in healthcare research helps us to understand the interpersonal and intergroup dynamics in healthcare interactions both between patients and healthcare staff and between different healthcare specialties. Understanding these dynamics is critical if researchers are to understand how an effective interaction plays out and why, and what participants evaluate as effective (see Watson, Jones, and Hewett 2016). This focus is the direction of the next phase of CAT research.

Communication Privacy Management Theory

Maria Brann, Jennifer Bute, and Sandra Petronio

Origins and Central Concepts

Communication privacy management (CPM) theory was first developed and introduced in 2002 by Professor Sandra Petronio. CPM theory is evidenced-based and, accordingly, provides a dependable understanding of how decisions are made regarding disclosing and protecting private information. CPM theory is based on a communicative-social behavioral perspective and not necessarily a legal point of view. This theory uses plain language to understand privacy management in everyday life and in contexts such as health communication, face-to-face interactions, social media, and dyads or group interactions. CPM theory illustrates that privacy is not paradoxical but is sustainable through the process of a privacy management system used in everyday life.

CPM theory proposes that individuals believe they rightfully own their private information and uses the metaphor of boundaries to illustrate where a person's private information resides. Privacy boundaries can be thick, with impermeable membranes that are closed to most or all others as illustrated by secrets. On the other side of this spectrum, privacy boundaries can be very permeable where the information flows almost unchecked as is seen with complete openness. There are gradations of boundary types in between, and they can shift and change dependent on the needs of the "information owner." When private information is shared, the information transitions from an individual privacy boundary to a collective boundary (Petronio 1991). The perception of owning private information leads individuals to assume they have the right to control their private information.

People develop privacy rules to guide whether and how they choose to reveal or conceal private information. According to the theory, privacy rules are based on gendered expectations, assessments of risk versus benefit, motivations for disclosing (or not disclosing), and contextual criteria that can prompt the creation or revision of privacy rules (Petronio 2002). Co-owners of information might form the privacy rules that should be followed through negotiation in explicit conversations. While negotiation is one way to understand how individuals come to know privacy rules, individuals also learn privacy rules through socialization. Because privacy management is complex, occasions arise where information owners or their authorized co-owners experience privacy turbulence. Because individuals do not live in a perfect world, incidents occur where there are differences, disruptions, and breakdowns in the way private information is handled. Individuals either intentionally or unintentionally violate privacy rules, leading to potential changes. For instance, research in the context of infertility suggests that members of married couples might disclose their fertility problem at levels that diverge from the practices of their partner, which could be a sign of mismatched or misunderstood privacy rules (Steuber and Solomon 2011).

Applications of CPM

Originally applied to personal relationships, CPM theory is also well-positioned to explore a variety of health-related issues. Kathryn Greene and colleagues (2003) recognized the value of this by applying CPM theory to understand disclosure and privacy of HIV in interpersonal relationships with partners, family members, friends, colleagues, and healthcare providers. Since its inception and this early noteworthy application to health, CPM theory has been applied in multiple health contexts about numerous health topics. For example, scholars have explored health-related relationships such as patient–provider (Petronio and Sargent 2011), interprofessional (Lindsay et al. 2019), and various family relations (e.g. Bute, Petronio, and Torke 2015; Ebersole and Hernandez 2016).

Two areas that have benefited from a CPM exploration are patient care and stigmatized health issues. For example, with healthcare becoming ever more present in the online world, researchers have explored eHealth through a CPM lens and have discovered the practical application of boundary coordination in computer-mediated interactive health communication (Jin 2012). Concerning stigmatized health issues, multiple topics have benefited from a CPM perspective. For example, recent research has explored how individuals identifying as lesbian, gay, or bisexual manage the disclosure of their sexual orientation to their healthcare providers (Hudak and Carmack 2018). Bute and Brann (2015; Bute, Brann, and Hernandez 2019) have explored the stigmatized topic of miscarriage and assessed not only how couples manage their privacy around their experience but also how society as a whole influences how and what we talk about related to miscarriage. Other taboo health topics studied using CPM theory include alcoholism (Byrnes-Loinette and Brann 2019), genetic testing (Weiner, Silk, and Parrott 2005), and obesity (Polk and Hullman 2011). Finally, a growing trend ripe for CPM exploration is mental health. Thus far, scholars have examined mental health using CPM theory in contexts such as military couples' disclosure strategies of post-traumatic stress disorder (Cox and Albright 2016), parental disclosures of children's autism (Hays and Butauski 2018), and student disclosures of mental health counseling to instructors (Price, Carmack, and Kuang 2020) among others.

Appraisal of CPM

As noted, in its relatively short history, CPM theory has generated a wealth of health communication research spanning a range of contexts. The theory offers heuristic value and "a reliable set of tools" (Petronio 2013,

p. 12) for explaining complex social phenomena (Petronio and Durham 2014), while advancing practical implications for patients, their families, and health care providers. Moreover, CPM theory is flexible in the sense that both interpretive (Bute, Petronio, and Torke 2019) and post-positivist (Lewis, Matheson, and Brimacombe 2011) scholars have employed the framework; thus, the theory is not bound to a particular set of methodological expectations. Although Petronio expanded upon particular aspects of the theory, including core and catalyst criteria, in a 2013 status report on the theory and its applications, there is still room for scholars to challenge, refine, and expand upon the theory in novel applications of its tenets. Petronio and Durham (2014) have also called for the development of a diagnostic tool to evaluate incidents of boundary turbulence, which would surely be useful for scholars of health communication, particularly scholars interested in the emotional and relational effects of such turbulence (e.g. Aloia 2018).

Theory of Negotiated Morality

Maureen Keeley

Negotiated morality theory (NMT) (Waldron and Kelley 2008) provides a framework for examining how individuals negotiate the moral concerns that are inherently a part of health in their personal relationships. The communication that occurs within relationships reveals and shapes people's moral standards and values (Waldron and Kelley 2015). Moreover, issues pertaining to morality are often present within health contexts beginning with conception and ending with death, with a lifetime of ethical concerns in-between. In almost every health scenario, there is some degree of value judgment that must be negotiated amongst relevant participants. Lifestyle behaviors are entangled with health moral standards as can be seen through the communication regarding healthy actions (e.g. exercise, moderation in food and alcohol, etc.) versus unhealthy behaviors (e.g. overweight, drug and alcohol use, failure to take prescribed medications regularly, and risk-taking behaviors) (Parrot 2009). Furthermore, moral discourse within relationships and families often dictates how individuals cope with serious and life-threatening illnesses (Fischer and Wolf 2015). The negotiation about the correct course of action may be morally correct because it is health-promoting, but it may be morally wrong because it does not take into consideration the family values (such as quality of life) or perhaps the patient's adjustment to the illness and/or assessment of the risks associated with the medical treatment (Fischer and Wolf 2015). Exploring the moral aspect of health issues may elucidate how and why individuals make health decisions that are not always congruent with the standard ways of behaving (Fischer and Wolf 2015). Thus, utilizing NMT, scholars are provided a new framework for examining complex health issues and the negotiations that occur within relationships and families in the midst of health issues.

Originally, NMT (Waldron and Kelley 2008) was based on eight principles, but the theory has evolved and is now grounded upon four core principles (Waldron and Kelley 2017). First, shared moral duties is an important driving force for communication in the family and in health contexts. Second, verbal and nonverbal communication are used to calibrate beliefs and actions when ethical stability is threatened. Third, moral violations trigger negative emotions that can include anger, guilt, hurt, outrage, regret and shame; alternatively, compliance of moral values can trigger positive emotions that include respect, increased self-esteem, gratification, and unity. Fourth, strong emotions help family members legitimize, regulate, and challenge moral actions. Bear in mind that when issues of morality exist at multiple levels (i.e. family, institutions, society, culture) the communication necessarily becomes more complex.

Moral standards are originally learned in the family, within the context of multifaceted levels of influence that include institutions (e.g. education, health, legal, political, and religion), society (e.g. socioeconomic, race, gender, sexual orientation), and culture (e.g. traditions, expectations) (Waldron and Kelley 2015). Families in the midst of health crises view moral standards as right or wrong, good or bad, adaptive or maladaptive, worthy or unworthy of the behavior and choices (Fischer, and Wolf 2015). As with most things that involve communication, moral standards are fluid in so much as they are defined, then reconsidered and adapted to meet the ever-changing needs of the participants and the situation, and evolve as new information is learned, new technology is created, and new perspectives are revealed (Parrott 2009). Medical advancements prolong life, but often at the cost of the quality of life (Johnson 2008).

NMT infers that dyadic communication is the means by which individuals are held accountable (themselves and their partners), as well as how they resolve any tensions that are created by the different moral values of the participants (Waldron and Kelley 2008). The goal of these negotiations is to establish how individuals "should" behave (Fischer and Wolf 2015). Specifically, regarding health (wellness and illness), judgment is often an inherent part of the discussion. Regarding wellness, individuals in relationships and/or are beginning a family are often given rewarding and/or punishing messages indicating that it is time to stop selfish behaviors that risk their health (e.g. smoking, participating in extreme sports, or risky, health threatening, social behaviors) for the protection of the relationship/family (Parrott 2009). During times of illness, individuals often communicate judgment by highlighting bad health habits (e.g. overweight, lack of exercise, level of alcohol use, failure to get appropriate and timely medical tests), emphasizing how they should have behaved, resulting in a value assessment of responsibility (Broom and Whitaker 2004). Further, individuals often put pressure on their loved ones to do everything that is possible to fight the illness/disease saying they should want to live because the family members want them to do so, but it may be at the cost of the individuals' experience of pain and/or quality of life (Fischer and Wolf 2015). Additionally, the expectation for having positive health outcomes is often tied up with family expectations of staying positive, thus denying individuals the opportunity to discuss their fears; they may be forced to eliminate any negative talk (Fischer and Wolf 2015).

Individuals' need to preserve their moral code motivates a wide variety of communication behaviors such as communicating forgiveness versus accusations of blame (Waldron and Kelley 2008), discussing medical dilemmas (e.g. sharing of private medical information, right to life, right of women to have a say over their own bodies, use of experimental treatments; Parrott 2009), and communicating/negotiating health decisions (e.g. suicide-euthanasia versus right to die, comfort care versus treatment of the disease; Keeley and Generous 2017). Ultimately, negotiated morality aims to value the dignity of both people, increase their well-being, and ultimately to repair and strengthen their relationship (Waldron and Kelley 2017). Thus, adding NMT to the discussions concerning health has the potential to add to the explanation of how and why people make the health decisions that they do.

Some Comparisons and Contrasts

Importantly, the three theories discussed in this chapter all take a dyadic approach to our understanding of interpersonal communication in healthcare. Early work in interpersonal communication and in health communication tended to take a more simplistic, one-way view of the communicative process. This was oft-criticized, and appropriately so.

Communication is a dyadic process and can only be understood by looking at both participants as they interact together. None of the theories are simplistic; they all demonstrate the requisite complexity and variety necessary to understand health communication. All three of these theories can and have been applied to address important communication problems. They all have multiple applications in the healthcare context. Additionally, all of the theories have important implications for values and emotions as they pertain to the interpersonal dimensions of health communication. The theory of negotiated morality most directly addresses ethical concerns, but ethics also underlie notions of convergence/divergence inherent in CAT and privacy issues in CPM.

The three theories all recognize in their own ways the complexity of healthcare (group relations, decision-making and information-sharing, and moral judgments). The recognition of the roles played by status, hierarchical structures, and stigmatized groups is explicit in each theory and also introduces implicit issues as well. How are moralistic decisions made around who receives treatment and when it is decided that further treatment represents futile care? This is especially relevant because decisions about lifestyle behaviors are often left to the majority or more powerful group. Passive participation can be encouraged because of a patient's group membership. In today's world where refugees strive for any healthcare at all and need interpreters, where do their rights to privacy begin and end? Is it even considered?

Each theory focuses on more than just the message; none of them is focused on message design. Instead they are highly focused on the individual and their individual and group level variables that predict a successful interaction, whether that be encouraging a patient to disclose vital information or a doctor communicating in an appropriate and effective manner. This relates to patient-centered care (see Chapter 6), such that the theories focus on communication adaptations that strive to provide care that is satisfactory to each patient. This is relevant be it maintaining a space for private disclosures, validating patient emotions, or considering the whole patient taking a biopsychosocial approach thinking about lifestyle in morality and ethics.

Blending the distinctive perspectives of these three theories expands our understanding of the ongoing and sometimes insurmountable problems in healthcare around the world. Interpersonal communication can occur in nearly all health communication contexts. Whether communicating with a healthcare provider about symptoms you are experiencing, a family member about health choices they are making, a Facebook friend about a celebrity's endorsement of a health product, or a co-worker about the public health messaging being disseminated at work, interpersonal communication is at play in each health communication context. Even when focusing on mass-mediated health communication or public or organizational health messaging, we often turn to confidantes to interpersonally discuss what we learn, read, see, and do. The three interpersonal communication theories presented in this chapter help explain the communicative processes we use when communicating in various health contexts. Utilizing interpersonal communication theories in health communication contexts helps us make sense of some of our most important interactions.

Note

*Authors are listed alphabetically except within sections

References

Aloia, L. S. (2018). The emotional, behavioral, and cognitive experience of boundary turbulence. *Communication Studies, 69*(2), 180–195. doi:10.108 0/10510974.2018.1426617

Angus, D., & Gallois, C. (2017). New methodological approaches to IGC. In H. Giles & J. Harwood (Eds), *Oxford encyclopedia of intergroup communication* (Vol. 2, pp. 163–179). New York, NY: Oxford University

Baker, S. C., & Watson, B. M. (2015). How patients perceive their doctors' communication: Implications for patient willingness to communicate. *Journal of Language and Social Psychology, 34*, 621–639. doi:10.1177/02619 27X15587015

Bartunek, J. M. (2010). Intergroup relationships and quality improvement in healthcare. *British Medical Journal: Quality and Safety, 20*, i62–i66.

Beisecker, A. E., & Beisecker, T. D. (1993). Using metaphors to characterize doctor–patient relationships: Paternalism versus consumerism. *Health Communication, 5*, 41–58. doi:10.1207/s15327027hc0501_3

Broom, D., & Whittaker, A. (2004). Controlling diabetes, controlling diabetics: Moral language in the management of diabetes type 2. *Social Science & Medicine, 58*, 2371–2382. doi:10.1016/j. socscimed.2003.09.002

Bute, J. J., & Brann, M. (2015). Co-ownership of private information in the miscarriage context. *Journal of Applied Communication Research, 43*(1), 23–43. doi:10.1080/00909882.2014.982686

Bute, J. J., Brann, M., & Hernandez, R. (2019). Exploring societal-level privacy rules for talking about miscarriage. *Journal of Social and Personal Relationships, 36*(2), 379–399. doi:10.1177/0265407517731828

Bute, J. J., Petronio, S., & Torke, A. M. (2015). Surrogate decision makers and proxy ownership: Challenges of privacy management in health care decision making. *Health Communication, 30*(8), 799–809. doi:10.1080/104 10236.2014.900528

Byrne, D. (1969). Attitudes and attraction. In L. Berkowitz (Ed.), *Advances in experimental social psychology* (Vol. 4, pp. 35–89). New York, NY: Academic Press.

Byrnes-Loinette, K., & Brann, M. (2019). Using CPM to understand (im)permeable boundaries: Stories of adult children of alcoholics. In S. L. LeBlanc (Ed.), *Casing the family: Theoretical and applied approaches to understanding family communication* (pp. 243–254). Dubuque, IA: Kendall Hunt.

Chevalier, B., Watson, B., Falconer, N., & Cottrell, N. (2017, June). Educating pharmacy students to speak with patients about their medications – a novel use of CAT. Presented at *International Symposium on Intergroup Communication*, Thessaloniki, Greece.

Coupland, N., Coupland, J., Giles, H., & Henwood, K. (1988). Accommodating the elderly: Invoking and extending a theory. *Language in Society, 17,* 1–41. doi:10.1017/S0047404500012574

Cox, J. A., & Albright, D. L. (2016). Can you keep a secret? Examining military couples' disclosure through the lens of communication privacy management theory. *Journal of Military and Government Counseling, 4*(1), 12–21.

Ebersole, D. S., & Hernandez, R. A. (2016). "Taking good care of our health": Parent–adolescent perceptions of boundary management about health information. *Communication Quarterly, 64*(5), 573–595. doi:10.1080/01463 373.2016.1176939

Eley, V., Callaway, L., van Zundert, A., Lipman, J., & Gallois, C. (2017). Interpretations of care guidelines for obese women in labor: Intergroup language and social identity. *Journal of Language and Social Psychology, 36,* 388–414. doi:10.1177/0261927X16668564

Farzadnia, S., & Giles, H. (2015). Patient–provider interaction: A communication accommodation theory perspective. *International Journal of Society, Culture, and Language, 3,* 17–34.

Fiol, C. M., Pratt, M. G., & O'Connor, E. J. (2009). Managing intractable identity conflicts. *Academy of Management Review, 34,* 32–35. doi:10.5465/ amr.2009.35713276

Fischer, C., & Wolf, B. (2015). Morality and family communication when coping with cancer. In V. Waldron & D. Kelley (Eds.), *Moral talk across the lifespan: Creating good relationships. Lifespan communication.* New York, NY: Peter Lang.

Gallois, C., Ogay, T., & Giles, H., (2005). Communication accommodation theory: A look back and a look ahead. In W. Gudykunst (Ed.), *Theorizing about intercultural communication* (pp. 121–148). Thousand Oaks, CA: Sage.

Gallois, C., Watson, B. M., & Giles, H. (2018). Intergroup communication: Identities and effective interactions. *Journal of Communication, 68,* 309–317. doi:10.1093/joc/jqx016

Gallois, C., Wilmott, L., White, B., Winch, S., Parker, M., Graves, N., . . . Close, E. (2015). Futile treatment in hospital: Doctors' intergroup language. *Journal of Language and Social Psychology, 34*(6), 657–671. doi:10.1177/02619 27x15586430

Gasiorek, J. (2016). Theoretical perspectives on interpersonal adjustments in language and communication. In H. Giles (Ed.), *Communication accommodation theory; Negotiating personal relationships and social identities across contexts* (pp. 13–35). Cambridge, UK: Cambridge University Press.

Giles, H. (1977). Social psychology and applied linguistics: Towards an integrative approach. *ITL – International Journal of Applied Linguistics, 35*, 27–42.

Giles, H. (2016). *Communication accommodation theory: Negotiating personal relationships and social identities across contexts*. Cambridge, UK: Cambridge University Press.

Giles, H., Mulac, A., Bradac, J. J., & Johnson, P. (1987). Speech accommodation theory: The first decade and beyond. In M. McLaughlin (Ed.), *Communication yearbook* (Vol. 10, pp. 13–48). Beverly Hills, CA: Sage.

Giles, H., & Powesland, P. F. (1975). *Speech style and social evaluation*. London, UK: Academic Press.

Greene, K., Derlega, V. J., Yep, G. A., & Petronio, S. (2003). *Privacy and disclosure of HIV in interpersonal relationships. A sourcebook for researchers and practitioners*. Routledge. doi:10.4324/9781410607706

Harwood, J., Gasiorek, J., Pierson, H., Nussbaum, J. F., & Gallois, C. (2019). *Language, communication, and intergroup relations*. New York, NY: Routledge.

Hays, A., & Butauski, M. (2018). Privacy, disability, and family: Exploring the privacy management behaviors of parents with a child with autism. *Western Journal of Communication, 82*(3), 376–391. doi:10.1080/10570314.2017.1398834

Hewett, D. G., Watson, B. M., Gallois, C., Ward, M., & Leggett, B. A. (2009). Intergroup communication between hospital doctors: Implications for quality of patient care. *Social Science and Medicine, 69*, 1732–1740. doi:10.1016/j.socscimed.2009.09.048

Homans, G. C. (1961). *Social behavior*. New York, NY: Harcourt, Brace & World.

Hudak, N. C., & Carmack, H. J. (2018). Waiting for the doctor to ask: Influencers of lesbian, gay, and bisexual identity disclosure to healthcare providers. *Qualitative Research in Medicine & Healthcare, 2*(1), 20–29. doi:10.4081/qrmh.2018.7157

Jin, S-A. A. (2012). "To disclose or not to disclose, that is the question": A structural equation modeling approach to communication privacy management in e-health. *Computers in Human Behavior, 28*(1), 69–77. doi:10.1016/j.chb.2011.08.012

Johnson, C. S. (2008). Aging and healthy life expectancy: Will the extended years be spent in good or poor health? *Journal of the Indian Academy of Geriatrics, 4*(2), 64–67.

Johnson, M. E., & Hauser, P. M. (2001). The practices of expert psychiatric nurses: Accompanying the patient to a calmer personal space. *Issues in Mental Health Nursing, 22*, 651–668. doi:10.1080/01612840117788

Jones, L., Woodhouse, D., & Rowe, J. (2007). Effective nurse parent communication: A study of parents' perceptions in the NICU environment.

Patient   Education   and   Counseling,   69,   206–212.   doi:10.1016/j.
pec.2007.08.014

Keeley, M. P., & Generous, M. A. (2017). Final conversations: Overview and practical implications for patients, families and healthcare workers. *Behavioral Sciences, 7*(2), 1–9. doi:10.3390/bs7020017

Lagacé, M., Tanguay, A., Lavallée, M. L., Laplante, J., & Robichaud, S. (2012). The silent impact of ageist communication in long term care facilities: Elders' perspectives on quality of life and coping strategies. *Journal of Aging Studies, 26,* 335–342. doi:10.1016/j.jaging.2012.03.002

Lewis, C. C., Matheson, D. H., & Brimacombe, C. E. (2011). Factors influencing patient disclosure to physicians in birth control clinics: An application of the communication privacy management theory. *Health Communication, 26*(6), 502–511. doi:10.1080/10410236.2011.556081

Lindsay, D., Brennan, D., Lindsay, D., Holmes, C., & Smyth, W. (2019). Conceal or reveal? Patterns of self-disclosure of long-term conditions at work by health professionals in a larger regional Australian health service. *International Journal of Workplace Health Management, 12*(5), 339–351. doi:10.1108/IJWHM-05-2018-0071

Parrott, R. L. (2009). *Talking about health: Why communication matters.* Oxford: Wiley Blackwell.

Petronio, S. (1991). Communication boundary management: A theoretical model of managing disclosure of private information between marital couples. *Communication Theory, 1*(4), 311–335. doi:10.1111/j.1468-2885.1991.tb00023.x

Petronio, S. (2002). *Boundaries of privacy. Dialectics of disclosure.* Albany, NY: State University of New York Press.

Petronio, S. (2013). Brief status report on communication privacy management theory. *Journal of Family Communication, 13*(1), 6–14. doi:10.1080/15267431.2013.743426

Petronio, S., & Durham, W. T. (2014). Communication privacy management theory: Significance for interpersonal communication. In D. O Braithwaite & P. Schrodt (Eds.), *Engaging theories in interpersonal communication: Multiple perspectives* (2nd ed., pp. 335–348). Thousand Oaks, CA: Sage. doi:10.4135/9781483329529

Petronio, S., & Sargent, J. (2011). Disclosure predicaments arising during the course of patient care: Nurses' privacy management. *Health Communication, 26*(3), 255–266. doi:10.1080/10410236.2010.549812

Pines, R., Giles, H., & Watson, B. (2019, July). Addressing patient aggression and violence in a hospital setting: Developing competent accommodation among health professionals. *Presented at the Asian Association of Social Psychology 13th Biennial Meeting.* Taipei, Taiwan.

Pitts, M. J., & Harwood, J. (2015). Communication accommodation competence: The nature and nurture of accommodative resources across the lifespan. *Language and Communication, 41,* 89–99. doi:10.1016.j.langcom.2014.10.002

Polk, D. M., & Hullman, G. W. (2011). Weight-related stigma as a predictor of self-disclosure patterns in women. *The Open Communication Journal, 5,* 1–10. doi:10.2174/1874916X01105010001

Price, S. F., Carmack, H. J., & Kuang, K. (2020). Contradictions and predicaments in instructors' boundary negotiations of students' health disclosures. *Health Communication*. Advance online publication. doi:10.1080/10410236.2020.1712525

Setchell, J., Leach, L. E, Watson, B. M., & Hewett, D. G. (2015). Impact of identity on support for new roles in health care: A language inquiry of doctors' commentary. *Journal of Language and Social Psychology, 34,* 672–686. doi:10.1177/0261927x15586793

Sheeran, N., Jones, L., & Rowe, J. (2013). The relationship between maternal age, communication and supportive relationships in the neonatal nursery for mothers of pre-term infants. *Journal of Neonatal Nursing, 19,* 327–336. doi:10/1016/j.jnn.2013.01.006

Soliz, J., & Bergquist, G. (2016). Methods of CAT inquiry: Quantitative studies. In H. Giles (Ed.), *Communication accommodation theory; Negotiating personal relationships and social identities across contexts* (pp. 36–59). Cambridge, UK: Cambridge University Press.

Steuber, K. R., & Solomon, D. H. (2011). Factors that predict married partners' disclosures about infertility to social network members. *Journal of Applied Communication Research, 39*(3), 250–270. doi:10.1080/00909882.2011.585401

Street, R. L. (2003). Interpersonal communication skills in health care contexts. In J. O. Greene & B. R. Burleson (Eds.) *Handbook of communication and social interaction skills* (pp. 909–933). Mahwah, NJ: Erlbaum.

Tajfel, H., & Turner, J. C. (1986). The social identity theory of intergroup behavior. In S. Worshel & W. Austin (Eds.), *The psychology of intergroup relations* (pp. 7–24). Chicago, IL: Nelson-Hall.

Waldron, V. R., & Kelley, D. L. (2015). *Moral talk across the lifespan: Creating good relationships (Lifespan communication).* New York, NY: Peter Lang.

Waldron, V., & Kelley, D. (2017). Negotiated morality theory: How family communication shapes our values. In D. Braithwaite, E. Suitor, & K. Floyd (Eds.), *Engaging theories in family communication* (2nd ed.). New York, NY: Routledge.

Waldron, V. R., & Kelley, D. L. (2008). *Communicating forgiveness.* Thousand Oaks, CA: Sage.

Watson, B. M., Jones, E., & Hewett, D.G. (2016). Accommodating health. In H. Giles (Ed.) *Communication accommodation theory: Negotiating personal relationships and social identities across contexts* (pp. 152–168). Cambridge, UK: Cambridge University Press.

Watson, B. M., & Gallois, C. (1998). Nurturing communication by health professionals toward patients: A communication accommodation theory approach. *Health Communication, 10,* 343–55. doi:10.1207/s15327027hc1004_3

Watson, B. M., & Gallois, C. (1999). Communication accommodation between patients and health professionals: Themes and strategies in satisfying and unsatisfying encounters. *International Journal of Applied Linguistics, 9,* 167–184. doi: 10.1111/j.1473-4192.1999.tb00170.x

Watson, B. M., & C. Gallois. (2004). Emotional expression as a sociolinguistic strategy: Its importance in medical interactions. In S. H. Ng, C. N. Candlin & C. Y Chiu (Eds.), *Language matters: Communication, culture and identity* (pp. 63–84). Hong Kong: City University of Hong Kong Press.

Watson, B. M., Hewett, D., & Gallois, C. (2012). Intergroup communication and healthcare. In H. Giles (Ed.), *The Routledge handbook of intergroup communication* (pp. 293–305). Abingdon, UK: Routledge.

Watson, B. M., Jones, L., & Cretchley, J. (2014). Time as a key topic in health professionals' perceptions of clinical handovers. *Global Qualitative Nursing Research, 1,* 1–11. doi:10.1177/2333393614550162

Weatherall, A., Watson, B., & Gallois, C. (Eds.). (2007). *Language, discourse and social psychology.* Springer.

Weiner, J. L., Silk, K. J., & Parrott, R. L. (2005). Family communication and genetic health: A research note. *Journal of Family Communication, 5*(4), 313–324. https://doi.org/doi:10.1207/s15327698jfc0504_5

Williams, A., Giles, H., Coupland, N., Dalby, M., & Manasse, H. (1990). The communicative contexts of elderly social support and health: A theoretical model. *Health Communication, 2,* 123–143. doi: 10.1207/s15327027hc0203_1

Young, T. J., Manthorp, C., Howells, D., & Tullo, E. (2011). Developing a carer communication intervention to support personhood and quality of life in dementia. *Aging & Society, 31,* 1003–1025. doi:10.1017/S0144686X10001182

5

Families Interacting in the Healthcare Context

Maureen Keeley and Hannah Jones

A common communicative process that families face is healthcare and healthcare decisions. For example, one in five adults in America is the primary caregiver for family members who are disabled or have chronic health problems (CDC 2018). Family members manage household tasks, perform personal care assistance (CDC 2018), complete medical/nursing tasks, as well as advocate for the medical care recipient (AARP 2015). Consequently, family members are the first (and sometimes last) line of defense for illness and health crises for the patient. Therefore, it is important to explore how communication impacts all members of the family during health crises.

To explain how families manage these communicative processes, family and health communication researchers have developed different models and theories to provide explanations and predictions concerning healthcare issues. This chapter examines four models and theories which highlight the role that our interpersonal and familial relationships play in the healthcare process: double ABCX model of family stress and coping, Olson's circumplex model of marital and family systems, inconsistent nurturing as control theory, and affection exchange theory. These

Health Communication Theory, First Edition. Edited by Teresa L. Thompson and Peter J. Schulz.
© 2021 John Wiley & Sons, Inc. Published 2021 by John Wiley & Sons, Inc.

theories are important for addressing the complexities that are inherent when exploring families and healthcare processes. For examples, families in the midst of health crises must deal with multiple issues, including physical, emotional, psychological, and relational challenges (Manne and Badr 2010). Financial strain, changes in quality of life, and disruption of daily routines can also impact health and family outcomes (Horan et al. 2009). Family members in the midst of health crises face changes in affection (Floyd 2014), alterations in family roles, and power shifts (Le Poire, Hallett, and Erlandson 2000). Lastly, difficult health challenges create communication burdens that must be addressed by family and health communication experts (Wittenberg et al. 2017). Each of these four models and theories focuses on one or more of these diverse and complicated challenges when dealing with health communication in the family.

Double ABCX Model of Family Stress and Coping

The Double ABCX Model of Family Stress and Coping (Double ABCX; McCubbin and Patterson 1983a) is an extension of the ABCX family stress model (ABCX; Hill 1958). Initially, scholars explore what pre-crisis factors impact how families deal with stressful life events (Hill 1958) through the consideration of four pre-crisis factors ABCX (Hill 1958). The "a" factor is the stressor/hardship that creates pressure on the family system (e.g. diagnosis of metastatic cancer of one parent, unexpected death in the family). The "b" factor includes existing resources that the family has to manage the stressor (e.g. insurance to cover the medical bills, secondary income for financial support, a network to support the family [tangibly, financially, emotionally]). The "c" factor encompasses perceptions of a family member's ability to cope with the stressor (e.g. "we will get through this together," versus "there is only so much we can do,"). The "x" factor shows how much stress and adjustment occurs in family roles and structure and stability resulting in the event being manageable or unmanageable. The original ABCX is a deterministic and linear model that only accounts for pre-crisis variables; it infers that while all "x" factors can become a crisis for a family, they do not always become a crisis.

The Double ABCX extends the original theory because it recognizes that stressful events have long-term impacts on the family which makes it necessary for members to continue to make adjustments and adaptations to their original response to the stressor. The post-crisis components include an extension and renaming of the four original pre-crisis factors, as well as an additional interaction (xX) component (McCubbin and Patterson 1983a). In the Double ABCX, the a, b, and c component become aA, bB, and cC respectively with addition of the uppercase letters to symbolize the additional stressors in the model. The first component (aA) includes the original crisis, *plus additional strains and stressors* (also referred to as the "pile-up") that accumulate as a result of the crisis (e.g. depression, changes in family duties and responsibilities, reduced availability of money). The second component (bB) focuses on family attempts to *produce, acquire, and utilize new resources* to deal with the crisis (e.g. new roles assimilated in the family, closer relationships with extended family and friends, support groups, food stamp programs). The final component (cC) reveals the *reassessment of family perceptions* of the situation that often reframes the dilemma (e.g. "we are stronger because of our experience" or "we're overwhelmed, stuck, and we keep losing ground"). All these factors (aA + bB + cC) interact to impact how the family copes with the stressor, resulting in the xX component exposing how effectively the family adapts and handles the crisis overall (McCubbin and Patterson 1983a). The range of adaptation highlighted in the Double ABCX includes very successful adaptation (bonadaptation) where the family comes out of the crisis stronger, resilient, and more confident in their abilities to handle crisis, versus unsuccessful adaptation (maladaptation) where the family is left poorer, weaker, and more unstable (McCubbin and Patterson 1983b). The extended model (pre-crisis and post-crisis) presents a more comprehensive, realistic, and long-range picture of how families cope with stressors.

Application to Health Communication

Due to the complexity of health crises, the Double ABCX effectively explains how families cope, adjust, and ultimately adapt or suffer with their new reality. Health crises may include permanent health issues such as families with children with disabilities (Xu 2007), autism spectrum disorders (Pickard and Ingersoll 2016), and intellectual disabilities (Park et al. 2018), as well as Alzheimer's (Famighetti 1986), sudden onset health crises such as strokes (Hesamzadeh et al. 2015), and physical disabilities (Florian and Dangoor 1994). While not exhaustive, this list is representative of many chronic health issues that would cause a family a great deal of disruption and stress, thereby triggering coping and adaptive responses. The outcome (xX) is greatly impacted by the available resources (bB) and by the family's perception of the chronic health issue (cC). Scholars using the Double ABCX find value in its ability to describe and explain coping responses used when dealing with on-going, chronic health challenges.

Communication is especially valuable as a resource (bB) for creating positive outcomes within family system resources (Famighetti 1986). Four specific areas have been highlighted: open dialogue, honest feedback, recognition and acknowledgement of resiliency in the face of crisis, and perceived appropriate and effective social support (McCubbin and Patterson 1983b). First, open dialogue allows members to learn effective problem-solving. Second, honest feedback (verbal and nonverbal responses) can help family members adjust coping methods. Third, recognizing and acknowledging family members' resiliency and perseverance in the face of the crisis increases their self-esteem and belief that they can get through the situation. Fourth, with open communication, members of the family network can provide the most appropriate and needed types of social support. Thus, creating open communication, implementing successful problem-solution plans amongst family members, and utilizing existing support within networks (i.e. family, friend, and community) is essential for family members to offset the degree of negative stress experienced, thereby manifesting a greater sense of self and family efficacy (Han, Yang, and Hong 2017).

Limits/Merits

The limitations of this model include measurement issues, design concerns, and a lack of predictive ability. Specifically, the measurement of model variables (e.g. aA, bB, cC) is not clear. The aA (i.e. additional stressors) has been measured as a single variable, which is not an accurate reflection of the pile-up impact of aA (Park et al. 2018). In many cases, measured outcome variables are not consistent with the intervention variables (Pickard and Ingersoll 2017). The cC (i.e. various revised family assessments) variable has primarily been defined and measured individually as opposed to the whole family. In addition, the model is primarily focused on cognitive factors instead of communication. Finally, the model has not been tested longitudinally; if scholars want to understand the impact of long-term stress as a result of chronic health issues, they will need to see how families adjust to the stress throughout time (Frishman et al. 2017). Because of these limitations, the Double ABCX is descriptive and explanatory, but not predictive. Given that there are many variables involved in the model, it often becomes almost impossible to make a clear prediction for families in general. In other words, predictions could be made for each family observed; however, this prediction would only be successful for that one observed family.

The Double ABCX gives valuable descriptions of numerous factors that impact family members' abilities to cope and adapt amid health crises. These descriptions can lead to more effective interventions and should focus on external factors (e.g. friends, church support systems, community resources, cultural norms), as well as internal factors (e.g. redefine needs, refocus strengths and weaknesses, redirect energies; Xu 2007). These interventions could be utilized by health practitioners, social workers, and family and/or health scholars, to improve the family's ability to adapt to a wide range of health crises (Florian and Dangoor 1994). Additionally, interventions can be assessed for their success or failure regarding the family's long-term ability to adapt during health crises to maximize health outcomes (Pickard and Ingersoll 2017). The Double ABCX highlights that families are dynamic, interrelated systems, rather than static (Hesamzadeh et al. 2015). Lastly, increased awareness about the factors of the model empowers families to help themselves build resiliency to overcome challenges (Xu 2007).

While this model is useful for exploring how stressors can impact a family's healthcare experience, the model tends to focus more on cognitive factors and not communication. Olson's circumplex model of marital and family systems focuses directly on communication structures and processes.

Olson's Circumplex Model of Marital and Family Systems

Olson's circumplex model (Olson 1993, 2000) explores how family behavior impacts family functioning across three dimensions: adaptability, cohesion, and communication (Olson 1993). Adaptability encompasses a family systems' ability to change its relational rules, roles, and power structure, as well as exists on a continuum (Olson 1993, 2000). There are four different levels of flexibility/adaptability within the model: rigid, structured, flexible, and chaotic. Rigid families are at the base with low levels of adaptability. These families tend to possess authoritarian leadership and utilize strict discipline. Additionally, family roles seldom vary and there is little overall change within the family. Next, structured families will sometimes share leadership among individuals and democratic discipline starts to occur. Roles tend to be stable, but the family can change when absolutely needed. Moving up, flexible families possess slightly higher levels of adaptability, tend to share leadership, and are considered egalitarian. Additionally, they engage in democratic discipline and utilize more implicit than explicit rules. Roles are shared between individuals and families can enact change when necessary. Chaotic families exist at the most extreme level of adaptability. These families tend to lack leadership, discipline is lenient or chaotic, and family members possess poor negotiation and problem-solving skills. Chaotic families are very prone to change, and dramatic role shifts between members.

The second dimension of the model, cohesion, focuses on emotional bonding and the individual autonomy individuals experience within their family (Olson 1993, 2000). Like adaptability, cohesion exists on a continuum with four different levels: disengaged, separated, connected, and enmeshed. Disengaged families possess the lowest levels of cohesion. These families are very individual and independent, members possess little closeness and there tends to be a lack of loyalty. Separated families are slightly more cohesive than disengaged families. These families fluctuate between low to moderate levels of cohesion and have low to moderate levels of emotional bonding and closeness. Members are more independent than dependent and there is little loyalty. Connected families possess moderate to high levels of cohesion, some loyalty exists within the family, and members are more dependent on each other. Lastly, enmeshed families possess extreme levels of cohesion and are very close with one another. Enmeshed families display high levels of loyalty and dependence.

Communication, also known as the facilitating dimension in the model, allows families to shift their levels of adaptability and cohesion (Olson 1993, 2000). When situations arise as families develop, it is often necessary for adaptability and cohesion levels to shift to ensure proper functioning. For example, expressive communication can lead to positive family functioning whereas communication centered around traditionalism and conflict avoidance is negatively associated with a family's ability to facilitate cohesion and adaptability (Schrodt 2005). If families are unable to alter their communication, they tend to remain at static levels of adaptability and cohesion; this could ultimately lead to dysfunction within the family.

Application to Health Communication

Adaptability and cohesion have been utilized to explain a wide array of physical and mental health-related outcomes. For example, greater perceptions of family cohesion have been linked to increased communication and coping during stressful situations as well as survivorship care (e.g. if an individual survives cancer and they exhibit positive familial interactions, their partner may not feel burdened communicating cancer-related issues with them). These interactions are positively associated with one's physical health (Lim and Shon 2018). Additionally, increased levels of cohesion and flexibility within families have been positively linked with information sharing about cancer risk and more frequent communication about cancer within extended families (Rodriguez et al. 2016). This health information sharing with the family could potentially allow for earlier discoveries of cancer or other health-related issues.

Olson's circumplex model has also been utilized to explain mental health-related outcomes within families (Berryhill, Harless, and Kean 2018). For example, families who possess cohesive levels of flexible family functioning (i.e. moderate levels of adaptability and cohesion) are more likely to engage in positive family communication. This family communication has been positively linked to self-compassion within parent-child relationships, such that when college-aged children experienced self-compassion, they were more likely to experience lower levels of anxiety and depression (Berryhill et al. 2018).

Lastly, caregiving in the healthcare context impacts family's levels of adaptability and cohesion. Increased time spent as a caregiver leads to lower levels of adaptability within families (e.g. if an individual is the main caregiver for a family member, they are more likely to exhibit high levels of distress and perceive their family to be less flexible given the caregiving is not shared equally, or at all, between members; Crowe and Lyness 2014). Additionally, when one individual experiences a chronic mental illness, family members are likely to experience lower levels of adaptability and cohesion, and these levels will decrease throughout the illness journey (Crowe and Lyness 2014). Specifically, when comparing families experiencing chronic mental illnesses, with those families where one member has experienced a first episode of psychosis, chronic illness families are less likely to be able to adapt to change, more likely to engage in limited negotiation with other members, and become very dependent on and reactive to one another (Kourta et al. 2014).

Limits/Merits

The critiques of the model include faulty research designs (e.g. problematic measurement scales; Burr and Lowe 1987), inconsistent research findings (curvilinear vs linear outcomes; Schrodt 2005), conflicting perspectives (i.e. adolescent vs parent, family member vs rater; Perosa and Perosa 2001), and a lack of longitudinal studies that could reveal whether superficial changes or true structural changes occur in the family based on their family communication processes (Schrodt 2005). The merits of the Olson's circumplex model include its explanatory value by highlighting important communication frameworks and processes (Schrodt 2005), and its heuristic value, as it is used to explain family functioning in numerous and a wide variety of contexts (Olson 2000).

Beyond family functioning, researchers exploring the family healthcare context should consider examining the role of direct verbal and nonverbal communication between the primary family caregiver and the afflicted family member when navigating difficult health situations.

Inconsistent Nurturing as Control

Inconsistent nurturing as control theory explores consistent and inconsistent messages that occur amongst the primary dyad within the family.

With inconsistent nurturing as control (INC) theory, functioning family members manage competing goals of nurturing the afflicted person (i.e. caring for their distressed family member) while trying to control their negative behaviors (i.e. punishing the undesirable behaviors; Le Poire 1992, 1995). INC emphasizes the critical role that family members play when dealing with chronic health issues in so much as family members are the frontline defense for afflicted family members. INC posits that family members often unconsciously use inconsistent communication that backfires and often leads to greater occurrences of undesirable behaviors (Le Poire 1995).

INC suggests that prevalent patterns of communication commonly exhibited within this health/family context are problematic because the behavior is inconsistent (i.e. nurturing and controlling) and intermittent (i.e. erratic depending upon the behavior of the afflicted and the family member's level of frustration and despair; Le Poire 1995). Both indirect and direct communication and verbal and nonverbal cues are examined in INC (Le Poire 1992). Specifically, examples of reinforcing nonverbal behaviors that demonstrate involvement and caring by the functioning family member include a kind tone of voice, increased eye contact, and positive forms of touch. Punishing nonverbal communication behaviors include the use of the silent treatment, increased use of space, less eye contact, and less physical touch. These conflicting nonverbal behaviors are often used to try to reward good behavior and punish problematic behavior (Burgoon and Newton 1991). Nonverbal cues are often considered more indirect communication strategies, while verbal messages are more direct.

Verbal strategies are also used to reinforce positive actions and punish problematic behaviors. Newton and Burgoon (1990) highlight three verbal reinforcing strategies; these include content validation, supportive messages, and self-assertions. Content validation consists of a description of the issue, agreement on the topic, summarization of a problem, problem-solving, and positive questioning to seek new information. Support messages include acknowledgement of positive steps taken, supporting the other person or relationship, complimenting the other person, accepting responsibility, and conceding to the other person. Self-assertion messages are those that include assertion of claims, making wish statements, self-disclosing, making needs and wants known, and other types of statements that validate or promote the self.

Three verbal punishing strategies consist of content invalidation, other accusations, and defensive talk (Newton and Burgoon 1990). Content invalidation includes rejection of claims and evidence through tactics such as disagreement, vagueness, exaggeration, correction, and fake-accommodation. Accusations disconfirm and invalidate the other person through criticism, making fun of the person, making allegations, blaming, threatening, negative information-seeking, advising, and acting superior. Self-defense strategies include denials, excuses, and self-justifications.

Research findings suggest that the direct and consistent verbal messages are more effective for predicting INC outcomes than nonverbal communication (Duggan and Le Poire 2006). Particularly, consistent verbal punishment regarding substance abuse usually results in lower relapse, while verbal messages that nurture and support the substance-abusing partner inadvertently reinforce the negative behavior and result in greater relapse. Indirect, nonverbal messages often give contradictory messages that result in intermittent reinforcement and punishment, which ultimately strengthens the behavior the partner is trying to extinguish (Duggan and Le Poire 2006).

There are three phases of discussion (verbal and nonverbal communication) identified as the prelabel, postlabel, and postfrustration phases (Le Poire, Erlandson, and Hallett 1998). The prelabel phase includes communication that reinforces the problematic behavior because the behavior is not yet labeled as a health threat. The postlabel phase involves communication that punishes the behavior to try to get the person to modify or stop the behavior. Due to previous, unsuccessful attempts to curb problematic behavior during the first two phases, the postfrustration phase comprises inconsistent messages of reinforcement and punishing. INC also highlights the paradox of an ongoing exchange of control between the functioning family member and the afflicted family member (Le Poire et al. 2000). While at times the functioning family member has control since s/he does not have the health affliction and has the ability to reward and punish the afflicted family member; the afflicted family member also has periods of control both when s/he resists efforts to curtail the behavior (Le Poire et al. 2000), and when the functioning family member adapts and adjusts his/her life to accommodate the needs of the afflicted family member (Duggan, Dailey, and Le Poire 2008).

Application to Health Communication

A selection of the application of INC in family and health communication includes drug addiction (Le Poire et al. 2000), general substance abuse (Duggan et al. 2008), problematic drinking (Glowacki 2016), smoking and drinking (Glowacki and Donovan 2018), depression (Duggan and Le Poire 2006; Duggan et al. 2008), sex addiction (Wright 2011; Glowacki 2017), and eating disorders (Prescott and Le Poire 2002). The commonality of these health issues is that they are chronic, compulsive, and progressively destructive and more stressful on the family.

Consistent with INC, the use of inconsistent messages of nurturing/reinforcing and punishing behaviors does not curtail dysfunctional behavior. There is, however, a difference between outcomes of addiction health issues versus depression health issues. Expressly, consistently punishing substance abuse and/or the addict are more effective for curtailing addiction (Duggan et al. 2008), whereas utilizing consistently validating, supporting, or nurturing behaviors are more effective for managing depression (Duggan and Le Poire 2006).

Family members often unwittingly possess conflicting goals with the afflicted person, which ultimately leads the unafflicted family member to intermittently reinforce and/or punish the afflicted person during their interactions. For example, the unafflicted family member may give up his or her own needs and goals during the crisis (e. g. struggling for rent money while the substance abuser spends money on drugs or alcohol), may choose to nurture the partner during a crisis (e.g. take care of their son/daughter in the midst of the physical consequences of the overdose), as well as use threats to try to change the unacceptable behavior (e.g. "I'm going to tell mom/dad about your problem unless you fix this problem"; Duggan et al. 2008).

Unafflicted family members who consistently punish substance abuse (e.g. threaten to leave, call police) and reinforce non-substance abuse behaviors (e.g. attend AA meetings, get physically healthy) have greater success and less recidivism (Le Poire et al 2000). On the other hand, contradictory messages that intermix reinforcing/nurturing messages and punishing messages are less persuasive and less effective (e.g. "You have this, you are strong." with "Why can't you just stop this behavior for our family?") How many times are you going to lie? I know that you are still using."; Le Poire 2000).

Limits/Merits

Much of the research using INC has focused on the romantic/spousal family dyad, therefore little is known about the impact of other family members' communication on the afflicted person (e.g., parent–child, child–parent, sibling–sibling; Duggan et al. 2006). Exploration of INC has been primarily conducted through retrospective interviews (Duggan et al. 2006; Glowacki 2017; Glowacki and Donovan 2018) and would benefit from a diary method whereby participants can report the interaction immediately following the event. In addition, quantitative testing of INC is necessary for generalizability. Additionally, it would be beneficial to gather dyadic data to gain insight from both parties' perspectives and conduct longitudinal studies to examine the long-term impact of communication and health outcomes.

INC is a strong theory for highlighting the important role that verbal and nonverbal communication have in health contexts. It also illustrates great potential for the creation of practical applications of training programs for family members to teach them to utilize effective and consistent types of communication to help their afflicted family member overcome health issues. Relational partners and other family members need to be able to recognize when they are inadvertently reinforcing negative behaviors through communication, as well as be taught what types of behavior (nurturing or punishing) are best given the type of illness. There have been consistent findings amongst a growing body of INC scholarship demonstrating the impact of communication on health outcomes. However, there is still much research that needs to be done to effectively use communication in these challenging family/health contexts, as well as numerous other chronic health conditions that require consistent healthy choices for the best possible health outcomes (i.e. diabetes, high blood pressure, etc.,) and require the person with the illness to choose healthy behaviors (i.e. taking medication regularly, choosing healthy diets and lifestyles).

Affection Exchange Theory

The previous three theories have sought to explain different contexts within the family healthcare experience. The final theory, affection exchange theory, takes this a step further and looks at the role of biology as it relates to families and healthcare.

Affection exchange theory (AET; Floyd 2001, 2006) argues that affectionate communication is an adaptive behavior that is linked to humans' motivations for fertility and health (Floyd 2014). AET is rooted in evolutionary theory, but distinct in that it aims to explore affection as adaptive for survival of species by describing biological (trait and physiological) and environmental ways affection can positively and negatively serve individuals (Floyd 2006). AET is comprises five main claims.

First, individuals have an inborn need and capacity for affection (Floyd 2006). Essentially, this claim argues that an individual's need for affection is rooted in internal rather than behavioral experiences. Fulfilling this need for affection can be beneficial to one's physical and mental well-being by impacting biological factors such as oxytocin, dopamine, serotonin, and norepinephrine levels to induce feelings of safety and warmth (Floyd 2006). Additionally, affection can be replicated intergenerationally within families (e.g. uncle–nephew), and is subject to environmental conditioning, modeling, and reinforcement in one's social environment (Floyd 2006).

Second, while affectionate feelings and expressions can work together, they are distinct experiences and will not always concurrently occur (Floyd 2006). Individuals can inhibit, simulate, intensify, deintensify, or mask affectionate feelings. This can be done to hide true feelings or to match what an individual believes is expected in social situations

(Floyd 2006). When affectionate feelings and expressions do not match, this can cause one's relational partner to feel unfilled in their need for affectionate behavior or can falsely initiate or accelerate relational development (Floyd 2006).

Third, Floyd (2006) argues that the benefits of affection for survival and procreation are true for both senders and receivers. Affectionate communication promotes the sexual and platonic creation and maintenance of human relationships, which can contribute to long-term viability (Floyd 2006). Through the lens of Darwinism, this can be thought of as procreation selection, in so much as highly affectionate behavior illustrates an individual's emotional capacity to be a competent parent and increases opportunities for successful reproduction. Therefore, highly affectionate individuals would be more likely to be in long-term romantic relationships with another individual (Floyd 2006).

Fourth, individuals have varying optimal tolerances for affection and affectionate behaviors (Floyd 2006). Attachment styles, early family experiences, and communication environments impact these variations in the expression of affection, but are not the only sources of variation. Individuals' tolerance for affection and affectionate behavior are constrained by their required and wanted levels of affectionate emotion and behavior, otherwise known as their need and desire thresholds: minimum (i.e. does not meet basic affection need) and maximum (i.e. affection received surpasses the level with which s/he is comfortable) thresholds (Floyd 2006). When an individual experiences affection within needed and desired levels, this can stimulate hormonal rewards, increase immunity, or minimize stress and subsequent stressors. When this affectionate communication occurs, it can enhance reproductive success by contributing to health and viability of one's offspring (Floyd 2006).

Fifth, when affectionate behavior violates one's optimal tolerance, this initiates a nervous system arousal and a cognitive appraisal of the behavior (Floyd 2006). Violating one's needed and desired levels of affectionate behavior creates a threat to the body causing a fight-or-flight response via increased pupil dilation, respiratory and heart rates, blood pressure and blood sugar levels (Floyd 2006). Therefore, when individuals send or receive an affectionate behavior or message that is not within their optimal tolerance, they will assess their physiological arousal as a result of the behavior before assessing the behavior itself. Unlike the evolutionary perspective, AET proposes that any violation of the optimal behavior range will produce a negative outcome for an individual. A violation below the minimum need threshold will result in perceptions of physical and mental problems, threatening the health of an individual. A violation above the maximum desire threshold initiates a stress response that can threaten an individual's success at procreation. These violations are often subconsciously accounted for and can be seen as distressing to the receiver (Floyd 2006).

Application to Health Communication

AET is often utilized to explain the impact affection has on an individual's health via stress-alleviating effects and one's reproductive ability. For example, affectionate communicators are likely to be less stressed, depressed, and have better mental health (Floyd 2002). Additionally, affectionate communicators are more likely to recover quickly from stress and have lower cholesterol levels (Floyd et al. 2007). When individuals receive affectionate communication from their spouse, they are better able to regulate hormonal stress (Floyd and Riforgiate 2008).

While the positive benefits of affectionate communication and behaviors are frequently reported, affectionate behaviors can also trigger negative health-related outcomes. For example, intimate affectionate behaviors such as kissing can expose individuals to diseases and infections, such as the Epstein-Barr virus (Floyd et al. 2014). Consequently, there are certain instances where expressing affection with a partner might not be beneficial for individuals.

Affection deprivation has also been directly linked with health outcomes, specifically mental and physical health (Floyd 2014). For example, a lack of affection is often connected with experiences of physical pain (e.g. immune disorders: Floyd 2014; or bodily pain: Floyd 2016) and lowered levels of sleep quality (e.g. higher levels of sleep disturbances and daytime disfunction; Floyd 2016).

Limits/Merits

Three limitations of the theory have been identified. First, there is currently limited knowledge about how affectionate communication contributes to an individual's physical health (Floyd, Hesse, and Generous 2015). While AET can help to generally identify and explain the benefits, as of now the predictive ability of the theory in this context is limited (Floyd et al. 2015). Second, while the evolutionary perspective asserts that behavior violations can have positive and negative effects on an individual, AET argues that these effects will always be negative. Third, affection is viewed differently across culture, potentially limiting generalizability of current studies utilizing AET.

AET also possesses many merits, namely, AET is strongly studied in different familial contexts. For example, researchers have utilized AET with both heterosexual and homosexual couples, platonic and non-platonic couples, parents and children with both sexes, siblings-in-law, and grandparents and grandchildren. There is also great potential for more examination of AET in different health contexts (e.g. increased touch during cancer treatments, for premature babies, at the end of life). AET is widely studied and has offered unique implications for health and familial communication.

Summary

In sum, both unexpected and expected health stressors inevitably cause disruptions in the family. From the very young to the very old, every family member is touched by the experience. The Double ABCX model highlights both the pre- and post-crisis aspects of the stress event and illuminates the complexity of coping with health crises for the family. Thus, the Double ABCX model is valuable for describing the multitude of factors that impact the family's health crises. Olson circumplex model focuses on structures that the family has in place as it faces and manages health crises. The extremes of rigidity and chaos within family structures often make the health crisis worse given that they limit the family's ability to effectively adjust to health challenges. As well, too much autonomy or too much embeddedness within the family exacerbate health issues because too much independence often leads to a lack of trust and/or willingness to be an active participant in the family crisis. Finally, too much cohesion can restrict the ability for people outside the family to help in the time of need and would suggest greater co-dependence amongst family members. Inconsistent nurturing as control theory focuses on the actual communication (verbal and nonverbal) that occurs in response to the person with the chronic and challenging health issues. Inconsistent and intermittent nurturing and punishing communication is problematic, is often done without awareness by the unafflicted family member, and can have a tremendous impact on whether the afflicted person can cease the destructive behavior. Lastly, affection exchange theory focuses on the nonverbal and verbal expression of affection (receiving and giving) that occurs within the family regarding its mutual impact on family members' general levels of health at the hormone and physiological response level. Thus, the models/theories focus on different aspects of the family, different levels of emphasis about the role/impact of communication, and different types of health outcomes measured/described. All four models/theories are similar in that they provide opportunities to develop effective interventions that can be implemented by health professionals, social workers, health educational programs, and campaigns for better health outcomes for family members. The interventions that result from examining health issues within the family context will be diverse because the models/theories highlight very different aspects of the complex contexts of health and families.

References

AARP. (2015). *Research report: Caregiving in the U.S*. Retrieved May 27, 2019 from https://www.caregiving.org/wpcontent/uploads/2015/05/2015_CaregivingintheUS_Final-Report-June-4_WEB.pdf

Berryhill, M. B., Harless, C., & Kean, P. (2018). College student cohesive-flexible family functioning and mental health: Examining gender differences and the mediation effects of positive family communication and self-compassion. *The Family Journal: Counseling and Therapy for Couples and Families, 26*, 422–432. doi:10.1177/1066480718807411

Burgoon, J. K., & Newton, D. A. (1991). Applying a social meaning model to relational message interpretations of conversational involvement: Comparing observer and participant perspectives. *Southern Communication Journal, 56*, 96–113. doi:10.1080/10417949109372822

Burr, W. R., & Lowe, T. A. (1987). Olson's circumplex model: A review and extension. *Family Science Review, 1*, 5–22.

CDC. (2018, August). *Caregiving*. Retrieved May 27, 2019 from https://www.apa.org/pi/about/publications/caregivers/faq/cdc-factsheet.pdf

Crowe, A., & Lyness, K. P. (2014). Family functioning, coping, and distress in families with serious mental illness. *The Family Journal: Counseling and TherapyforCouplesandFamilies,22*,186–197.doi:10.1177/1066480713513552

Duggan, A., Dailey, R. M., & Le Poire, B. (2008). Reinforcement and punishment of substance abuse during ongoing interactions: A conversational test of inconsistent nurturing as control theory. *Journal of Health Communication, 13*, 417–433. doi:10.1080/10810730802198722

Duggan, A., & Le Poire, B. A. (2006). One down; two involved: An application and extension of inconsistent nurturing as control theory to couples including one depressed individual. *Communication Monographs, 73*, 379–405. doi:10.1080/03637750601024149

Famighetti, R. A. (1986). Understanding the family coping with Alzheimer's disease. *Clinical Gerontologist, 5*, 363–384. doi:10.1300/J018v05n03_09

Floyd, K. (2001). Human affection exchange: I. Reproductive probability as a predictor of men's affection with their sons. *Journal of Men's Studies, 10*, 39–50. doi:10.3149=jms.1001.39

Floyd, K. (2002). Human affection exchange: V. Attributes of the highly affectionate. *Communication Quarterly, 50,* 125–152. doi:10.1080/01463370209385653

Floyd, K. (2006). *Communicating affection: Interpersonal behavior and social context.* Cambridge, UK: Cambridge University Press.

Floyd, K. (2014). Relational and health correlates of affection deprivation. *Western Journal of Communication, 78,* 383–403. doi:10.1080/10570314.2014.927071

Floyd, K. (2016). Affection deprivation is associated with physical pain and poor sleep quality. *Communication Studies, 67,* 379–398. doi:10.1080/10510974. 2016.1205641

Floyd, K., Hesse, C., Boren, J. P., & Veksler, A. E. (2014). Affectionate communication can suppress immunity: Trait affection predicts antibodies to latent Epstein-Barr virus. *Southern Communication Journal, 79,* 2–13. doi:10.10 80/1041794X.2013.858178

Floyd, K., Hesse, C., & Generous, M. A. (2015). Affection exchange theory: A bio-evolutionary look at affectionate communication. In D. O. Braithwaite & P. Schrodt (Eds.), *Engaging theories in interpersonal communication* (2nd ed., pp. 309–313). Thousand Oaks, CA: Sage.

Floyd, K., Mikkelson, A. C., Tafoya, M. A., Farinelli, L., La Valley, A. G., Judd, J., . . . Wilson, J. (2007). Human affection exchange: XIII. Affectionate communication accelerates neuroendocrine stress recovery. *Health Communication, 22,* 123–132. doi:10.1080/10410230701454015

Floyd, K., & Riforgiate, S. (2008). Affectionate communication received from spouses predicts stress hormone levels in healthy adults. *Communication Monographs, 75,* 351–368. doi:10.1080//03637750802512371

Florian, V., & Dangoor, N. (1994). Personal and familial adaptation of women with severe physical disabilities: A further validation of the Double ABCX model. *Journal of Marriage and Family, 56,* 735–746. doi:10.2307/352882

Frishman N., Conway, K. C., Andrews, J., Oleson, J., Mathews, K., Ciafaloni, E., . . . Romitti, P. (2017). Perceived quality of life among caregivers of children with a childhood onset dystrophinopathy: A double ABCX model of caregiver stressors and perceived resources. *Health and Quality of Life Outcomes 15,* 1–12. doi:10.1186/s12955-017-0612-1

Glowacki, E. M. (2016). Communication about problematic drinking between young adults and their parents: An application of inconsistent nurturing as control theory. *Health Communication 31,* 1135–1144. doi:10.1080/104102 36.2015.1045578

Glowacki, E. (2017). Examining sibling communication about problematic drinking: An application of Inconsistent Nurturing Control Theory. *Journal of Family Communication, 17,* 65–87. doi:10.1080/15267431.201 6.1251919

Glowacki, E. M., & Donovan, E. E. (2018). Predicting reinforcement and punishment behaviors in college students coping with substance misuse: An application of inconsistent nurturing as control theory. *Communication Quarterly, 66,* 541–556. doi:10.1080/01463373.2018.1466345

Han, K. S., Yang, Y., & Hong, Y. S. (2017). A structural model of family empowerment for families of children with special needs. *Journal of Clinical Nursing, 27,* 831–843. doi:10.1111/jocn.14195

Hill, R. (1958). Generic features of families under stress. *Social Casework, 49*, 139–150. doi:10.1177/1044389458039002-318

Hesamzadeh, A., Dalvandi, A., Khoshknab, M., & Fazlollah A. (2015). Family adaptation to stroke: A metasynthesis of qualitative research based on double ABCX model. *Asian Nursing Research 9*, 177–184. doi:10.1016/j.anr.2015.03.005

Horan, S. M., Martin, M. M., Smith, N., Schoo, M., Eidsness, M., & Johnson, A. (2009). Can we talk? How learning of an invisible illness impacts forecasted relational outcomes. *Communication Studies, 60*, 66–81. doi:10.1080/10510970802623625

Kourta, K., Triliva, S., Roumeliotaki, T., Stefanakis, Z., Basta, M., Lionis, C., & Vgontzas, A. N. (2014). Family functioning in families of first-episode psychosis patients as compared to chronic mentally ill patients and healthy controls. *Psychiatry Research, 219*, 486–496. doi:10.1016/j.psychres.2014.06.045

Le Poire, B. A. (1992). Does the codependent encourage substance-dependent behavior? Paradoxical injunctions in the codependent relationship. *The International Journal of the Addictions, 27*, 1465–1474. doi:10.3109/10826089209047363

Le Poire, B. (1995). Inconsistent nurturing as control theory: Implications for communication-based research and treatment programs. *Journal of Applied Communication Research, 22*, 60–74. doi:10.1080/00909889509365414

Le Poire, B. A., Erlandson, K. T., & Hallett, J. S. (1998). Punishing versus reinforcing strategies of drug discontinuance: Effect of persuaders' drug use. *Health Communication, 10*, 293–316.

Le Poire, B. A., Hallett, J. S., & Erlandson, K. T. (2000). An initial test of inconsistent nurturing as control theory: How partners of drug abusers assist their partners' sobriety. *Human Communication Research, 26*, 432–457. doi:10.1111/j.1468-2958.2000.tb00764.x

Lim, J., & Shon, E. (2018). The dyadic effects of family cohesion and communication on health- related quality of life: The moderating role of sex. *Cancer Nursing, 41*, 156–165. doi:10.1097/ncc.0000000000000468

Manne, S. L., & Badr, H. (2010). Intimate relationships and cancer. In K. T. Sullivan & J. Davila (Eds.), *Support processes in intimate relationships* (pp. 240–263). New York, NY: Oxford University Press.

McCubbin, H. I., & Patterson, J. (1983a) The family stress process. *Marriage & Family Review, 6*, 7–37. doi:10.1300/J002v06n01_02

McCubbin, H. I., & Patterson, J. (1983b). The family stress process: The double ABCX model of adjustment and adaptation. In H. McCubbin, M. Sussman, & J. Patterson (Eds.), *Social stress and the family: Advances and developments in the family stress theory and research* (pp. 7–37). New York, NY: Haworth Press.

Newton, D. A., & Burgoon, J. K. (1990). The use and consequences of verbal influence strategies during interpersonal disagreements. *Human Communication Research, 16*, 477–518. doi:10.1111/j.1468-2958.1990.tb00220.x

Olson, D. H. (1993). Circumplex model of marital and family systems: Assessing family functioning. In F. Walsh (Ed.), *Normative family processes* (pp. 104–137). New York, NY: Guilford.

Olson, D. H. (2000). Circumplex model of marital and family systems. *Journal of Family Therapy, 22*,144–167. doi:10.1111/1467-6427.00144

Park, J., Chun, J., Park, H.-C., Lee, E.-J., & Ivins-Lukse, M. (2018). Factors affecting perceived stress among Korean caregivers of transition-age youth with intellectual and developmental disabilities using the double ABCX model. *Journal of Rehabilitation, 84*, 5–12. doi:10.1080/20473869.2019.1633166

Perosa, L. M., & Perosa, S. L. (2001). Adolescent perceptions of cohesion, adaptability, and communication: Revisiting the circumplex model. *The Family Journal: Counseling and Therapy for Couples and Families, 9*, 407–419. doi:10.1177/1066480701094008

Pickard, K. E., & Ingersoll, B. R. (2017). Using the double ABCX model to integrate services for families of children with ASD. *Child Family Studies, 26*, 810–823. doi:10.1007/s10826-016-0605-4

Prescott, M. E., & Le Poire, B. (2002). Eating disorders and mother–daughter communication: A test of inconsistent nurturing as control theory. *The Journal of Family Communication, 2*, 59–78. doi:10.1207/S15327698JFC0202_01

Rodriguez, V. M., Corona, R., Bodurtha, J. N., & Quillin, J. M. (2016). Family ties: The role of family context in family health history communication about cancer. *Journal of Health Communication, 21*, 346–355. doi:10.1080/10810 730.2015.1080328

Schrodt, P. (2005). Family communication schemata and the circumplex model of family functioning. *Western Journal of Communication, 69*, 359–376. doi:10.1080/10570310500305539

Wittenberg, E., Borneman, T. Koczywas, M., Del Ferraro, C., & Ferrell, B. (2017). Cancer communication and family caregiver quality of life. *Behavioral Sciences, 17*, 1–16. doi:10.3390/bs7010012

Wright, P. J. (2011). Communicative dynamics and recovery from sexual addiction: An inconsistent nurturing as control theory analysis. *Communication Quarterly, 59*, 395–414. doi:10.1080/01463373.2011.597284

Xu, Y. (2007). Empowering culturally diverse families of young children with disabilities: The double ABCX model early childhood. *Education Journal, 34*, 431–437. doi:10.1007/s10643-006-0149-0

6

Theoretical Frameworks of Provider–Patient Interaction

Peter J. Schulz and Shaohai Jiang

Some qualities make patient–provider communication a unique and special form of human communication. Among these are a long history and fixed roles, which can never be switched. Moreover, medical consultations are of different relevance to providers and patients. For the latter, they may be a matter of life and death, while for the physicians, however compassionate they may be, they are just a job. We will begin this chapter with some considerations of what makes medical consultations differ from other forms of communication. The considerations relate to the status of theory in the field, to the co-existence of prescriptive or normative theory on the one side and analytical theory on the other, and to attempts to structure the field. They can be considered as early forms of theory, as something from which proper theories develop. We refer to them as proto-theories, using as the prefix the Greek term for "first."

The second, much longer part of the chapter introduces theories relevant to provider–patient interaction in healthcare. The theories introduced belong to two traditions on which this field was built: a linguistic perspective dealing with the principal code used for communication – language – and a behavioristic perspective with roots in psychology, communication

Health Communication Theory, First Edition. Edited by Teresa L. Thompson and Peter J. Schulz.
© 2021 John Wiley & Sons, Inc. Published 2021 by John Wiley & Sons, Inc.

and elsewhere, and concerned with individual and social processes with tangible consequences for human health and beyond. But we shall first return to the special features of provider–patient communication.

Proto-Theory in Studies of Provider–Patient Communication

Status of Theory in Research on Provider–Patient Interaction

There is a clear atheoretical streak to much of the research on provider–patient interaction, as has been noted by other scholars (e.g. Watson & Gallois 1998). Either there is no reference to theory at all in published research papers, or the reference to theory is somewhat arbitrary.

The absence of a convincing theoretical grounding of much research in provider–patient communication might be a consequence of some special features of the medical consultation: its potential seriousness for the patient, the provision for confidentiality, the gap in expertise between the two communication partners, or the asymmetry between the routine with which a physician conducts such communication, while many consultations will not be routine for the patient at all. These features make the provider–patient situation so special that researchers abstain from referring to general communication theory when specific communication between physician and patient is to be explained (e.g. Roter & Hall 2006). And, secondly, a theory is more valuable if it has a broader area of application. As it is unlikely that theories of medical consultation will have much potential to be applied elsewhere, building such theory might be perceived as not worth the effort.

The practitioner–patient communication literature does not – and is not intended to – offer much in terms of theory. Instead, it tends to be practically oriented and provides theoretical contributions, for example on the significance of race, ethnicity, and/or gender concordance between providers and patients. There are scholars who consider the applicable theoretical contributions that emerge from this research as one of its main assets, while the often weak theoretical basis is seen as no loss.

Normative Theory

The difference between normative and empirical or analytical theory is a crucial one in epistemology. Normative theory tells what should be done, while analytical theory explains what is being done, and why. The idea of empirically testing theory belongs to the analytical category of theory. The testing of general communication theories has rarely been undertaken with data gained from medical consultation. Theory testing begins with hypotheses or research questions being deduced from theory. Choice and application of some appropriate methodology follows, whereby the hypotheses are tested and the research questions, one hopes, are answered. The classical model of empirical research thus begins with a problem in the realm of theory, and the ultimate conclusions pertain to theory as well. Besides this grand research design, there are a number of ways to make research more systematic and, consequently, to make it look "more" theoretical, by providing one's hypotheses with clear and sound rationales, making efforts to choose the best design for one's research, using theory to interpret results, and reflecting upon possible impact of the research along with critical reflection upon methodology. The latter proposal was followed for instance by Street et al. (2009), who presented and discussed seven different variables that could function as mediator variables in an attempt to explain the correlation between high-quality physician–patient communication and favorable health outcomes. Strictly speaking, this is not theory, but only good research design, which yet might pave the way for constructing theories.

Normative theory is always close at hand when the unquestionable good of health is in the background. That the good functioning of communication in medical consultation is a valuable property has been oft-argued: "Interpersonal communication between health care providers and consumers clearly plays an important role in health care delivery . . . Effective communication can promote the delivery of high quality health care, while ineffective communication can seriously deter the quality of health care delivery" (Kreps 1988, p. 344; see also Kreps and Thornton, 1984; Ong et al. 1995). Thompson and Parrott (2004, p. 680) some time ago noted, "interpersonal research in the health care context has impacts on diagnosis, adherence to treatment regimens, patient recovery and pain, and malpractice suits. Medical errors are frequently communication issues rather than just errors in judgment or negligence." This might be so evident that the necessity of theory may just not figure prominently in researchers' thinking. Yet there are attempts at theorizing these consultations. Examples include the work of Sharf (1990), who conceptualized physician-patient communication as interpersonal rhetoric, and Mauksch et al. (2008), who developed a model of physician–patient communication based on a review of literature considering effectiveness.

The distinction between normative and empirical theory is not absolute. It is rather that theories relevant to patient–provider interaction have stronger or weaker normative components. Many studies address issues of quality of patient–provider interaction and are therefore concerned with normative theory. Graham and Smith (2016), for example, reviewed studies on provider–patient interaction in routine cases in emergency departments (EDs). Their systematic search identified 55 studies. They deduce from their review a normative theoretical framework for guiding behavior in the ED, which is also suited as a theoretical frame for studying communication of teams of providers and patients or as criteria for the quality of physician conduct. The framework is a long and differentiated list of maxims, rules of conduct and problem areas, structured in "three overarching themes" (p. 210) – team, interpersonal, and situation, referred to by the acronym T.IP.S.

The Ideal of Patient-Centered Communication

In affluent societies at least, the ideal relationship in patient–provider communication is often given the label "patient-centered." Its opposite pole used to be called "provider-centered," but that is not advocated any more. The notion of patient-centeredness has a strong normative element. The next two sections describe the functions of patient-centeredness and the pathways by which consequences for patient health are achieved.

Functions of Patient-Centered Communication

The Institute of Medicine (2001) underscored the importance of patient-centered care, and stated that patients' needs, values, and preferences should be adequately respected and responded. Furthermore, doctors' clinical decisions should be guided by patients' values. Epstein and Street (2007) further proposed a framework for patient-centered communication that is organized around six core communication functions: fostering healing relationships, exchanging information, responding to emotions, managing uncertainty, making decisions, and enabling patient self-management.

Fostering healing relationships is characterized by trust, rapport, respect, and understanding of each other's roles and responsibilities. The healing relationship emphasizes providing support, care, and mutual understanding. There are several critical steps to foster healing relationships, such as valuing a non-judgmental emotional connection, managing doctors' powers in ways that could benefit patients most, and showing a commitment to caring for patients.

Exchanging information is achieved when doctors adequately respond to patients' informational needs, understand what patients know and believe about their health, communicate clinical information in ways that are clear and understandable, and share bad news and prognostic information in an appropriate way.

Responding to emotions is accomplished when doctors can respond to patients' fear, anger, sadness and even depression and anxiety in a timely manner. If patients fail to resolve their emotional burdens, they will often encounter difficulties in making medical decisions and meeting the needs of treatment. Thus, doctors should recognize the cues provided by patients regarding their emotional concerns.

Managing uncertainty is important for quality care. Patients inevitably experience uncertainty for a couple of reasons. For example, health symptoms are unpredictable; patients often have questions about recurrence; and the course of care involves an unknown future. In medical encounters, doctors provide explanations about treatment, answer questions in an understandable way, check for questions or concerns, and thus facilitate effective uncertainty management.

Making medical decisions is a significant element of high-quality care. In the current health care system, it is difficult for patients to make informed decisions by themselves. This is frequently due to a lack of equipment and mechanisms to inform patients in a timely and accurate way. To overcome this limitation, scholars highlight the importance of information exchange (e.g. sharing of both patient and doctor points of view), deliberation (e.g. finding common ground, reconciling doctor–patient differences), and shared decision-making (e.g. assisting the patient to understand their health conditions, and participating in decision-making).

Enabling self-management aims to activate patients and facilitate self-care skills that are important for managing health after leaving clinical visits. An important element of self-management communication focuses on navigating and assessing health resources. Doctors should provide useful health resources to patients and help them navigate the resources, offering easy and affordable care (e.g. supporting patient autonomy, introducing self-help resources, utilizing social support groups, and providing opportunities to answer patients' questions).

Pathways Linking Communication to Health Improvement

Street and colleagues (2009) proposed pathways that include both direct and indirect effects of medical communication on health improvement (see Figure 6.1). In some situations, patient-centered communication may have direct effects on people's health. A doctor who encourages, reassures, and offers clear and understandable explanations may reduce a patient's anxiety level, help the patient sleep better, or have an enhanced appetite immediately after the medical consultation. Doctors' talk to validate patients' concerns could also help improve their psychological well-being as well as physical health. However, in most situations, communication affects health indirectly, mediated by proximal outcomes and intermediate outcomes. The proximal outcome is the immediate effect of doctor–patient communication. Proximal outcomes may include better understanding of medical treatment, satisfaction with care, reaching doctor–patient agreement, increased patient trust in doctors, the patient's feeling of being known and cared about, the patient's sense of getting involved, and rapport and motivation to adhere to treatment. Proximal outcomes are mediators of the relationships between communication and intermediate and health outcomes. For example, when a doctor clearly explains treatment and expresses support (communication behavior), a patient might have a better understanding of his or her health condition, and feel greater trust toward the doctor (proximal outcomes). The intermediate outcome is the mediator

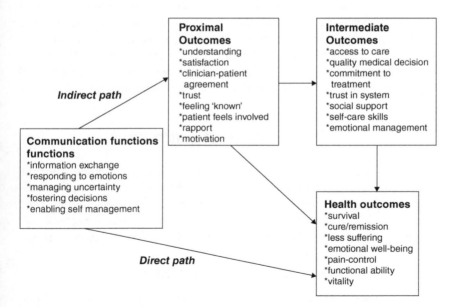

Figure 6.1 Communication pathways to improved health outcomes (adapted from Street et al. 2009).

between proximal outcome and health outcome. Intermediate outcomes may include access to care, high-quality medical decision, commitment to treatment, social support, self-care skills, and adherence to medications. For example, when patients have a clear understanding of medical treatment (proximal outcomes), they will follow through with the recommended therapy (intermediate outcomes), which in turn, improves a particular health outcome.

Researchers have only started to model pathways through which patient-centered communication contributes to better outcomes during recent years. A study among colorectal cancer patients found that patient-centered communication was positively associated with the perceived quality of doctor-patient relationship (proximal outcome), which in turn positively influenced adherence to colonoscopy (intermediate outcome), and finally increased the rate of colorectal cancer screening (health outcome; Underhill and Kiviniemi 2012). Another study of cancer survivors showed that doctors' decision-making style was associated with two proximal outcomes – the patient's self-efficacy and trust in doctors. The increased self-efficacy and patient trust then both significantly predicted two intermediate outcomes, better personal control as well as lower uncertainty, which resulted in better health-related quality of life (Arora et al. 2009). A more recent study among 2729 American adults illustrated another pathway from patient-centered communication to patient satisfaction (proximal outcome), to emotion management (intermediate outcome), and finally to emotional well-being (health outcome). This study also indicated that communication could enhance health via the proximal outcome, without the mediator of intermediate outcome (Jiang 2017).

The Heritage of Antiquity

There are two, maybe three areas of thinking, which originate from the Greek and Roman civilizations, but still provide tools to analyze patient–provider interaction to this very day. They are narration (including rhetoric) and argumentation. Following the idea of a continuum between a linguistic and a behavioral dimension, the antique traditions belong to the linguistic pole.

Narrative Medicine and Rhetoric

The key idea of narrative medicine is to make use of the widespread narrative competence (Montello 1997) among humans for health-related purposes (see also Ch. 3, this volume). Narrative competence includes the capacity to understand stories, to see events from the point of view of other people (preferably more than one), to form impressions and expectations of individual persons, and to reflect on one's own experience (Charon 2000, 2001, 2006). Narrative competence has been shown to improve health outcomes (Franke 2009). Physicians can learn new aspects about a patient's condition if they can get the patients to tell stories.

A comprehensive overview of the relevance of narratives for health communication is offered by Bosticco and Thompson (2008).They discuss social functions of narration as well as specific applications for health, healing, illness, and coping. Narration is treated as a force that helps physicians and researchers to understand patients and health conditions and plays a role in patients' self-identification and their efforts in coping and healing. Beyond that it helps us understand the nature of health and illness, and teaches us how to live.

Narration can play a role in diagnosis, therapy choice, the education of both physicians and patients, and in adaption of clinical practice to changed contexts. In diagnosis it provides material to a physician for anamnesis and may encourage empathy, understanding, and reflection. In therapy, it has a potential for helping to provide a more holistic picture and may help to find alternatives to the therapies selected for application. In education, it may support memory and generate trust, as narration appears to be rooted in real experience. And in practice it might challenge tradition and encourage innovation (Greenhalg and Hurwitz 1999). Narrative medicine has been used to help healthcare staff to adapt to increasing involvement of patients as well as their families in healthcare decision-making and practice (Dickey et al. 2011).

This short list makes clear that narration is nothing that has to be artificially added to healthcare in general and physician–patient consultation in particular. It is rather that an element of narration is likely to be present in all the situations mentioned, without anyone having to propagate it. Yet, efforts to add further narrative elements might further improve healthcare. A study of 50 patient encounters with gastroenterologists about ulcerative colitis, for instance, concludes: "By giving greater attention to how narratives and knowledge are co-constructed in negotiated interactions between physicians and patients, it is possible to continue to improve the physician–patient relationship and thereby derive improved healthcare outcomes" (Franke 2009, p. 280).

According to Fisher (1987), narration provides people with good reasons for doing or not doing something. To be rhetorically effective, a story must be coherent, that is, free of contradictions, and must possess fidelity, that is, it must sound realistic. Kleinmann (1988) emphasized the differences between the way health care providers and consumers are bound to narrate the same disease.

A concise yet comprehensive overview of the role of narration was published by Gray (2009). It presents evidence for the efficacy of narration and describes theories that have a potential to explain the effects. Both themes are discussed for three settings: (i) professional medical training, (ii) patient-doctor consultations, and (iii) patient education in a clinical context. Obviously, the second setting is of interest here, but the third focus on clinical counseling has to be examined as well. In consultation, narrative activities make patients as well as doctors reflective, which may have therapeutic effects and may improve well-being in patients. Patients are more satisfied with doctors who listen to the stories they have to tell.

For patient education in the consultation, persuasive materials that use narrative techniques have generally been found to be more efficacious than persuasive communication using statistical evidence. That phenomenon is known in other contexts than health, and is known under different labels, such as exemplars. The explanations that come with it can be summarized as exemplification theory (Zillmann 2002), which can be traced back to the cognitive shortcuts that have come to be known as heuristic processing. In particular, the representative heuristic (one case stands for a whole class) and the availability heuristic (the mind judges what is closest) are relevant (Kahneman, Slovic, and Tversky 1982). Other attempts explain the efficacy of narrative elements by their vividness and salience.

Transportation theory holds that targeted individuals have to be drawn into a narrative by a promise of enjoyment or some functional equivalent for the narrative to be effective (Green and Brock 2002). Green (2006) describes the central concept of transportation as absorption, or the experience of becoming completely immersed in a story, much like the experience of flow, the complete immersion into an activity as described by Csikszentmihalyi (1990). The experience is measurable and can be induced in humans to a degree. Women experience it as often as men, and several psychological variables facilitate its occurrence. Transportation functions through identification with characters, the presentation of model behavior, norms, and emotions. Narration and transportation can overcome resistance against changing one's views fairly easily. One condition of success is the degree of realism of a narration: if the world in which a story takes place has no connection to ours, it will be hard to make sense of it. On the other hand, the events in a narration must be unusual or else they will fail to catch attention, or no one will bother to tell the story. Fictional narration, due to its malleability, might be more useful for changing behavior than factional.

As to theories, stress reduction as a consequence of engaging in narration is described in Lazarus and Folkman's (1984) *ipsative-normative model of transactional coping*, which is the cornerstone of one version of the theory of stress and coping with stress. According to this theory, people perceive their life as stressful when their resources are not sufficient to meet the demands with which they are faced. Coping mechanisms, of which narration is one, are then developed to deal with the situation. More recently, and in a broader approach, Lazarus has emphasized four elements in his theory of emotions: appraising, coping, flow of actions and reactions, and relational meaning. Coping, in this approach, is considered the most decisive element, and emotions are best determined by narration.

The oldest human cultures knew narration, as we know from epic literature that was handed down through the centuries. And we must assume that its potential to help make sense of the world was already at work at the time when the ancient narrations were compiled. Gray (2009) expresses the point well: "Storytelling has been a way to communicate information, learn about life, transmit culture, make sense of experience, and express one's emotions since primitive forms of language emerged ages ago" (p. 259).

Argumentation Theory

That argumentation should be discussed in relation to patient–provider communication might come as a surprise, largely because the term "argumentation" is often associated with quarrelling and conflict. The traditional notion of patient–doctor communication encompasses information transfer, first from the patient to the doctor (symptoms, family history, etc.), then vice versa, when the doctor informs the patient of the diagnosis and the treatment (Walton 1985). This is as outdated as it is incomplete because argumentative elements are also necessary in consultation communication. Examples include:

- a diagnosis has to be justified,
- a treatment and/or further examination has to be justified,
- the patient's erroneous notions of the disease and the treatments have to be corrected, and

- the patient's worst worries and fears have to be put in perspective (Schulz and Rubinelli 2008; see also Brashers et al. 2006; Goodnight 2006; Rubinelli and Schulz 2006).

These elements all contain a change in views, opinions, and (though not in the brief list above) behavior. Yet it is not the occurrence of change alone that is of interest to argumentation theorists; they are also concerned with the way the change is brought about. That is, argumentation strives for change for good reasons. This intention is captured in this definition, influenced by the pragma-dialectical school of argumentation theory (van Eemeren and Grootendorst 2004): Argumentation "refers to a joint effort of dialogical partners to resolve a difference of opinion by rationally convincing the other party of the acceptability of one's treatment preference by means of advancing arguments" (Labrie and Schulz 2014, p. 997).

One of the central elements of argumentation theory is, therefore, the distinction between cogent or valid and fallacious arguments. This differentiation and other concepts developed within the framework of argumentation theory can be used to describe the reality and quality of argumentation as it occurs, and they can be used to help people find and formulate good arguments. Argumentation theory can therefore be used descriptively and proscriptively, linking it to the tradition of normative theory.

The subjects of research on argumentation in doctor–patient communication are more frequently chosen from open questions in argumentation than from intentions directed at medical consultations, as a fairly recent systematic review shows (Labrie and Schulz 2014). Examples include the utility of argumentation theory for better understanding medical consultations (Brashers et al. 2006; Goodnight 2006; Rubinelli and Schulz 2006: Schulz and Rubinelli 2008), the consequences of argument use, the importance of teaching argumentation in medical training (Rubinelli and Zanini 2012), and the development of instruments for analyzing argumentation (e.g. Zanini and Rubinelli 2012).

Relational Models

Relational models pertain to dyads of patients and physician, but mostly to any other pair of human beings as well, provided they communicate. The focus of relational models is on the relationship that develops from communicative acts in the past. A relationship at a given point in time is the result of any number of communicative incidences. Relationships acquire some consistency and stability even though they can be assumed to result from volatile momentary interactive behavior. It is evident that these models belong to the behavioristic side of the structuring continuum.

Relational Communication Model

This theoretical concept has stronger roots in the general communication literature than most others introduced here. The relational communication model does not focus on two actors, the patient and physician in our case, but on the unit or dyad they both form, developing patterns of activities, negotiating and defining the direction they are to go. A central notion in this model is that of relational control, defined by Millar and Rogers (1987, p. 120) as the "process of establishing the right to define, direct, and delimit the actions of the dyad at the current moment." The idea builds on the work of Watzlawick and colleagues (1967) and their differentiation of communication and meta-communication. This view is frequently referred to as the pragmatic or interactional perspective. Every utterance, according to this view, has a content aspect, that which is overtly communicated, and a relationship aspect in that it defines the relationship between the two dialogue partners. A harsh order to close a window not only says something about the speaker and their dissatisfaction with the current state of the window, but also something about the claim of the speaker to be entitled to boss the other person around. Most of the relational and meta-communicative aspect is in the non- or para-verbal elements of talk. The relational aspect is meta-communicative insofar as it defines and often restricts or constrains reactions and subsequent behaviors. A relational communication control coding system (RCCCS) was developed for measuring the placement of dyads with regard to relational control (Rogers and Farace 1975).

Research in the area is diverse, covering theoretical (Friederichs-Fitzwater and Gilgun, J. 2001; Shay et al. 2012) as well as specific empirical aspects (Step et al. 2009). Empirically, the approach allows the study of relational control acivities in patient/physician dyads. In terms of health outcomes, patients showed high compliance with treatment recommendations when physicians are less assertive and patients less submissive (Cecil 1998).

Relational Health Communication Competence Model

With the relational communication model in mind, and in search for a unified theoretical framework for the patient–physician encounter, researchers moved communication competence into the center of attention. One task in this endeavor was to define the components of competence. Work by Cegala et al. (1996) asked patients as well as doctors to assess their and their counterpart's competence and also asked for the reasons why they gave that assessment. The results indicated two components reminiscent of the content and the relational aspect in Watzlawick's pragmatic theory. The two components were information exchange and relational development. Most elements of competence could be subsumed under the two labels. Information exchange was considered the more important one and the responsibility for the relational tasks was mostly the doctor's.

The earliest suggestions for a relational health communication competence originated from the work of Gary L. Kreps, who presented such a model in 1988. His starting point was a relative neglect of the relational dimension of doctor–patient communication. The model itself is a continuation of a related model published some years earlier (Kreps and Thornton 1984). Both models present the patient as the hub of a wheel and the spokes as different healthcare providers. The concept of health communication competence has fallen out of fashion since the models were published. Their place has been taken by the concept of health literacy, which is both an extension and a restriction of the older term. It is an extension because health communication competence was restricted to dyadic consultation while health literacy also includes skills in media use, which now especially pertains to the internet. It was a limitation because competence also referred to the physician's communication skills while literacy excludes these.

Building on the notion of the relational perspective, Ashley Duggan (2006) reviewed work in interpersonal communication in healthcare that focused on the relationship between the healthcare provider and the health care consumer. This focus is not treated as a formal theory, which deduces assumptions about relationships from fundamental concepts and axioms. The review finds that patient involvement improves health outcomes, that an increased attention to communication training in professional medical education is necessary, and that patients, too, need some training. The potential success of the communicative competence perspective therefore rests on the ability and willingness to maintain or, better still, advance medical communication competence, foremost but not completely in health professionals (e.g. Duggan, Bradshaw, and Altman 2010). It also focuses on the teaching of communication skills (Shue 2010), including ways of examining these (Spagnoletti et al. 2009) and skill training via the web (Van Zanten et al. 2007).

Dialectical Tensions

The theory of dialectical tensions, first formulated by Baxter (1990; Baxter and Montgomery,1996 and formerly called *relational dialectic*) is more than a communication theory; it is a theory of action and relationships. It intends to describe how contradictions in social situations or ongoing dyads such as husband and wife or physician and patients influence the development of the respective relationships. It understands social interactions as taking place in fields of opposing forces, which establish, dissolve, or maintain interpersonal relationships. Baxter and Montgomery (1996) point out three key dimensions: (i) integration, with the opposing poles of autonomy and connectedness; (ii) certainty, with the poles of stability and change; and (iii) expression, with the poles of candor and discretion. Individuals act between these tensions in different ways. People may generally prefer one pole over the other, switch between them according to situation or context, or attempt to cater to both at the same time. Research often focuses on identifying abstract dimensions of dialectic tensions from concrete information given by research subjects. Dialectical tensions are not conceptualized as something to overcome or avoid, but rather the force that moves the relationship on. They are "inherent to social life" (Brann et al. 2010, p. 324).

The theory has been applied to non-medical relationships, such as couples, and to medical subjects, as well. Among these, work has been done on families who are caring for someone, on end-of-life-communication, on consultation in emergency departments, and a number of other contexts. The theory was applied to doctor–patient relationships (e.g. Dean and Oetzel 2014), or such application was recommended (Rimal 2001). The theory of dialectical tensions was applied to healthcare staff interactions (Apker, Propp, and Zabava Ford 2005), reactions to sexual harassment, informed consent to radiological treatment (Olufowote 2011), and end-of-life care (Amati and Hannawa 2014; Hsieh, Shannon, and Curtis 2006; Miller and Knapp 1986). Almost as a rule, these studies change, rename, or complement the original three dimensions pointed out by Baxter and Montgomery (1996). The theory is somewhat watered down by this, as the level of abstraction of some of the additions is not similar to the original level. For instance, Hsieh and colleagues add to their analysis the conflict between the dying person's and the relatives' preferences, or among different versions of a deceased person's wishes. Not every conflict, however, is suited to constitute a meaningful dialectical difference. Considine and Miller (2010) add a dimension defined by the poles of life and death, which, however, appear to be too much removed from everyday human decision-making and action to be treated on the same level as the classic dimensions of integration, certainty, and expression. The same study moreover introduces leading and following as new poles, making an addition close to the level of abstraction of the original dialectical poles.

If scholars, as they apparently do, feel free to alter the dialectical poles that form the central part of the dialectical tensions approach, and still be true to the theory, then the content of the poles cannot be considered the essence of this approach. This leaves the form of having a space defined by dialectical poles, which are interchangeable, as the core of this theory. This also means that the theory cannot be falsified by empirical findings that clash with the theory's predictions, because the results might be based on the wrong poles. The worth of the theory is assessed by feasibility in use, not by validity per se.

Social and Public Conduct

The theories mentioned under this heading refer to everyday behavior in social or public situations, or at the border between private and public. They reach far beyond medical consultation, but have been used in this area or adapted for it. The approaches take us still further away from the linguistic and towards the behavioristic pole of our structure, touching disciplines such as psychology, social psychology, or sociology.

Politeness Theory

Politeness theory was first introduced by Brown and Levinson (1987). It is concerned with the ways people react if their own or their communication partner's face is threatened. As Yin et al. (2012) define it, "politeness is the intentional, strategic behavior of an individual wishing to satisfy the needs of the face of both self and others in cases of threat" (p. 535). The theory is derived from a series of general assumptions about human motives and behavior, among them compliance, efficiency, and maintaining face. People are concerned about their own face as well as that of their communication partner. Face is the image a person wishes to leave with his or her fellow humans. The concept draws heavily on Goffman's (1967) term facework, except that Brown and Levinson (1987) consider the threat of losing face a permanent danger. In order of increasing politeness, the strategies for keeping face are, in the original version, (i) bald on-record or little consideration of face; (ii) positive face, or the desire to bond with others, (iii) negative face, or the desire for autonomy, (iv) off-record or dealing with diverse face threatening in groups of people with different values or tastes, and (v) maximum politeness by not making requests, that is by not demanding anything from the other person, bearing in mind that a demand can be understood as expression of dissatisfaction with something within the other person's reach or competence.

Applications in the field of patient–provider interaction mainly aim at identifying politeness strategies in particular groups. For instance, Yin et al. (2012) studied communication between pediatricians, parents, and patients in clinics in Taiwan. Results indicate that physicians use bald on-record and negative politeness strategies more often than patients. While physicians show less politeness, patients' parents offer more support. Kosmoski (2009) used politeness theory for developing a tool to be used in conversations between doctors and patients about prescription medication directly advertised to consumers.

Robins and Wolf (1988) put untrained medical students in a situation where communication between a patient and a physician broke down. They recognized that face saving and politeness was necessary and used their everyday communication experience for doing it. Politeness theory would help, if students were to be trained for such situations, to provide frames for interpreting the situation.

Stigma and Stigma Management Communication Theory

The inclusion of stigma at this place might come as a surprise as the term is most often associated with public opinion rather than the privacy of the doctoral consultation. Yet stigma has a broad potential to impair interpersonal communication (Smith 2007; Smith and Baker 2012), which is why it (also) belongs here. There are in fact three different situations that might bring stigma management close to medical consultations. One is patients' possible hesitancy of revealing a stigmatizing condition to their physician, which might become a problem when the physician is new; a second situation occurs when a physician has to confront a patient with a diagnosis of a condition that is often stigmatized. Yet another possibility occurs when the healthcare provider treats the patient differently than he or she otherwise would because of the stigma associated with the patient's illness or condition.

Some authors have tried to define stigma by lists of content attributes the existence of which make a stigma of a particular mark or sign (Ablon 1981; Mahajan et al. 2008; Meisenbach 2010). A more promising theoretical approach to stigma was formulated by Rachel Smith (2007). Stigma is defined there as "a simplified, standardized image of the disgrace of certain people that is held in common by a community at large" (p. 464). The crucial concept in Smith's approach is stigma communication, which is characterized by four attributes: (i) it carries cues about an alleged difference between people with and without a particular mark or quality; (ii) it understands the two groups of people as separate; (iii) it suggests the existence of the stigmatized is a danger; and (iv) that the stigmatized group itself is to blame for their position vis-à-vis the majority of unstigmatized persons. This type of communication is held to create or perpetuate stigmas, and reactions to this kind of communication have been shown to be in line with the theory (Smith 2012, 2014). Yet in another sense, one could also say that the fact that such communication occurs *is* the stigma.

That stigmas are hard to bear for the stigmatized is self-evident. But from the point of view of unstigmatized individuals, interacting with the stigmatized can also create feelings of uncertainty, discomfort, and anxiety. Negative feelings such as these have different origins, and they clash with prevailing social norms that the stigmatized be treated normally yet kindly. The non-stigmatized person's unawareness of the stigma creates a situation in which self-disclosure emerges as a viable alternative to keeping silent. Self-disclosure may have the potential to reduce the negative implications of carrying a stigma and might be a potentially successful stigma management strategy. Empirically Thompson and Seibold (1978) found some support for this assumption.

Conclusion

The frameworks that have been specifically designed for use in health communication introduced in the chapter could not be more diverse. Some reach back to the beginning of human thinking; others reflect up-to-date theory construction, borrowing from the methods and substance of theory-building in communication, but also in such eminently modern disciplines as sociology and psychology. Most of the frameworks were not introduced with health communication in view. They rather had a much broader focus, but were later found to be applicable in the study of health communication, or, even more specifically, of the communication between healthcare provider and patient. The variety of theoretical approaches with many different origins may sometimes appear to many of us as a troublesome condition. Yet it is an asset, and not only because we have a high number of theories to choose from when it comes to seeking a frame for a piece of research. The rich and divers traditions in theory-building are themselves an object of research. We hope to read more about it in the not-too-distant future.

References

Ablon, J. (1981). Stigmatized health conditions. *Social Science & Medicine, 15B*, 5–9.

Apker, J., Propp, K., & Zabava Ford, W. (2005). Negotiating status and identity tensions in healthcare team interactions: An exploration of nurse role dialectics. *Journal of Applied Communication Research, 33*, 93–115.

Arora, N. K., Weaver, K. E., Clayman, M. L., Oakley-Girvan, I., & Potosky, A. L. (2009). Physicians' decision-making style and psychosocial outcomes among cancer survivors. *Patient Education and Counseling, 77*, 404–412.

Baxter, L. A. (1990). Dialectical contradictions in relationship development. *Journal of Social and Personal Relationships, 7*, 69–88.

Baxter, L. A., & Montgomery, B. M. (1996). *Relating: Dialogues and dialectics*. New York, NY: Guilford.

Bosticco, C., & Thompson, T. L. (2008). *Let me tell you a story: Narratives and narration in health communication research*. In H. M. Zoller & M. J. Dutta (Eds.), *Emerging perspectives in health communication: Meaning, culture, and power* (pp. 39–62). New York, NY: Routledge.

Brann, M., Leezer Himes, K., Dillow, M. R., & Weber, K. (2010). Dialectical tensions in stroke survivor relationships. *Health Communication, 25*, 323–332.

Brashers, D. H., Rintamaki, L. S., Hsieh, E., and Peterson, J.(2006). Pragma-dialectics and self-advocacy in physician-patient interactions. In P. Houtlosser & A. Van Rees (Eds.), *Considering pragma-dialectics* (pp. 23–34). Mahwah, NJ: Erlbaum.

Brown, P., & Levinson, S. C. (1987). *Politeness: Some universals in language usage*. New York, NY: Cambridge University Press

Cecil, D. W. (1998). Relational control patterns in physician-patient clinical encounters: Continuing the conversation. *Health Communication, 10*, 125–149.

Cegala, D. J., McGee, D. S., & McNeilis, K. S. (1996). Components of patients' and doctors' perceptions of communication competence during a primary care medical interview. *Health Communication, 8*, 1–27.

Charon, R. (2000). Medicine, the novel, and the passage of time. *Annals of Internal Medicine, 132*, 63–68.

Charon R. (2001). Narrative medicine: A model for empathy, reflection, profession and trust. *JAMA, 286*, 1897–902.

Charon, R. (2006). *Narrative medicine: Honoring the stories of illness*. New York, NY: Oxford University Press.

Considine, J., & Miller, K. (2010). The dialectics of care: Communicative choices at the end of life. *Health Communication, 25*, 165–174.

Csikszentmihalyi, M. (1990). *Flow: The psychology of optimal experience*. New York, NY: Harper and Row.

Dean, M., & Oetzel, J. G. (2014). Physicians' perspectives of managing tensions around dimensions of effective communication in the emergency department. *Health Communication, 29*, 257–266.

Dickey, L. A., Truten, J., Gross, L. M., & Deitrick, L. M. (2011). Promotion of staff resiliency and interdisciplinary team cohesion through two small-group narrative exchange models designed to facilitate patient-and family-centered care. *Journal of Communication in Healthcare, 4*, 126–138.

Duggan, A. (2006). Understanding interpersonal communication processes across health contexts: Advances in the last decade and challenges for the next decade. *Journal of Health Communication, 11*, 93–108.

Duggan, A., Bradshaw, Y. S., & Altman, W. (2010). How do I ask about your disability? An examination of interpersonal communication processes between medical students and patients with disabilities. *Journal of Health Communication, 15*, 334–350.

Epstein, R. M., & Street R. L. (2007). *Patient-centered communication in cancer care: Promoting healing and reducing suffering*. Bethesda, MD: National Cancer Institute.

Fisher, W. R. (1987). *Human communication as narration: Toward a philosophy of reason, value and action*. Columbia, SC: University of South Carolina Press.

Franke, D. (2009). Patterns of communication between gastroenterologists and patients suffering from ulcerative colitis. *Journal of Communication in Healthcare, 2*, 274–281.

Friederichs-Fitzwater, M. M. von, & Gilgun, J. (2001) Relational control in physician-patient encounters, *Health Communication, 13*, 75–87.

Goffman, E. (1967). *Interaction ritual: Essays on face to face behavior*. New York, NY: Anchor Books.

Goodnight, G. T. (2006). When reasons matter most: Pragma-dialectics and the problem of informed consent. In P. Houtlosser & A. van Rees (Eds.), *Considering pragma-dialectics* (pp. 75–85). Mahwah, NJ: Erlbaum.

Graham, B., & Smith, J. E. (2016). Understanding team, interpersonal and situational factors is essential for routine communication with patients in the emergency department (ED): A scoping literature review and formation of the

"T. IP. S" conceptual framework. *Journal of Communication in Healthcare, 9,* 210–222.

Gray, J. B. (2009). The power of storytelling: Using narrative in the healthcare context. *Journal of Communication in Healthcare, 2,* 258–273.

Green, M. C. (2006). Narratives and cancer communication. *Journal of Communication, 56,* S163–S183.

Green, M., & Brock, T. C. (2002) In the mind's eye: Transportation-imagery model of narrative persuasion. In M. C. Green, J. J. Strange, &. T. C. Brock, (Eds.), *Narrative impact: Social and cognitive foundations* (pp. 315–341). Mahwah, NJ: Erlbaum.

Greenhalg, T., & Hurwitz, B. (1999) Narrative based medicine. *British Medical Journal, 318,* 48–50.

Hsieh, H. F., Shannon, S. E., & Curtis, J. R. (2006). Contradictions and communication strategies during end-of-life decision making in the intensive care. *Journal of Critical Care, 21,* 294–304.

Institute of Medicine (2001). Crossing the quality chasm: A new health system for the 21st century. Retrieved from https://iom.nationalacademies.org/Reports/2001/Crossing-the-Quality-Chasm-A-New-Health-System-for-the-21st-Century.aspx

Jiang, S. (2017). Pathway linking patient-centered communication to emotional well-being: Taking into account patient satisfaction and emotion management. *Journal of Health Communication, 22,* 234–242.

Kahneman, D., Slovic, P., & Tversky, A. (Eds.). (1982), *Judgment under uncertainty: Heuristics and biases.* New York, NY: Cambridge University Press.

Kleinman, A. (1988). *The illness narratives: Suffering, healing and the human condition.* New York, NY: Basic Books

Kosmoski, C. L. (2009) Breaking the ice: Toward a conversation tool for use in discussions between patients and health care providers about direct-to-consumer advertised prescriptions. *Dissertation Abstracts International Section A: Humanities and Social Sciences* (Vol. 70; pp. 4102).

Kreps, G. L. (1988), Relational communication in health care. *Southern Speech Communication Journal, 53,* 344–359.

Kreps, G., & Thornton, B. (1984). *Health communication: Theory and practice.* New York, NY: Longman.

Labrie, N., & Schulz, P. J. (2014) Does argumentation matter? A systematic literature review on the role of argumentation in doctor–patient communication. *Health Communication, 29,* 996–1008.

Lazarus, R. S., & Folkman, S. (1984). *Stress, appraisal, and coping.* New York, NY: Springer.

Mahajan, A. P., Sayles, J. N., Patel, V. A., Remien, R. H., Ortiz, D., Szekeres, G., & Coates, T. J. (2008). Stigma in the HIV-AIDS epidemic: A review of the literature and recommendations for the way forward. *AIDS, 22*(Suppl. 2), S67–S79.

Mauksch, L. B., Dugdale, D. C., Dodson, S., & Epstein, R. (2008). Relationship, communication, and efficiency in the medical encounter: Creating a clinical model from a literature review. *Archives of Internal Medicine, 168,* 1387–1395.

Meisenbach, R. J. (2010). Stigma management communication: A theory and agenda for applied research on how individuals manage moments of stigmatized identity. *Journal of Applied Communication Research, 38,* 268–292.

Millar, F. E., & Rogers, L. E. (1987). Relational dimensions of interpersonal dynamics. In M. Roloff & G. Miller (Eds.), *Interpersonal processes: New directions in communication research* (pp. 117–139). Newbury Park, CA: Sage.

Miller, V. D., & Knapp, M. L. (1986). Communication paradoxes and the maintenance of living relationships with the dying. *Journal of Family Issues, 7*(3), 255–275.

Montello, M. (1997). Narrative competence. In H. L. Nelson, *Stories and their limits: Narrative approaches to bioethics* (pp. 185–97). New York, NY: Routledge.

Olufowote, J. O. (2011). A dialectical perspective on informed consent to treatment: An examination of radiologists' dilemmas and negotiations. *Qualitative Health Research, 21,* 839–852.

Ong, L. M., De Haes, J. C., Hoos, A. M., & Lammes, F. B. (1995). Doctor-patient communication: A review of the literature. *Social Science & Medicine, 40,* 903–918.

Rimal, R. N. (2001) Analyzing the physician–patient interaction: An overview of six methods and future research directions. *Health Communication, 13,* 89–99.

Robins, L. S., & Wolf, F. M. (1988). Confrontation and politeness strategies in physician-patient interaction. *Social Science & Medicine, 27,* 217–221.

Rogers, L. E., & Farace, R. V. (1975). Analysis of relational communication in dyards: New measurement procedures. *Human Communication Research, 1,* 222–239.

Roter, D. L., & Hall, J. A. (2006). *Doctors talking with patients/patients talking with doctors: Improving communication in medical visits* (2nd ed.). Westport, CT: Praeger Publishers.

Rubinelli, S., & Zanini, C. (2012). Teaching argumentation theory to doctors: Why and what. *Journal of Argumentation in Context, 1,* 66–80.

Rubinelli, S., & Schulz, P. J. (2006). Let me tell you why! When argumentation in doctor–patient interaction makes a difference. *Argumentation, 20*(3), 353–375.

Schulz, P. J., & Rubinelli, S. (2008). Arguing "for" the patient: Informed consent and strategic maneuvering in doctor–patient interaction. *Argumentation, 22*(3), 423–432.

Sharf, B. F. (1990). Physician-patient communication as interpersonal rhetoric: A narrative approach. *Health Communication, 2,* 217–231.

Shay, L. A., Dumenci, L., Siminoff, L. A., Flocke, S. A., & Lafata, J. E. (2012). Factors associated with patient reports of positive physician relational communication. *Patient Education and Counseling, 89,* 96–101.

Shue, C. K. (2010). Accrediting and licensing standards as evidence of impact. *Health Communication, 25,* 563–564.

Smith, R. A. (2007). Language of the lost: An explication of stigma communication. *Communication Theory, 17*, 462–485.

Smith, R. A. (2012). An experimental test of stigma communication content with a hypothetical infectious disease alert. *Communication Monographs, 79*, 522–538.

Smith, R. A. (2014). Testing the model of stigma communication with a factorial experiment in an interpersonal context. *Communication Studies, 65*, 154–173.

Smith, R. A., & Baker, M. (2012). At the edge? HIV stigma and centrality in a community's social network in Namibia. *AIDS Behavior, 16*, 525–534.

Spagnoletti, C. L., Bui, T., Fischer, G. S., Gonzaga, A. M. R., Rubio, D. M., & Arnold, R. M. (2009). Implementation and evaluation of a web-based communication skills learning tool for training internal medicine interns in patient-doctor communication. *Journal of Communication in Healthcare, 2*, 159–172.

Step, M. M., Hannum Rose, J., Albert, J. M., Cheruvu, V. K., & Siminoff, L. A. (2009). Modeling patient-centered communication: Oncologist relational communication and patient communication involvement in breast cancer adjuvant therapy decision-making. *Patient Education and Counseling, 77*, 369–378.

Street, R. L., Makoul, G., Arora, N. K., & Epstein, R. M. (2009). How does communication heal? Pathways linking clinician-patient communication to health outcomes. *Patient Education and Counseling, 74*, 295–301.

Thompson, T. L., & Parrott, R. (2004). Interpersonal communication and health care. In M. L. Knapp & J. A. Daly (Eds.), *Handbook of interpersonal communication* (3rd ed.; pp. 680–725). Beverly Hills, CA: Sage.

Thompson, T. L., & Seibold, D. R. (1978). Stigma management in "normal"-stigmatized interactions: Test of the disclosure hypothesis and a model of stigma acceptance. *Human Communication Research, 4*, 231–242.

Underhill, M. L., & Kiviniemi, M. T. (2012). The association of perceived provider–patient communication and relationship quality with colorectal cancer screening. *Health Education & Behavior, 39*, 555–563.

van Eemeren, F. H., & Grootendorst, R. (2004). *A systematic theory of argumentation: The pragma-dialectical approach*. Cambridge, UK: Cambridge University Press.

van Zanten, M., Boulet, J. R., & McKinley, D. (2007) Using standardized patients to assess the interpersonal skills of physicians: Six years' experience with a high-stakes certification examination. *Health Communication, 22*(3), 195–205.

Walton, D. N. (1985). *Physician–patient decision making. A study in medical ethics*. Westport, CT: Greenwood.

Watson, B., & Gallois, C. (1998). Nurturing communication by health professionals toward patients: A communication accommodation theory approach. *Health Communication, 10*, 343–355.

Watzlawick, P. F., Bavelas, J., & Jackson D. (1967). *Pragmatics of human communication*. New York, NY: Norton.

Yin, C. P., Hsu, C. W., Kuo, F. Y., & Huang, Y. T. (2012). A study of politeness strategies adopted in pediatric clinics in Taiwan. *Health Communication, 27,* 533–545.

Zanini, C., & Rubinelli, S. (2012). Using argumentation theory to identify the challenges of shared decision-making when the doctor and the patient have a difference of opinion. *Journal of Public Health Research, 1,* 165–169.

Zillmann, D. (2002). Exemplification theory of media influence. In J. Bryant & D. Zillmann (Eds.), *Media effects: Advances in theory and research* (pp. 19–41), Mahwah, NJ: Erlbaum.

PART III

Perspectives on Influence Processes

7

Information-Processing and Cognitive Theories

Monique Mitchell Turner, Youjin Jang, and Shawn Turner

"We are addicted to our thoughts. We cannot change anything if we cannot change our thinking."

Santosh Kalwar, Author

In health and risk contexts, what we perceive and believe about messages, provider interactions, our susceptibility to disease(s), or treatment options can have a direct effect on our health behaviors. Both the content of our thoughts and the distinct way we process health-related information matter when making health judgments.

Research aimed at understanding relationships between messages and effects is an important area of academic inquiry. This chapter, however, deals with the *underlying cognitive mechanisms* that mediate and moderate our responses to health and risk communication messaging.

Many health communication theories attempt to account for underlying cognitive mechanisms like perceived severity, susceptibility, and subjective norms. By testing and validating perceptual variables, scholars have demonstrated that what audiences think or believe will, in many cases, ultimately have an impact on health outcomes. As such,

Health Communication Theory, First Edition. Edited by Teresa L. Thompson and Peter J. Schulz.
© 2021 John Wiley & Sons, Inc. Published 2021 by John Wiley & Sons, Inc.

when campaign designers develop health communication messages to change behaviors, they are, in effect, attempting to change how and what target audiences think about the health issue and the related behaviors. If health communication professionals can change what target audience members *think*, they can likely change what they *do*.

We begin with an examination of information processing through a dual processing model. The multiple motive heuristic systematic model (HSM) suggests that persuasive information is processed in either the systematic or heuristic route based on the individual's level of motivation and perceived capability.

We will then explore two theoretical frameworks for cognition and health behavior – attribution theory and the health belief model. These theories take a unique view of how our thoughts impact behaviors. The health belief model assumes that a rational person considers multiple aspects of the health context she is dealing with – including benefits and barriers, severity and susceptibility, and efficacy. Attribution theory, on the other hand, centers on curiosity and, as Heider noted in 1944, the belief that people are motivated by a desire to understand the causes that underly events.

Finally, we turn to information seeking models that elucidate our understanding of how people come to be informed (or misinformed) about their health. The risk perception attitude (RPA) framework argues that threat causes anxiety, and that anxiety affects the depth of message processing. The risk information seeking and processing (RISP) model explores factors that predict differential use between seeking and processing risk information. The planned risk information seeking model (PRISM) addresses the importance of attitude and behavior intention in risk related information-seeking.

The models and theories selected herein represent an established but still growing body of research aimed at expanding our understanding of information seeking, health beliefs, information processing, and the resultant impact on attitudes and behaviors.

Information Processing

The Multiple Motive Heuristic Systematic Model

Origins and central concepts

It is relatively well understood that receiving health-related messages can change the way people behave, but it's important to understand why. Dual-processing models of persuasion illuminate causal factors by focusing on the nature of cognitive processing that occurs after persuasive message exposure. Most critically, these theories argue that the manner in which individuals process information predicts the likelihood that they will sustain the attitudes or behaviors encouraged by the persuasive message.

The two most dominant dual-processing models in the persuasion literature, which are often adopted by health communicators, are the elaboration likelihood model (ELM; Cacioppo and Petty 1984) and the heuristic systematic model (HSM; Eagly and Chaiken 1993). Both models argue that there are two distinctive routes to attitude change via message processing: (i) the peripheral (ELM) or *heuristic* (HSM) route and (ii) the central (ELM) or *systematic* (HSM) route. Here, we will adopt the terminology of the HSM.

The basic premise of the HSM is that messages can be processed by scrutinizing arguments and engaging in careful, in-depth processing of the relative logic of a message. This mode of processing is known as systematic processing, whereby people pay attention to the arguments presented in the message. But messages can also be processed by examining superficial cues present in messages (i.e. heuristics) such as the attractiveness or credibility of the source, or whether a friend is persuaded by the message. Heuristics are "simple decision-making cues" that are learned knowledge structures stored in memory (Chaiken, Liberman, and Eagly 1989).

The HSM proposes that whether people engage in systematic processing, heuristic processing, or both is highly dependent on their ability and motivation to engage in processing. Ability refers to the cognitive resources available for processing a message and can be impacted by several factors, including health and scientific literacy, numeracy (ability to understand numbers), and language of origin. Distraction and mood have also been shown to affect individuals' ability to process persuasive messages for argument quality versus other kinds of heuristics. Motivation is affected by one's perceived outcome involvement in the topic. When people believe that a persuasive health topic affects an outcome in their own lives, they are more likely to spend time carefully reading the arguments and judging them for credibility.

We earlier noted that people can engage in systematic *or* heuristic processing. HSM proposes that systematic *and* heuristic processing can co-occur in certain instances. In what is called the additivity hypothesis, Chen and Chaiken (1999) outlined several patterns of cognition where people add heuristic information to the argument-based information. For example, people could be exposed to a persuasive message that suggests that 12-year-old girls should get vaccinated for cervical cancer.

The arguments in the message may be sound and logical; however, the message receivers then realize that the message source is Khloe Kardashian, who they may perceive to be a celebrity with low credibility on issues related to health. This heuristic information could weaken the overall persuasiveness of the message. Moreover, when people process persuasive health messages, they may be driven by particular motivations. Chaiken 1980 referred to this tendency as motivated processing and there are three forms. Audiences may approach the message with *accuracy motivations* whereby they engage in an open-minded, even-handed treatment of the arguments in a message. Here, the audience wants to know the "truth" about the topic. Contrast this motivation with *defense motivations*. People with defense motivations desire to have attitudes that are harmonious with their prior attitudes or interests. In other words, they may scrutinize the message for arguments that support them or their stance on the issue. *Impression motivations* refer to the desire to hold attitudes that will satisfy social goals (Chen and Chaiken 1999). Thus, they process the message for information that will allow them to get along with others.

The HSM also posits that people tend to be economy-minded when engaging in message processing. The sufficiency principle holds that people will vary in the amount of time, or processing, they need to feel sufficiently informed about a given issue. According to Chaiken, Giner-Sorolla, and Chen (1996), the basis for this principle is that people "strike a balance" between minimizing cognitive effort on the one hand and meeting their goals for sufficient information on the other.

Applications

There are numerous applications for the HSM in health and risk communication. Importantly, how people process messages is predictive of longer-term behavior change. When people engage in systematic processing, they are more likely to make a behavioral decision that is thoughtful and evidence based. As such, they are more likely to stick with that choice. This implies that as health communication professionals, we should design messages that promote systematic message processing. For example, Steginga and Occhipinti (2004) studied 111 men who had recently been diagnosed with prostate cancer. Men with more uncertainty, which may lower the ability to process, were more likely to rely on the expert opinion heuristic. Men with a strong internal locus of control (discussed below in the section "Attribution theory") were more likely to desire involvement in the decision process. Kim, King, and Kim

(2018) examined how people process advertising and social media messages. Their data showed that people with accuracy motivations were more likely to engage in both systematic and heuristic processing, whereas defense motivated people sought specific kinds of information regardless of their level of motivation. Also, Zuckerman and Chaiken (1998) applied the HSM to the effectiveness of warning labels. They noted that the likelihood of paying attention to the actual warning labels is dependent on the presence of heuristic cues like the color of the text, the presence of a signal word like "warning," or the presence of a signal graphic, for example a skull and crossbones. Warning labels represent an area where additive processing (co-processing) is advantageous.

Beliefs and Health Behaviors

Attribution Theory

Origin and central concepts

Attribution theory dates to the early twentieth century (Heider 1958). Fritz Heider's dissertation in the 1920s argued that people made sense of the world by understanding causal attributions, as in "How did this come to happen?" Heider fundamentally believed that people act as naïve psychologists, trying to make sense of their social world by asking themselves, "Why would someone do that?" or "How did this come to happen?"

In the original iteration of attribution theory, two forms of attribution were proposed: internal and external attributions. *Internal attributions* (or dispositional) are causes that come from within us (e.g. I did well on the test because I studied hard) and *external attributions* (or situational) are those causes that happen outside of us (e.g. I did poorly on the test because the noise outside the room distracted me). It is important to note how these constructs correspond with the notion of locus of control. All other things being equal, when individuals believe that that they maintain the locus of control over their health behavior, their self-efficacy (confidence in their ability to deal with a problem) increases.

Heider also noted a fundamental attribution error that humans make. When explaining the behaviors of others, we tend to rely on internal attributions. For example, people with obesity are often assumed by observers to be lazy (which has ultimately led to the stigmatization of people with the disease; see Puhl and Heuer 2009, 2010 for further review). Yet, when people assign causality to their own weight, they may be more likely to assign external attributions, such as, "I cannot afford fancy health foods" or "I am genetically big-boned." The fundamental attribution error shines a light on the notion that when individuals are observing others' behaviors, they often neglect to consider external causes – people are angry because they are "awful" people, not because something awful might have happened to them earlier in the day. This finding is sometimes referred to as the "actor/observer difference" that our attributions of causality tend to be dependent on whether we are explaining our own behavior (we are the actor) or whether we are observing others' behaviors. Indeed, causal attributions tend to have a self-serving bias. When we (the actor) fail, then we tend to attribute the cause to external factors; when we succeed, we tend to assign attribution to internal factors.

There are several distinct explanations for the self-serving bias. One explanation is that people are inherently motivated to protect their self-image as a defensive mechanism. A second explanation is based on expectation violations. When we expect to do well because of some inherent trait we believe we have (e.g. intelligence) and a different outcome occurs (e.g. poor grade on a test), then we need an explanation for that outcome that lies outside of us (e.g. distraction).

The self-serving bias helps us to understand the defensive attribution hypothesis. That is, when something bad happens we do not want to be assigned with the blame; rather, we prefer to assign blame to others. This phenomenon may be particularly relevant when individuals witness a negative event such as a car accident or an assault. The optimism bias has been argued to be an example of defensive attribution. When people hold an optimism bias, they believe (implicitly or explicitly) that negative events are more likely to happen to other people than to themselves. In addition, the just-world hypothesis falls under the categorization of defensive processing. This hypothesis would argue that "good things happen to good people." Problematically, this type of causal reasoning can lead to serious problems such as "people contracted the Ebola virus and died because they made the gods angry." In such cases, it is difficult to persuade people to change habits or lifestyles because they do not believe those factors to be part of the causal equation.

Applications

Attribution theory has been applied to health communication and health psychology more broadly. Attribution theory provides a clear explanation for the stigmatization of persons with obesity.

Studies find that when explaining other people's weight issues, people tend to rely on internal attributions, like laziness or lack of self-control. Yet, studies also find that numerous factors outside of one's control have an impact on individuals' weight. These factors include living in a food desert, income, and having experienced trauma or adverse childhood experiences (ACEs). Diet-based and obesity-related communication can exacerbate these issues. Messages can imply that if one simply ate more vegetables or drank more water, one's weight problems would disappear. Although caloric intake is clearly predictive of weight gain, these messages imply a strong internal locus of control over one's weight and deny epigenetics or structural factors. One study found that people often attribute juvenile diabetes to the child's internal factors (Vishwanath 2014). Indeed, this study revealed that outsiders will use pejorative terms to describe juveniles with diabetes, such as lazy, unhealthy, or refusing to exercise.

Attribution theory has also been applied across cancer types. For example, leukemia is attributed to external causes, while lung cancer is assigned internal attribution – thus leading to less sympathy and more stigmatization (Marlow, Waller, and Wardle 2010). Yet, not all lung cancers are caused by one's smoking. It has long been known that second-hand and tertiary causes may be responsible for several lung diseases. One qualitative study interviewed lung cancer patients for their own causal attributions for their lung cancer (Faller, Schilling, and Lang 1995). The most common external attribution was smoking in the workplace. More importantly, perhaps, is that patients who made internal attributions had greater emotional distress, were more depressed, and were less hopeful than other patients. The authors also suggested that patients making internal, or psychosocial, attributions were more likely to use maladaptive ways to cope with their illness.

There are major implications to the findings reported above. The ways in which people assign causality to disease affects how we see them and treat them. Moreover, the ways in which people assign causality to their own health issues can have negative ramifications on their coping behaviors. Therefore, health communicators (including providers) must be conscientious about these fundamental attribution errors that could be inherent in the language they use with patients or target audiences.

Health Belief Model

Origin and central concepts

The health belief model (HBM) was developed in the early 1950s at the US Public Health Service (USPHS) to explain the adoption and maintenance of preventive health behaviors (Janz and Becker 1984; Rosenstock 1974). The basic assumption of the HBM is individuals' beliefs play a critical role in health intentions and decisions (Rosenstock 1974). At the time, social psychologists working at the USPHS were perplexed by people's non-adherence to medical regimens and desired to develop stronger models explaining such behaviors. Being informed by both stimulus-response and cognitive learning theories, they reasoned that human behavior is a function of reinforcements (events that reinforce a behavior), values (whether we value getting well or being healthy), and expectations (our reasoning about what will happen if we engage in behavior). Ultimately, theorizing of this sort led to the HBM (see Champion and Skinner 2008).

The fundamental constructs comprising the HBM are perceptions of severity, susceptibility, self-efficacy, benefits, and barriers (Janz and Becker 1984). The theory also includes external cues to action.

Perceived susceptibility refers to the subjective possibility of exposure to the risk, that is, the likelihood of experiencing the health issue. Perceived severity is defined as the subjective magnitude of the risk and the subjective degree of effect of the risk on their own lives, including social, personal, mental, and economic aspects. In other words: How bad would it be to be affected by this health problem? Perceived benefits refer to people's beliefs about the potential benefits of engaging in health behaviors. And, perceived barriers are the potential negative aspects or barriers to engaging in specific behaviors. Self-efficacy refers to the personal confidence the audience has in their ability to engage in the recommended behavior. For example, when considering electronic cigarettes or vaping behaviors, first, the audience has to believe that vaping can lead to serious negative health effects like lung disease (severity). This audience also must believe that they are susceptible to the possible harms of vaping – that these negative impacts could happen to them (susceptibility). Next, the audience must believe that quitting vaping has benefits such as reducing the likelihood of lung disease, saving money, or making friends happy and relieved. The audience also must minimize the beliefs that there are barriers to quitting, such as believing they will gain weight if they stop vaping or they will not seem as interesting and cool to their friends. Finally, the audience member must have confidence that they can easily quit. Self-efficacy is reduced when people are addicted to behaviors, have low self-esteem, perceive other structural barriers to behavior change, or do not understand the steps to engage in a healthy behavior.

According to Carpenter's 2010 meta-analysis, the HBM is a good predictor of future behavior. Notably, the most powerful predictors of behavioral intention were barriers and benefits (Carpenter 2010). The data also showed that perceived susceptibility and perceived severity had only modest impacts on longer-term behavior (Carpenter 2010). The results also showed that the length of time between the initial measure of the HBM variables and measurement of behavior, as well as the health topic, were significant moderating variables of the model. For example, the size of the effects for benefits and barriers were stronger when the outcome was preventing a negative health outcome than when it was treating an existing one.

Cues to action are another predictor of health behavior intention. They occur when certain events or motivations to act influence preventive behaviors. Cues to action can be divided into internal (e.g. a realization of the disease, change in one's health status) and external cues (e.g. health intervention, interpersonal communication, exposure to the media). Regardless of type, the HBM predicts that cues to action motivate one to adopt discrete health behaviors. Meanwhile, self-efficacy, which refers to a belief in one's own ability to realize the positive outcome of one's behavior, was added to HBM to increase the model's predictive power (Bandura 1997; Janz and Becker 1984). Self-efficacy is regarded as an important determinant of long-term behavior change (Rosenstock, Stretcher, and Becker 1988). Although HBM had been expanded with self-efficacy added, HBM was found to be less effective at predicting health behavior than other models such as the theory of reasoned action, and social cognitive theory (Harrison, Mullen and Green 1992; Zimmerman and Vernberg 1994).

Applications

The HBM is one of the most used theories to explicate one's health behavior (Glanz and Bishop 2010). There have been numerous applications of the HBM in various contexts not only to predict one's health behavior but also to design health interventions. As mentioned, a meta-analysis (Carpenter 2010) showed that perceived benefits and barriers were the strongest predictors of one's behaviors, whereas perceived severity and susceptibility were found to be weakly associated with behaviors and not associated with behaviors, respectively. Perceived benefits and barriers predicted the behavior better, especially when the behavior is preventive rather than curative.

Meanwhile, Jones, Smith, and Llewellyn (2014) conducted a systematic review to investigate the utility of the HBM in designing interventions to increase patients' adherence to medical advice. The results showed that only one-third of studies targeted all the components of the HBM. A commonly targeted component was perceived susceptibility, even though Carpenter (2010) found it to be modestly related to behavior. They concluded that the successes of interventions for adherence were not linked to the HBM.

The HBM has been often criticized as it only focuses on the cognition process in decision-making. That is, it is not appropriate for explaining habitual behaviors that do not require any cognitive processes or forced behaviors (Janz and Becker 1984).

Health Risk Information Seeking

If the number of theories seeking to explain a given behavior is any indication of the importance of that behavior, information seeking is clearly a chief interest among scholars. Today, there are at least a half dozen information-seeking theories and models; there continues to be a significant amount of new research in this area. In this section, we will review three dominant theories in the area: risk perception attitude (RPA) framework (Rimal and Real 2003), risk information seeking and processing model (RISP) (Griffin, Dunwoody, and Neuwirth 1999), and planned risk information seeking model (PRISM) (Kahlor 2010). The general premise is that people should, to varying extents, be informed on the health risks they face and that being informed should be positively related to making health-protective decisions. More pertinent, perhaps, is that risk communication is an interactive process of sharing knowledge and understanding about risks so that consumers arrive at well-informed decisions (Turner, Skubisz, and Rimal 2011). The goal of risk communication is to foster a better understanding of the actual and perceived risks, the possible solutions, and the related issues and concerns regarding the risk (Oleckno 1995). Unfortunately, though, most people passively consume risk and health information. It would be a false understanding of human behavior to believe that all people want to be informed about their health and health risks. Nonetheless, if risk communication is interactive, then scholars of risk should have a good understanding of the precursors to risk information seeking.

In fact, information seeking has been linked to engaging in preventive behaviors (Rimal, Flora, and Schooler 1999), using improved coping mechanisms (Brashers, Neidig, and Goldsmith 2004; Carver, Scheier, and Weintraub 1989; Folkman and Lazarus 1980; Kalichman et al. 2006), and improving one's quality-of-life (Ransom et al. 2005). These outcomes are dependent upon individuals' abilities and motivations to seek information, the depth of their processing of this information, and how those variables mediate the risk judgment and decision-making processes. We must understand risk information-seeking behaviors and what kinds of outcome seeking behaviors will lead to. Certainly, people vary in the extent to which they engage in risk information seeking; many people do not actively seek risk information because, for example, they do not believe the hazard to be relevant or of high priority for their lives.

Risk Perception Attitude Framework
Origins and central concepts

The risk perception attitude framework (RPA) was developed in the early 2000s to provide a parsimonious account of information seeking and its relationship to prevention-oriented behaviors (Rimal and Real 2003). Drawing from Witte's (1992) extended parallel process model, the RPA proposes that the most important predictors of risk information seeking are (i) risk perceptions and (ii) efficacy beliefs. More specifically, the RPA posits that the way perceived risk affects information seeking is dependent upon the level of efficacy people hold. In the RPA, risk perception refers to individuals' beliefs about their susceptibility to the risk and whether the consequences of risk are severe. Efficacy beliefs are defined as a composite measure including both self-efficacy (one's personal confidence in being able to execute certain health behaviors) and response efficacy, or the belief that a health behavior can help one avert risk. Using an audience segmentation approach, the RPA suggests that risk perception and efficacy can be used to create four distinct attitudinal groups that will have distinct information-seeking and health-related behaviors. Rimal and Real (2003) argued that information seeking can be viewed as a health-protective behavior; yet, they recognized that information seeking does not always translate into such behaviors. They reasoned that this may be due to the amount of knowledge *actually* gained when seeking information.

When the risk is perceived to be low (i.e. low severity and susceptibility), but efficacy is strong, individuals are predicted to have *proactive* attitudes. That is, they do not perceive they are in danger, but understand that there are behaviors they can engage in to maintain their low risk. They are not motivated by their perceived risk status, but rather by their desire to remain disease-free. Thus, they will engage in moderate information seeking and moderate levels of other health-protective behaviors.

When the risk is perceived to be low, and efficacy is low, the result will be an *indifferent* attitude. The RPA predicts that information seeking will not be different when comparing the proactive and indifferent audiences. They do not seek any risk information as they feel it is irrelevant to them.

However, when individuals perceive that risk is highly threatening, and they believe they can cope with the risk (i.e. high self- and response-efficacy), they will have *responsive* attitudes. The responsive group is predicted to engage in more health-protective behaviors than the other three groups – including information seeking.

When individuals' risk perception is high, but they do not think they have enough ability to deal with the risk, the original iteration of the RPA proposed them to have *avoidant* attitudes. These individuals are likely to experience conflicting motivations. On the one hand, their high level of risk perception likely makes them concerned about their health status, but on the other hand, their weak efficacy beliefs are likely to weaken their motivations. The avoidant group is likely to be motivated due to high-risk perception, but their motivation is dampened by their low level of efficacy belief simultaneously. As a result, they feel anxiety (i.e. affective interference) and have a lower level of motivation to adopt a recommended behavior compared to the responsive group. Turner, Rimal, Morrison, and Kim (2006) found that so-called avoidants were actually motivated to seek information. Still, their amount of information acquisition was low due to the high anxiety they felt. Turner et al. (2006) concluded that the primary motivation of information seeking for such individuals with high anxiety was reducing the level of anxiety. The high level of anxiety, however, hindered processing relevant information. That is, the avoidant group tends to seek information, but they do not have the ability to process information. As such, in later iterations of the RPA, this group is often labeled the "anxious" group instead of "avoidant."

Application

The RPA framework has been used for audience segmentations to design health interventions and tested in the various context of health risk such as cardiovascular diseases (e.g. Rimal 2001), cancers (Rimal and Juon 2010; Rimal and Real 2003; Turner et al. 2006), HIV (e.g. Rimal et al. 2009a; Rimal et al. 2009b), HPV (e.g. Katz et al. 2012; Pask and Rawlins 2016), and diabetes (e.g. Rains et al. 2019). For example, Rains et al. (2019) evaluated the RPA for its ability to be used as a message tailoring strategy. As such, they created messages that were consistent with the RPA categories and then randomly assigned individuals who had been previously categorized into the four groups to a message. Put simply, messages were most effective when they matched the individual's RPA category (e.g. when the responsive receives a responsive message).

A key application of the RPA is based on the knowledge generated about people who perceive serious threat but low efficacy. The RPA indicates that in such conditions, the ensuing anxiety may serve as a cognitive blocker and make it so that people cannot retain the information that they seek out. Clearly then, developing strong efficacy cues in messages is vital for information processing.

It should be noted that the RPA framework posits a moderated relationship between risk perception and efficacy beliefs. However, numerous studies have found only the main effects of risk and efficacy (Pask and Rawlins 2016). In fact, whether or not there are main effects or interaction effects of risk and efficacy may depend on the kind of study that was conducted. Survey studies measuring risk and efficacy yield different patterns in data than do experimental studies where risk and efficacy are manipulated (see Sullivan et al. 2008).

Risk Information Seeking and Processing Model

Origins and central concepts

The risk information seeking and processing (RISP) model (Griffin, Dunwoody, and Neuwirth 1999) evolved from a need for theories that could describe both information seeking and information processing. RISP describes the precursors of information seeking but is unique from the RPA in that it proposes that people can seek information heuristically or systematically. As such, the RISP is primarily based on dual-processing models (i.e. heuristic-systematic models) (Eagly and Chaiken 1993) and the theory of planned behavior (TPB) (Ajzen 1991).

The original RISP model proposed information insufficiency, perceived information-gathering capacity, and relevant channel beliefs as three primary factors influencing one's information seeking and processing behavior (Griffin et al. 1999). Other variables include individual characteristics, perceived hazard characteristics, affective response, and informational subjective norms.

The major proposition of the RISP model is that information insufficiency drives individuals to seek information related to risk. When individuals perceive a gap between information they need and their current knowledge (i.e. sufficiency threshold), they are motivated to seek relevant information. The perceived information insufficiency affects information seeking and processing behavior via perceived information-gathering capacity. The information insufficiency is influenced by one's informational subjective norms and affective response, such as worry or anger. Derived from the TPB's subjective norms concept, the RISP model defines informational subjective norms as one's perception regarding their significant others' expectation that he or she should hold a certain amount of knowledge about a risk (Griffin et al. 1999).

Information gathering capacity is one's efficacy belief in seeking and processing relevant information. Griffin et al. (1999) suggested that perceived information-gathering capacity mediates the effect of information insufficiency on one's information seeking/processing behavior, especially when it requires more effort to seek and process information. In other words, even though individuals feel the need for information seeking and processing due to their information insufficiency, if they perceive they do not have enough ability to seek/process information, they tend to seek less information compared to those who perceive themselves capable of seeking/processing relevant information. Relevant beliefs about the channel, another primary factor of the RISP model, include perceived trustworthiness and usefulness of channels. Based on this belief, one decides the channel they will use to find the needed information.

According to the RISP model, individuals will seek more actively and process information systematically, when (i) their information insufficiency is high, (ii) they perceive their information gathering capacity is high, and (iii) they believe the channels they use are trustworthy and useful.

Applications

The RISP model has been applied from the context of environmental risk such as water-related risks (e.g. Griffin et al. 2004; Kahlor et al. 2006) and climate change (e.g. Kahlor 2007; Yang and Kahlor 2013) to the context of health risk such as vaccination (e.g. Yang 2012) and cancer clinical trials (e.g. Yang et al. 2010a, 2010b, 2011). There also have been attempts to test the RISP model across different populations (e.g. ter Huurne, Griffin, and Gutteling 2009; Hovick, et al. Chervin 2011).

A meta-analysis (Yang, Aloe, and Feeley 2014), which excluded the relevant channel belief component due to the inconsistency of definitions across the RISP studies, showed that current knowledge and information subjective norms explained a large portion of the variance in the RISP model. Current knowledge, which consists of information insufficiency with information sufficiency threshold, was consistently found to influence the outcome variables. However, information insufficiency turned out to reduce the explanatory power of the RISP model in general. In other words, when individuals feel more need to seek or process information (i.e. high information insufficiency), the amount of the RISP model's explanatory power for information seeking and processing decreases. Given this result, Yang et al. (2014) concluded that the RISP model is less suitable to explain a situation when individuals are less familiar with risk.

This meta-analysis also showed that the explanatory power of the RISP decreased in heuristic processing. Heuristic processing, by definition, is a mode in which individuals analyze the information based on simple cues that are sometimes intuitive and emotional. However, the RISP model aims to depict the complicated process of how one seeks and processes information involving cognitive assessments such as perceived hazard characteristics, information insufficiency, informational subjective norms and relevant channel beliefs. Yang et al. (2014) pointed out that there might be "a mismatch in theorization of the RISP model and conceptualization of heuristic processing" (p. 35). Following this line of thinking, the RISP model might not be a proper model when one seeks information for less familiar risks and one processes information heuristically.

It is worth noticing that the RISP studies have tested the role of discrete emotions such as anger (e.g. Griffin et al. 2008), worry (e.g. Kahlor 2007), and negative affect in general (e.g. Yang et al. 2014), consistently showing that emotions influence not only one's information seeking but also information processing. These findings suggest the substantive importance of discrete emotions in one's information seeking and processing.

In general, the RISP model guides researchers and health communicators to understand what motivates individuals to seek more information and how they process information, especially for a risk that is familiar to audiences.

Planned Risk Information Seeking Model

Origins and central concepts

Although people often seek information in a spontaneous manner, there are also contexts in which people engage in planned information seeking. The planned risk information seeking model (PRISM; Kahlor 2010) is largely based on the TPB (Ajzen 1991) and the RISP (Griffin et al. 1999). As noted earlier, the RISP is also derived from the TPB in that it addresses the role of efficacy beliefs (i.e. perceived information gathering capacity) and subjective norms (i.e. informational subjective norms). Kahlor (2007), however, found that adding more components from TPB (i.e. attitude and behavior intention) into the RISP increased the explanatory power of the model. She added those two components in the model and proposed additional relationships between components in the RISP informed by other relevant theories such as extended parallel process model (EPPM; Witte 1992), health information acquisition model (HIAM; Freimuth, Stein, and Kean 1989), theory of motivated information management (TMIM; Afifi and Weiner 2004), and comprehensive model of cancer-related information seeking (Johnson and Meischke 1993).

For example, the RISP regarded the current knowledge as an exogenous variable, which is not influenced by other components in the model. Kahlor (2010) argued that past utility and experience related to information seeking (i.e. attitude toward seeking), informational subjective norms, and efficacy beliefs related to information seeking (i.e. perceived seeking control) affect one's perceived current knowledge based on the HIAM's propositions, that the cost and benefit analysis of pursing a goal plays a critical role in one's information seeking behavior. Derived from the EPPM research, Kahlor (2010) also added (i) the relationship between efficacy beliefs (i.e. perceived seeking control) and perceived knowledge insufficiency, and (ii) the relationship between the perceived threat (i.e. affective response to risk) and seeking intention in the model.

Recently, the PRISM has been developed into the planned risk information avoidance (PRIA) model (Deline and Kahlor 2019), which addresses how individuals decide to avoid information. The PRIA added perceived descriptive and injunctive norms, which refer to the perceived prevalence of behaviors and perceived (dis)approval of behaviors in one's reference group, respectively (Cialdini, Reno, and Kallgren 1990). Deline and Kahlor (2019) also added the sense of community (i.e. sense of belonging to the community) as a moderator of the effect of norms. To better explain one's decision for the closure of information, they included another concept, confidence in one's knowledge, instead of information insufficiency from the RISP. The model has not yet been tested; thus, we need empirical evidence for the PRIA.

Applications

The most tested context of the PRISM is cancer risks (e.g. Hovick, Kahlor, and Liang 2014; Hovick, Liang, and Kahlor 2014; Willoughby and Myrick 2016), followed by environmental risks such as climate change (Ho, Detenber, Rosenthal, and Lee, 2014), carbon capture and storage (CCS; Kahlor et al. 2020), and hydraulic fracturing (Eastin, Kahlor, Liang, and Ghannam 2015). The relationships between variables of the PRISM have varied across the contexts and samples. Willoughby and Myrick (2016) applied the PRISM to the context of cancer and sexual health with undergraduate students' samples. They compared their results with Kahlor's (2010) result that tested the PRISM in the context of general health. The findings show that the results were not consistent across the contexts. For example, they found the path from perceived control was not positively associated with seeking intention in both of the cancer and sexual health contexts, although Kahlor (2010) found they were related to each other. The results were also not consistent in terms of the relationships between subjective norms and knowledge insufficiency, the relationship between attitude and current knowledge, and the relationship between subjective norms and current knowledge across the contexts. Thus, they concluded that the PRISM should be adjusted based on the contexts.

There have been attempts to expand and develop the PRISM by adding more variables and combining it with other theories. For instance, Hovick, Kahlor, and Liang (2014) tested the extended PRISM by adding past seeking behaviors, source beliefs, and outcome expectancies. They, however, found that the inclusion of such variables increased only a small amount of explained variance in information seeking intention. In addition, the traditional PRISM was found to better fit with the data compared to the extended PRISM.

Another trend of the recent PRISM research is focusing on testing the role of affect and emotions in the PRISM (e.g. Ahn and Kahlor 2020). Although they did not test the full model, the result showed that the discrete emotion (e.g. anticipated regret) mediated the effect of informational subjective norms on one's perceived information insufficiency, which motivated one to seek the relevant information.

Previous studies showed the PRISM accounts for a significant amount of variance in seeking intention (e.g. Kahlor 2010; Hovick, Kahlor, and

Liang 2014), which indicates that the PRISM is useful to explain and predict one's information seeking intention. Still, some variables have been consistently found to predict one's seeking intention (i.e. subjective norms) (e.g. Ho et al. 2014; Hovick, Liang, and Kahlor, 2014; Kahlor et al. 2020; Willoughby and Myrick 2016), whereas others have not. Researchers may need to highlight consistent variables across the context, as Willoughby and Myrick (2016) suggested. Given the major criticism for the PRISM is its lack of parsimony, further research might be useful to reduce the model with only consistent variables. Health communicators should note that context matters when utilizing the PRISM to design interventions.

Conclusion

There is a wide range of theoretical perspectives on the cognitive processes preceding behavior. Information processing theories mainly focus on individual-level variables that account for the depth of processing in which people will engage. The HSM focuses on the importance of cognitive resources and motivation to process messages, both of which can be predicted by context and state as well as trait level characteristics.

Theories that focus on beliefs, like attribution theory and the health belief model, assume that people have already been exposed to messages and have processed[1] them. The real question for these two theories is how one's beliefs affect subsequent outcomes. The HBM assumes that individuals assess a health issue and form beliefs about the threat, their ability to cope with the threat, and benefits/barriers. Thus, it also assumes that people are rational – which is a limitation of the theory. In Chapter 8 in this volume, Nabi discusses the critical role of affect and emotion on health decisions – something the HBM seems to ignore. Attribution theory does not assume rationality. Indeed, this theory understands that people are flawed thinkers and regularly engage in erroneous and biased thinking.

We ended the chapter by discussing information seeking. It is critically important that we understand the circumstances in which people are exposed to and process health information. Where did they get the information? Why did they seek it out? These theories vary a great deal in the antecedent variables predicted to spark information seeking and/ or processing. Both PRISM and RISP take a dual-process perspective and apply the principles of the HSM. The RPA takes more of the HBM perspective – applying constructs like threat and efficacy. The RPA, however, does little to address processing information and rather focuses on the reception of the information. The caveat to this is the Turner et al. (2006) piece, which showed avoiders to have increased anxiety. This decreased the knowledge they gained from the messages sought.

One important issue with which we will conclude is the acknowledgment that across several theories efficacy appears to be critical. The HBM, RPA, and PRISM all make predictions about the role of efficacy. Dual-processing models, in an analogous fashion, discuss the role of the ability to process. One could argue that having increased ability gives people confidence that they can process the message – that is, they have message processing efficacy. Repeatedly, studies show that an individual's confidence that they can cope with a health threat, get the information they need, and process that information is fundamental to their engagement in life-saving health behaviors. It very well may be that efficacy is the single most efficacious cognitive quality one can have.

Note

1. Neither attribution theory nor the HBM was developed to explain the impacts of external messages. These theories explain how people's beliefs – created by messaging or not – affect outcomes.

References

Afifi, W. A., & Weiner, J. L. (2004). Toward a theory of motivated information management. *Communication Theory, 14*(2), 167–190.

Ahn, J., & Kahlor, L. A. (2020). No regrets when it comes to your health: Anticipated regret, subjective norms, information insufficiency and intent to seek health information from multiple sources. *Health Communication, 35*(10), 1295–1302

Ajzen, I. (1991). The theory of planned behavior. *Organizational Behavior and Human Decision Processes, 50*(2), 179–211.

Bandura, A. (1997). *Self-efficacy.* New York, NY: Worth Publishers.

Brashers, D. E., Neidig, J. L., & Goldsmith, D. J. (2004). Social support and the management of uncertainty for people living with HIV or AIDS. *Health Communication, 16*(3), 305–331.

Cacioppo, J. T., & Petty, R. E. (1984). The elaboration likelihood model of persuasion. *Advances in Consumer Research, 11*(1), 673–675.

Carpenter, C. J. (2010). A meta-analysis of the effectiveness of health belief model variables in predicting behavior. *Health Communication, 25*(8), 661–669.

Carver, C. S., Scheier, M. F., & Weintraub, J. K. (1989). Assessing coping strategies: A theoretically based approach. *Journal of Personality and Social Psychology, 56*(2), 267–283.

Chaiken, S. (1980). Heuristic versus systematic information processing and the use of source versus message cues in persuasion. *Journal of Personality and Social Psychology, 39*, 752–766. doi: 10.1037/0022-3514.39.5.752.

Chaiken, S., Giner-Sorolla, R., & Chen, S. (1996). Beyond accuracy: Defense and impression motives in heuristic and systematic information processing. In P. M. Gollwitzer & J. A. Bargh (Eds.), *The psychology of action: Linking cognition and motivation to behavior* (pp. 553–578). New York, NY: Guilford Press.

Chaiken, S., Liberman, A., & Eagly, A. H. (1989). Heuristic and systematic information processing within and beyond the persuasion context. In J. S. Veleman & J. A. Bargh (Eds.), *Unintended thought* (pp. 212–252). New York, NY: Guilford.

Champion, V., & Skinner, C. S. (2008). The health belief model. In K. Glanz, B. Rimer & K. Viswanath (Eds.), *Health behavior and health education* (4th ed.; pp. 45–65). San Francisco, CA: Jossey-Bass.

Chen, S., & Chiaken, S. (1999). The heuristic-systematic model in its broader context. In S. Chiaken, & Y. Trope (Eds.), *Dual-process theories in social psychology* (pp. 73–96). New York, NY: Guilford Press.

Cialdini, R. B., Reno, R. R., & Kallgren, C. A. (1990). A focus theory of normative conduct: Recycling the concept of norms to reduce littering in public places. *Journal of Personality and Social Psychology, 58*(6), 1015–1026.

Deline, M. B., & Kahlor, L. A. (2019). Planned risk information avoidance: A proposed theoretical model. *Communication Theory, 29*(3), 360–382.

Eagly, A. H., & Chaiken, S. (1993). Process theories of attitude formation and change: The elaboration likelihood and heuristic-systematic models. In A. H. Eagly & S. Chaiken, (Eds.), *The psychology of attitudes* (pp. 303–350). Orlando, FL: Harcourt Brace.

Eastin, M. S., Kahlor, L. A., Liang, M., & Abi Ghannam, N. (2015). Information-seeking as a precaution behavior: Exploring the role of decision-making stages. *Human Communication Research, 41*(4), 603–621.

Faller, H., Schilling, S., & Lang, H. (1995). Causal attribution and adaptation among lung cancer patients. *Journal of Psychosomatic Research, 39*(5), 619–627.

Folkman, S., & Lazarus, R. S. (1980). An analysis of coping in a middle-aged community sample. *Journal of Health and Social Behavior, 21*(3), 219–239.

Freimuth, V. S., Stein, J. A., & Kean, T. J. (1989). *Searching for health information: The cancer information service model.* Philadelphia, PA: University of Pennsylvania Press.

Glanz, K., & Bishop, D. B. (2010). The role of behavioral science theory in development and implementation of public health interventions. *Annual Review of Public Health, 31*(1), 399–418.

Griffin, R. J., Dunwoody, S., & Neuwirth, K. (1999). Proposed model of the relationship of risk information seeking and processing to the development of preventive behaviors. *Environmental Research, 80*(2), S230–S245.

Griffin, R. J., Neuwirth, K., Dunwoody, S., & Giese, J. (2004). Information sufficiency and risk communication. *Media Psychology, 6*(1), 23–61.

Griffin, R. J., Yang, Z., ter Huurne, E., Boerner, F., Ortiz, S., & Dunwoody, S. (2008). After the flood: Anger, attribution, and the seeking of information. *Science Communication, 29*(3), 285–315.

Harrison, J. A., Mullen, P. D., & Green, L. W. (1992). A meta-analysis of studies of the health belief model with adults. *Health Education Research, 7*(1), 107–116.

Heider, F. (1944). Social perception and phenomenal causality. *Psychological Review, 51*(6), 358–374. doi:10.1037/h0055425

Heider, F. (1958). *The psychology of interpersonal relations.* New York: Wiley.

Ho, S. S., Detenber, B. H., Rosenthal, S., & Lee, E. W. J. (2014). Seeking information about climate change: Effects of media use in an extended PRISM. *Science Communication, 36*(3), 270–295.

Hovick, S., Freimuth, V. S., Johnson-Turbes, A., & Chervin, D. D. (2011). Multiple health risk perception and information processing among African Americans and Whites living in poverty. *Risk Analysis: An International Journal, 31*(11), 1789–1799.

Hovick, S. R., Kahlor, L., & Liang, M.-C. (2014). Personal cancer knowledge and information seeking through PRISM: The planned risk information seeking model. *Journal of Health Communication, 19*(4), 511–527.

Hovick, S. R., Liang, M.-C., & Kahlor, L. (2014). Predicting cancer risk knowledge and information seeking: The role of social and cognitive factors. *Health Communication, 29*(7), 656–668.

Janz, N. K., & Becker, M. H. (1984). The health belief model: A decade later. *Health Education Quarterly, 11*(1), 1–47.

Johnson, J. D., & Meischke, H. (1993). A comprehensive model of cancer-related information seeking applied to magazines. *Human Communication Research, 19*(3), 343–367.

Jones, C. J., Smith, H., & Llewellyn, C. (2014). Evaluating the effectiveness of health belief model interventions in improving adherence: A systematic review. *Health Psychology Review, 8*(3), 253–269.

Kahlor, L. A. (2007). An augmented risk information seeking model: The case of global warming. *Media Psychology, 10*(3), 414–435.

Kahlor, L. (2010). PRISM: A planned risk information seeking model. *Health Communication, 25*(4), 345–356.

Kahlor, L., Dunwoody, S., Griffin, R. J., & Neuwirth, K. (2006). Seeking and processing information about impersonal risk. *Science Communication, 28*(2), 163–194.

Kahlor, L. A., Yang, J., Li, X., Wang, W., Olson, H. C., & Atkinson, L. (2020). Environmental risk (and benefit) information seeking intentions: The case of carbon capture and storage in Southeast Texas. *Environmental Communication, 14*(4), 555–572.

Kalichman, S. C., Cherry, C., Cain, D., Pope, H., Kalichman, M., Eaton, L., . . . Benotsch, E. G. (2006). Internet-based health information consumer skills intervention for people living with HIV/AIDS. *Journal of Consulting and Clinical Psychology, 74*(3), 545–554.

Katz, M. L., Kam, J. A., Krieger, J. L., & Roberto, A. J. (2012). Predicting human papillomavirus vaccine intentions of college-aged males: An examination of parents' and son's perceptions. *Journal of American College Health, 60*(6), 449–459.

Kim, K., King, K. W., & Kim, J. (2018). Processing contradictory brand information from advertising and social media: An application of the multiple-motive heuristic-systematic model. *Journal of Marketing Communications, 24*(8), 801–822.

Marlow, L. A., Waller, J., & Wardle, J. (2010). Variation in blame attributions across different cancer types. *Cancer Epidemiology and Prevention Biomarkers, 19*(7), 1799–1805.

Oleckno, W. A. (1995). Guidelines for improving risk communication in environmental health. *Journal of Environmental Health, 58*(1), 20–24.

Pask, E. B., & Rawlins, S. T. (2016). Men's intentions to engage in behaviors to protect against human papillomavirus (HPV): Testing the risk perception attitude framework. *Health Communication, 31*(2), 139–149.

Puhl, R. M., & Heuer, C. A. (2009). The stigma of obesity: A review and update. *Obesity, 17*(5), 941–964.

Puhl, R. M., & Heuer, C. A. (2010). Obesity stigma: Important considerations for public health. *American Journal of Public Health, 100*(6), 1019–1028.

Rains, S. A., Hingle, M. D., Surdeanu, M., Bell, D., & Kobourov, S. (2019). A test of the risk perception attitude framework as a message tailoring strategy to promote diabetes screening. *Health Communication, 34*(6), 672–679.

Ransom, S., Jacobsen, P. B., Schmidt, J. E., & Andrykowski, M. A. (2005). Relationship of problem-focused coping strategies to changes in quality of life following treatment for early stage breast cancer. *Journal of Pain and Symptom Management, 30*(3), 243–253.

Rimal, R. N. (2001). Perceived risk and self-efficacy as motivators: Understanding individuals' long-term use of health information. *Journal of Communication, 51*(4), 633–654.

Rimal, R. N., Böse, K., Brown, J., Mkandawire, G., & Folda, L. (2009a). Extending the purview of the risk perception attitude framework: Findings from HIV/AIDS prevention research in Malawi. *Health Communication, 24*(3), 210–218.

Rimal, R. N., Brown, J., Mkandawire, G., Folda, L., Böse, K., & Creel, A. H. (2009b). Audience segmentation as a social-marketing tool in health promotion: Use of the risk perception attitude framework in HIV prevention in Malawi. *American Journal of Public Health, 99*(12), 2224–2229.

Rimal, R. N., Flora, J. A., & Schooler, C. (1999). Achieving improvements in overall health orientation: Effects of campaign exposure, information seeking, and health media use. *Communication Research, 26*(3), 322–348.

Rimal, R. N., & Juon, H.S. (2010). Use of the risk perception attitude framework for promoting breast cancer prevention. *Journal of Applied Social Psychology, 40*(2), 287–310.

Rimal, R. N., & Real, K. (2003). Perceived risk and efficacy beliefs as motivators of change. *Human Communication Research*, *29*(3), 370–399.

Rosenstock, I. M. (1974). Historical origins of the health belief model. *Health Education Monographs*, *2*(4), 328–335.

Rosenstock, I. M., Strecher, V. J., & Becker, M. H. (1988). Social learning theory and the health belief model. *Health Education Quarterly*, *15*(2), 175–183.

Steginga, S. K., & Occhipinti, S. (2004). The application of the heuristic-systematic processing model to treatment decision making about prostate cancer. *Medical Decision Making*, *24*(6), 573–583.

Sullivan, H. W., Burke Beckjord, E., Finney Rutten, L. J., & Hesse, B. W. (2008). Nutrition-related cancer prevention cognitions and behavioral intentions: Testing the risk perception attitude framework. *Health Education & Behavior*, *35*(6), 866–879.

ter Huurne, E. F. J., Griffin, R. J., & Gutteling, J. M. (2009). Risk information seeking among U.S. and Dutch residents: An application of the model of risk information seeking and processing. *Science Communication*, *31*(2), 215–237.

Turner, M. M., Rimal, R. N., Morrison, D., & Kim, H. (2006). The role of anxiety in seeking and retaining risk information: Testing the risk perception attitude framework in two studies. *Human Communication Research*, *32*(2), 130–156.

Turner, M. M., Skubisz, C., & Rimal, R. N. (2011). Theory and practice in risk communication: A review of the literature and visions for the future. In T. L. Thompson, R. Parrott, & J. F. Nussbaum (Eds.), *The Routledge handbook of health communication* (2nd ed. pp. 146–164). New York, NY: Routledge

Vishwanath, A. (2014). Negative public perceptions of juvenile diabetics: Applying attribution theory to understand the public's stigmatizing views. *Health Communication*, *29*(5), 516–526.

Willoughby, J. F., & Myrick, J. G. (2016). Does context matter? Examining PRISM as a guiding framework for context-specific health risk information seeking among young adults. *Journal of Health Communication*, *21*(6), 696–704.

Witte, K. (1992). Putting the fear back into fear appeals: The extended parallel process model. *Communication Monographs*, *59*(4), 329–349.

Yang, Z. J. (2012). Too scared or too capable? Why do college students stay away from the H1N1 vaccine? *Risk Analysis: An International Journal*, *32*(10), 1703–1716.

Yang, Z. J., Aloe, A. M., & Feeley, T. H. (2014). Risk information seeking and processing model: A meta-analysis. *Journal of Communication*, *64*(1), 20–41.

Yang, Z. J., & Kahlor, L. (2013). What, me worry? The role of affect in information seeking and avoidance. *Science Communication*, *35*(2), 189–212.

Yang, Z. J., McComas, K., Gay, G., Leonard, J. P., Dannenberg, A. J., & Dillon, H. (2010a). From information processing to behavioral intentions: Exploring cancer patients' motivations for clinical trial enrollment. *Patient Education and Counseling*, *79*(2), 231–238.

Yang, Z. J., McComas, K., Gay, G., Leonard, J. P., Dannenberg, A. J., & Dillon, H. (2010b). Motivation for health information seeking and processing about clinical trial enrollment. *Health Communication, 25*(5), 423–436.

Yang, Z. J., McComas, K. A., Gay, G., Leonard, J. P., Dannenberg, A. J., & Dillon, H. (2011). Information seeking related to clinical trial enrollment. *Communication Research, 38*(6), 856–882.

Zimmerman, R. S., & Vernberg, D. (1994). Models of preventive health behavior: Comparison, critique, and meta-analysis. *Advances in Medical Sociology, 4*, 45–67.

Zuckerman, A., & Chaiken, S. (1998). A heuristic-systematic processing analysis of the effectiveness of product warning labels. *Psychology & Marketing, 15*(7), 621–642.

8

Theories of Affective Impact

Robin L. Nabi

It has become common practice to use emotional appeals, typically involving negative emotions, to motivate audiences to make changes to support better health and well-being. As such, theoretical frameworks to guide such efforts are of critical value. This chapter overviews theories of influence that address how affective arousal serves as the mechanism by which audiences are motivated to both accept messages and resist them. We begin with two theories drawn from the field of psychology that focus on psychological discomfort with affective roots – psychological reactance and dissonance – that have clear applicability to health message design. We then turn to theories of message influence that center on discrete emotional arousal, most notably fear but also anger and hope. The chapter concludes with discussion of more general theoretical frameworks of emotional influence to address the larger issue of how affect-based theories contribute to our understanding of effective health messaging.

Health Communication Theory, First Edition. Edited by Teresa L. Thompson and Peter J. Schulz.
© 2021 John Wiley & Sons, Inc. Published 2021 by John Wiley & Sons, Inc.

General Psychological Discomfort

Psychological Reactance

Psychological reactance theory (PRT; Brehm 1966; Brehm and Brehm 1981) was developed at a time when motivational theories of influence enjoyed great popularity. As a theory of resistance to influence, PRT asserts that people, driven by a desire for autonomy, resist attempts to restrict or eliminate their behavioral freedoms (i.e. freedom threats). In such circumstances, individuals will experience a drive called reactance, defined by Brehm (1966) as a motivation state directed toward the reestablishment of threatened or eliminated freedom. Reactance is argued to be intensified if the behavior is important to the individual (e.g. smoking to a smoker), is more strictly limited (e.g. a ban on smoking versus a restriction of location), or if there are no similar alternative behaviors to that being restricted (e.g. chewing gum is not similar to smoking), though limited research tests these assumptions. More substantial evidence supports the claim that the greater the perceived threat, the greater the aroused reactance (see Rosenberg and Siegel 2018, for a recent comprehensive review.)

Once aroused, reactance is predicted to motivate audiences to restore their desired freedom through a range of methods, including holding on to their initial beliefs more firmly, derogating the message source, and adopting the opposite behavior from the one advocated (Brehm and Brehm 1981). Given health messaging often focuses on instructing audiences on what they should or should not do, such messages run significant risk of evoking reactance, and thus undermining persuasive success. Indeed, the possibility of boomerang effects (i.e. encouraging the behavior one is hoping to dissuade) suggests reactance can be a significant barrier to message effectiveness.

Stemming from this dilemma, research has focused on addressing two key questions. First, how is reactance best conceptualized and measured? Second, how can messages be designed to mitigate reactance arousal? Regarding measurement, Brehm and Brehm (1981) suggested state reactance was unmeasurable. However, Dillard and Shen (2005) tackled this issue by first assessing multiple possible conceptualizations of reactance, including one based primarily on cognitions, one based primarily on negative affect, and combined models in which affect and cognition were either considered separate contributors or intertwined. The intertwined model was best supported by their data, suggesting reactance is appropriately measured by assessing both anger and negative cognitions (see Rosenberg and Seigel 2018, for a more detailed discussion of reactance measurement, and Rains 2013, for a meta-analytic review supporting the intertwined model).

As to message design, multiple approaches have been suggested to mitigate reactance response. In light of evidence that controlling language evokes reactance (e.g. Burgoon et al. 2002), avoiding controlling language (e.g. "must," "should") in favor of more autonomy supportive language (e.g. "might," "could") is recommended. The use of narrative has also become a popular method of health message delivery which, by transporting audiences into the story world, can promote identification with characters, which has been shown to reduce reactance (see Moyer-Guse and Nabi 2010). Other mitigation approaches include the inclusion of restoration of freedom postscripts in messages (e.g. "the choice is yours") to allow for direct expression of a recommended behavior while mitigating perceptions of threat (e.g. Miller et al. 2007), empathy arousal (e.g. Shen 2010), and including multiple behavioral options (i.e. choice clustering; Reynolds-Tylus, Gonzalez, and Quick 2019; see Quick, Shen, and Dillard 2013, for a review, and Quick et al., Chapter 2 in this volume, for a discussion of reactance proneness.) Finally, reactance can be harnessed as a persuasive strategy on its own. That is, if one evokes reactance against one's opposition, the motivation to resist the opposition will theoretically result in support for one's own position. The "truth" anti-tobacco campaign was in part motivated by this strategy (e.g. Farrelly et al. 2002).

In sum, reactance is a fundamentally affect-based theory that represents a well-documented and heavily studied phenomenon with significant implications for health message design. Although much attention has already yielded valuable insights, better understanding of the message features that both contribute to and mitigate reactance arousal, and how to harness reactance for persuasive gain continue to be fruitful avenues for future research.

Dissonance

Festinger's (1957) theory of cognitive dissonance maintains that when humans simultaneously hold two or more related, but inconsistent, cognitions or behaviors, they experience the psychologically uncomfortable sensation of dissonance. Dissonance is then hypothesized to motivate changes in attitudes or behaviors to eliminate the unpleasant psychological state when certain conditions are met. Those conditions are contingent on the two primary methods of dissonance evocation: counter-attitudinal advocacy or the hypocrisy paradigm.

Counter-attitudinal advocacy (CAA) involves advocating for a position or behavior inconsistent with one's existing cognitions or behaviors, typically by writing an essay, giving a speech, or making another type of declaration of the virtues of a behavior that one does not privately endorse. According to dissonance theory, such advocacy evokes psychological discomfort. This discomfort, in turn, motivates altering one's behaviors or attitudes to more closely align with the advocated behavior, but only if the advocacy is under individuals' volitional control, no external justification is available, and the physiological arousal is attributed to the advocacy (Cooper, Zanna, and Taves 1978). Classic research in this area supports this reasoning (Festinger and Carlsmith 1959), as does more contemporary research in domains such as disordered eating symptomology (see Stice et al. 2008 for a review).

A second dissonance-evoking technique, the hypocrisy paradigm, applies to contexts in which individuals hold desired attitudes but fail to act on them. This strategy evokes dissonance by encouraging voluntary public commitment to an attitude through some form of public advocacy, and then making the target mindful that their past behavior is inconsistent with their expressed attitude, usually by instructing participants to list reasons why they have previously failed to engage in the behavior. The resulting discrepancy between attitudes and behaviors is expected to induce dissonance, motivating individuals to bring their behaviors in-line with their attitude to restore their sense of integrity (Stone and Fernandez 2008; Stone et al. 1997).

The hypocrisy paradigm has been successfully used to motivate a variety of health-related behaviors (see Stone and Focella 2011, for a review). However, despite this resurgence of applied dissonance-based inquiry, the existing research is limited in multiple ways. Most critically, though the hypocrisy paradigm has been shown to generate desired behavior change immediately after the hypocrisy induction, there is little evidence that speaks to the longer term benefits of inducing dissonance via hypocrisy. In a rare exception, however, Nabi, Huskey, et al. (2019) provide some evidence that posting a melanoma awareness message to social media (public commitment) generated more sun safety behavior in the following week compared to non-posters.

As well, unlike reactance, for which a measure has been developed, a measure of dissonance is still elusive. That is, though it is hypothesized to be experienced, studies of dissonance do not actually measure its arousal. Future research might consider an approach similar to Dillard and Shen (2005) in which a combination of negative thoughts and affect (guilt specificaly) might capture dissonance arousal. Further, considering how exposure to multiple messages over time to chronically activate dissonant health attitudes and behaviors and thus promote more enduring change would be of great value.

Fear-Based Theories of Influence

The use of emotion to motivate desired health behaviors has a long history, with particular emphasis on fear. Fear is generally aroused when a situation is perceived as both threatening to one's physical or psychological self and out of one's control (Lazarus 1991). Based on the desire for protection, fear's action tendency is to escape from the threatening agent and, if realized, avoidance behavior results. As such, fear has been a popular strategy to discourage unhealthy behaviors or encourage healthy ones as a way of protecting oneself from negative health outcomes. However, a theory of fear-based messaging that is well supported by empirical evidence has been rather elusive.

Early Fear-Based Models

The fear-as-acquired drive model (i.e. the drive model) is the first model articulating the relationship between fear and persuasion, suggesting that stimuli that evoke fear result in a drive to avoid the unpleasant emotional state (Hovland, Janis, and Kelley 1953). If a message's behavioral recommendation, when cognitively rehearsed, provides relief from the fear arousal, that behavior will be seen as a functional or adaptive response to the threatening stimuli and be adopted. However, if the rehearsed message recommendation does not assuage fear, other strategies to reduce fear are adopted, such as source denigration or problem minimization. Such approaches may reduce fear, but are considered maladaptive as they do not address the existing threat. In light of these two possible outcomes, theorizing turned toward the idea that fear arousal has a curvilinear relationship with attitude change – too little is not sufficient to motivate change but too much fear pushes audiences toward maladaptive responses. As such, researchers spent the next decade searching for the optimal amount of fear arousal that would generate adaptive versus maladaptive responses (Janis 1967), though ultimately research did not support this predicted curvilinear relationship.

To explain the dual outcomes possible in response to fear appeals in light of growing evidence of a positive linear relationship between fear and persuasion, Leventhal (1970) presented the parallel process model (PPM), in which he proposed two possible responses to fear appeals – one based on cognition (danger control) and the other based on emotion (fear control). Specifically, he argued that if in response to a fear-based message a person focuses on managing the existing threat, they would engage in danger control, which would lead to adaptive outcomes (e.g. message-consistent attitude or behavior change.) However, if a person focuses on controlling their emotional arousal, fear control processes would be engaged, leading to such maladaptive outcomes as avoidance, denial, and reactance. Although conceptually appealing, the PPM did not specify the conditions under which individuals were more likely to rely on fear-control versus danger-control processes. Thus, the model proved less than helpful for both predicting responses to fear appeals as well as to fear appeal message design.

Protection Motivation Theory (PMT)

As cognitively based theories gained favor in psychology in the 1970s, the next major advance in fear appeal theorizing focused on the cognitive elements associated with fear appeal effectiveness. The protection motivation theory (PMT; Rogers 1975, 1983) elaborated on the danger-control branch of the PPM, explicating four different cognitive reactions to fear appeals. These included two perceptions related to the potential threat – threat severity and threat susceptibility – and two perceptions related to the advocated behavioral response – response efficacy, or the effectiveness of the target behavior for avoiding the threat, and self-efficacy, or the ability of the individual to enact the target behavior. Although the four cognitions identified in the PMT proved important to persuasive outcomes in response to fear appeals, the specific relationships among them as asserted by the theory were not fully supported by empirical evidence. Despite accumulating evidence that fear appeals could be persuasive, the field remained without a well-supported explanation for the mechanisms driving these message effects.

Extended Parallel Process Model (EPPM)

In light of the limitations of previous theorizing, and coinciding with an increased interest in affect and emotion in the psychology literature (Lazarus 1991), Witte (1992) proposed the extended parallel process model (EPPM), which in essence represents a merger of the PPM and the PMT with the advance of recentralizing the role of fear as an emotional state in the process of message influence. In essence, the EPPM posits that fear appeal effectiveness hinges on the relationship between threat appraisals and efficacy appraisals. Specifically, Witte argued that if a message contains information related to threat severity and susceptibility, fear will be aroused. Although fear may predispose audiences to engage in defensive motivations, it also prompts consideration of efficacy potential. As such, those experiencing message-induced fear will consider message content related to response and self-efficacy. If the threat appraisals (perceived severity and susceptibility) outweigh the efficacy appraisals (perceived response and self-efficacy), the unaddressed fear will trigger fear control, thus motivating maladaptive behaviors, such as message source denigration, problem minimization, or other forms of rationalizing unhealthy behaviors. However, if efficacy appraisals outweigh threat appraisals, individuals will quell their fear by engaging in danger control and adaptive responses, thus accepting the message recommendations.

The full model includes 12 propositions detailing numerous intricate relationships between these different types of cognitions, fear, and message effectiveness (Witte 1992). Visually, the EPPM is represented as a path model whereby the four message components in the external stimuli (i.e. self-efficacy, response efficacy, susceptibility, and severity) predict their related cognitive perceptions. These cognitive perceptions then form a feedback loop with fear, and interact with each other to either predict protection motivation (which results in message acceptance) or defensive motivation (which generates message rejection). From a message design standpoint, the EPPM suggests that fear-arousing messages should include both threat and efficacy information if they are to persuade audiences to take adaptive actions, as threat perceptions are necessary to elicit fear but efficacy perceptions are necessary to promote protection motivation.

Although it offers an appealing explanation for when fear appeals may be more or less persuasive, research has not supported the EPPM's key prediction. That is, though significant relationships between fear and persuasion have been identified and the four cognitions have been supported as relevant, meta-analyses have found only mixed support for the threat-efficacy interaction predicted by the EPPM (de Hoog, Stroebe, and de Wit 2007; Witte and Allen 2000). Further, the 12 propositions originally articulated within the EPPM (Witte 1992) have not been tested consistently, and two propositions regarding the effects of moderate and high perceived efficacy have yet to be tested at all (Popova 2012).

In sum, though meta-analyses of fear appeal research support the importance of the four cognitions identified in the PMT, and later the EPPM, to fear appeal effectiveness, no current fear appeal model has been fully endorsed as accurately capturing the process of fear's effects on decision-making and action (see Mongeau 2013; Popova 2012). Regardless, evidence does support a positive linear relationship between audiences' experience of fear and attitude, behavioral intention, and behavior change, and further, that fear appeals are more persuasive when efficacy components are included (Tannenbaum et al. 2015). Thus, to the extent message features in a fear appeal evoke perceptions of susceptibility to a severe health threat, fear may be aroused and in turn influence health behavioral outcomes in light of audiences' response efficacy and self-efficacy perceptions.

Given fear is undoubtedly a powerful tool in motivating health-related action, including information-seeking as well as performing prevention and detection behaviors, scholars continue to explore how fear-evoking messages may generate health behavior change. The most current work by Dillard and colleagues (e.g. Dillard et al. 2017) has cycled back to ideas originally proposed in the drive model, suggesting that a curvilinear relationship between fear arousal and persuasive outcomes may emerge when one looks at the experience of fear within (rather than between) subjects and over the course of message exposure. Although this perspective does not advance a new model of fear appeal effectiveness per se, it does highlight the importance of considering the dynamic experience of fear during message exposure, which speaks to the broader idea of how sequential emotional experiences may illuminate effective message design (see Nabi 2015, for detailed arguments on this point.)

A novel approach to understanding why fear appeal models have failed to fully capture the process of fear's influence I introduce here lies in moving away from models that balance threat and efficacy to one that considers thresholds. That is, models like the EPPM assume that efficacy must *outweigh* threat to motivate action. Yet, it is entirely plausible that efficacy need not outweigh threat but simply needs to reach a *necessary threshold* to translate fear into action. Indeed, one can point to a range of behaviors that people both fear and question their capacity to handle, yet do anyway, like needed medical procedures such as blood draws or MRIs. I argue that people do not only engage in feared behaviors because their belief in their own coping exceeds their fear but rather because their sense of efficacy is high enough that the discrepancy between threat and efficacy is within tolerable limits. Developing what I would call a threshold model of fear appeals, the field would move away from the more expectancy value-based models that have dominated the conversation to ones that allow for a more flexible way of understanding how threat and efficacy combine to motivate health behavior change.

Action Tendency Emotions

Other emotions beyond fear have been considered as motivators of behavior within persuasive message contexts which are pertinent to health message design. Although some theorizing of effects processes exists in some cases (e.g. anger, hope), they are mostly based on the fear-based models that posit emotional arousal should be followed by efficacy information. As well, limited empirical investigation of these approaches has been conducted. Also, other emotions, like guilt and amusement, have been incorporated into some messaging efforts, but theorizing is lacking. Below, each of these emotions is defined along with discussion of any theorizing addressing their persuasive effects and applications within health messaging.

Anger

Anger is generally evoked by situations in which either obstacles are perceived to interfere with goal-oriented behavior, or demeaning offenses against oneself or one's loved ones are perceived to have occurred (Lazarus 1991). Anger is believed to mobilize and sustain high levels of energy for the purpose of defending oneself, defending one's loved ones, or correcting some perceived wrong. When experiencing anger, attention is focused, and there is a desire to attack, strike out at, or in some way get back at the source of the offense. While intense forms of anger are often associated with impulsiveness and aggression, more mild manifestations of anger can benefit problem-solving with consequences generally more beneficial than harmful.

Anger is typically seen as a barrier to positive health-decision-making, as anger evoked in response to a health-promotion message is likely to be associated with reactance (as discussed above) and lead to message rejection. However, despite its generally negative consequences, anger may be productive in some health contexts. For example, anger may be harnessed to rally support for protest or policy change. As well, consistent with reactance theorizing, anger can be targeted toward an opponent's position to marshal support for one's own position. It is also possible that anger responses could prove useful in encouraging the more detailed processing of health information (Nabi 2002).

As to theorizing about anger's persuasive potential, the anger activism model (AAM; Turner 2007) stands as the only model specifically aimed at understanding the persuasive effect of anger-based messages. Like the EPPM, the AAM is rooted in the cognitive appraisal perspective, focusing specifically on how anger intensity and efficacy beliefs interact to produce distinct persuasive outcomes. Specifically, the AAM posits that anger, as a mobilizing force, can result in productive action only when coupled with high efficacy. As such, it seems closely modeled after the EPPM in its consideration of both emotional arousal and efficacy perceptions. Thus, to maximize effectiveness, persuasive messages should generate high levels of anger coupled with self-efficacy beliefs.

There have been only a few studies that have tested the AAM to this point and fewer that have applied it to a health context. However, one recent study indicated that individuals who experienced higher levels of anger and self-efficacy in response to an anti-smoking campaign expressed greater interest in taking action to stop smoking and were more likely to discuss the ad with others (Ilakkuvan et al. 2017). Further, a recent meta-analysis on anger-based persuasive appeals (Walter et al. 2019) found minimal effects of anger overall, but positive effects with the presence of strong arguments, relevant anger, and the inclusion of efficacy appeals. This is consistent with the tenets of both the AAM as well as the cognitive functional model (described below). Interestingly, the meta-analysis also suggested an inverse U-shaped relationship between anger intensity and attitude-related outcomes, such that moderate-high levels of anger result in lower persuasive effect.

In sum, scholars have overwhelmingly focused on the unintentional and counterproductive role of anger evocation in health messaging. However, some useful theorizing regarding how anger might be harnessed to generate positive action toward health goals has emerged. In light of the very limited extant empirical evidence, additional tests are needed to assess both the role of efficacy and depth of processing in tapping into anger's potential as a persuasive force.

Hope

Hope is the feeling of yearning for relief from a difficult situation or for a desired outcome in the face of discouraging odds (Lazarus 1991). Although theorists disagree about the extent to which an individual does or does not maintain a sense of control for the hoped-for outcome (e.g. Lazarus 1999; Snyder 2000), hopeful individuals are seen as determined to meet a goal and able to figure out how to do so. Thus, hope is believed to be associated with the motivation for and impetus for action toward important goals in light of some degree of uncertainty and/or adversity (Averill, Catlin, and Chon 1990; Lazarus 1991; Stotland 1969). Given the many health contexts in which the odds of success are, or seem, discouraging (e.g. quitting smoking, maintaining a healthy diet, surviving difficult treatments), hope is a particularly useful salve, both as a subjective experience and as a motivating force for action.

Despite the clear and direct relevance of hope to health contexts, there has been minimal theoretical or empirical attention given to hope in the context of health messaging. One exception is Chadwick's (2015) persuasive hope theory (PHT). Similar to the EPPM and AAM, it is rooted in cognitive appraisal theories with an emphasis on efficacy. Specifically, PHT asserts that messages that include components suggesting importance, goal congruence, positive future expectation, and possibility will generate both greater feelings of hope as well as greater message attention, interest, perceived message effectiveness, and behavioral intentions. PHT also predicts that message recommendations that boost response and self-efficacy influence subjective feelings of hope. Chadwick, however, leaves as a research question whether hope relates to persuasive outcomes (Chadwick 2015). Unfortunately, the first test of PHT (in the context of climate change) yielded mixed findings regarding predicted relationships and little insight into the actual role of felt hope on persuasive outcomes. Given PHT does not articulate how the emotion of hope might drive behavior, it is of limited value, in its current formulation, in shedding light on the persuasive effect of hope arousal.

Although not formulated as a theory per se, Nabi and Myrick (2018) argue that, within the context of fear appeals, efficacy information is likely to boost feelings of hope in that it can boost the perception of the likelihood of desired future outcomes. Felt hope, in turn, might directly motivate changes in behavior and/or interact with self-efficacy to generate more sustained behavioral change. That is, hope may intensify the benefits of self-efficacy. In their test of these ideas in the context of two studies on sun safety behavior, they found evidence that controlling for variables typically considered in fear appeal studies, felt hope explained unique variance in behavior intentions both alone and in combination with self-efficacy. Based on this evidence, theorizing that considers both a direct effect of hope on health behavioral intentions and behaviors as well as an interactive or reciprocal relationship with self-efficacy would be of value, regardless of any prior emotion that may be experienced (e.g. fear, guilt, anger, or none at all.) Given the association of hope with efficacy and the central role efficacy plays in behavior enactment, this is a very promising direction for future theorizing and research.

Other Action Tendency Emotions

Unlike anger and hope, there are no existing theories that address the persuasive effect of other discrete emotions (though see discussion of the cognitive-functional model below, Nabi 1999). This isn't to say that other emotions are not positioned to influence health decision-making and behavior. Rather, theorizing about their process of influence has yet to be specified, despite empirical attention to their effects. Two examples of such emotions include guilt and amusement.

Guilt. The persuasive influence of guilt arousal has received only sporadic attention over the years with just a handful of studies examining guilt in the context of health messaging. Guilt arises from one's violation of an internalized moral, ethical, or religious code, and, when aroused, motivates reparative behavior (Lazarus 1991). While O'Keefe's (2000) meta-analysis revealed that more explicit guilt-based appeals evoked stronger guilt, such messages were also found to have a negative linear relationship with persuasive outcomes (r = -.26), likely due to the concurrent arousal of anger evoked when audiences are primed to feel as though they have done something wrong. Interestingly, a recent meta-analysis (Xu and Guo 2018) examining the effect of guilt on health-related attitudes and intentions specifically found a strong, positive effect of guilt (r = .49). However, limitations to the study sample, including the dearth of studies that included different levels of guilt appeals or behavior measures, suggest we must be cautious in assuming that stronger guilt appeals are more effective than weaker ones.

Further, even if we can assume guilt can, in some circumstances, generate desired health behaviors, we are no closer in theorizing about the process of such effects. However, toward this end, we can draw from dissonance theory (Festinger 1957) in that the manipulations of dissonance that have been used in the past (e.g. lying) are also manipulations that have been used to evoke guilt in interpersonal compliance gaining studies. If we assume that some dissonance research may be capturing feelings of guilt (see O'Keefe 2000), then we gain potentially valuable insight into the possible theoretical process of guilt's influence in health settings. That is, we might assume that guilt can have a positive effect on behavior, but is so uncomfortable that it runs a great risk of rationalization tendencies. Thus, making the solution accessible and easy to enact quickly and with minimal effort may be especially important. Consistent with theorizing associated with fear and hope, then, guilt-based messages should likely contain the appraisals that underlie guilt arousal and offer effective solutions that can be performed easily (response and self-efficacy) and in the moment to translate guilt into behavior.

Amusement. Finally, humor, and its related affect of amusement, have received growing attention in health contexts. Amusement is associated with a sense of well-being, pleasure, and security, providing a respite from goal-driven activity and promoting playfulness and creativity (Lazarus 1991). Although amusement may not be associated strongly with action per se, it has been incorporated into health messaging sufficiently to warrant mention here. Recent meta-analyses of the persuasive effects of humor have shown a mix of findings. In the advertising literature, humor has been found to enhance message liking as well as psychological states associated with persuasion – attitudes and intentions specifically. However, humor has also been found to detract from source credibility, and there is no consistent evidence that humor impacts ad recall or purchase behavior (Eisend 2009). Thus, the use of humor to motivate positive health behaviors may be suspect.

Indeed, a more recent meta-analysis comparing humorous and non-humorous messages across a range of contexts, including education, marketing, political contexts, and health found, for health messages specifically, no appreciable effect on knowledge, attitudes, or behavioral intentions (Walter et al. 2018). Given topic-related humor and more moderate levels of humor seemed more effective across the data set, it may be that humor, incorporated judiciously, could enhance health message effectiveness. Perhaps more critically, if humor helps garner attention to messages beyond what serious messages might encourage, humorous messages might enjoy an inherent and substantial persuasive advantage over other message styles. Further, humorous messages are more likely to be socially shared than non-humorous ones, thus increasing their potential exposure and influence. Thus, the type of humor employed and its integration with message content become particularly important issues to consider as scholars work to specify a theoretical model articulating the conditions under which humor exerts positive influence via the arousal of amusement.

General Theories of Emotional Influence

Apart from the emphasis on understanding the influence of specific discrete emotions on the persuasive influence of health messaging, there has been some theorizing in the past 20 years that considers a range of discrete emotions under umbrella models of influence, though with varying degrees of empirical support. Three such models are discussed below.

Cognitive-Functional Model (CFM)

In response to the dearth of theorizing about emotional influence apart from fear, Nabi (1999) proposed the cognitive-functional model (CFM) to advance the literature on negative emotional appeals generally. Combining aspects of cognitive response theories of persuasion with the appraisal-based perspectives on emotion, the CFM focuses on the role of three concepts: motivated attention, motivated processing, and message expectations. *Motivated attention* refers to the degree of approach or avoidance response to the message based on the receiver's initial emotional response, *motivated processing* refers to how motivated the message receiver is to process the message carefully, and *message expectations* pertain to the audience's degree of certainty that the message will offer reassurance or not. In essence, the CFM suggests that negative emotions with avoidance tendencies (e.g. fear) would generate less careful processing unless the message had cues suggesting the message would offer reassurance and that reassurance is not easily gained via peripheral processing. Conversely, negative emotions with approach tendencies (e.g. anger, guilt) would associate with more careful processing unless the message contains cues suggesting the message is unlikely to offer reassuring information. In an initial test of the model, the predictions that fear promotes less careful message processing relative to anger and uncertainty of message reassurance results in more careful processing than certainty of reassurance were supported. However, the prediction that fear, but not anger, would be associated with less careful information processing when expectation of reassurance was high was not supported (Nabi 2002). More recently, a meta-analysis of anger appeals generally (Walter et al. 2019) suggested support for the CFM in that anger arousal was associated with persuasion in the presence of strong argument and efficacy information. Thus, though there have been few direct tests of the CFM, it has been useful in generating frameworks for thinking about how specific emotions influence health message processing and thus can inform both empirical work as well as the development of more specific models, such as the AAM.

Emotions as Frames Model (EFM)

A second more general approach to considering the influence of discrete emotions – both negative and positive – on persuasive outcome is the emotions-as-frames perspective (Nabi 2003, 2007). The EFM argues that an audience member's emotional state provides a lens through which individuals pay attention to and process message information. Rooted in appraisal theories of emotions (e.g. Lazarus 1991), the EFM argues that when a message contains information that is relevant to an emotion's core relational theme, or the essential perception that underlies an emotional experience, that particular emotion is aroused. For example, the core relational theme of fear is imminent threat. So, if an audience member appraises a message as representing an imminent threat to her own well-being, she will likely experience fear. The EFM then predicts that once an emotion is experienced, emotion-consistent information will be made accessible from memory. Additionally, audiences will be motivated to attend to message information that is consistent with the goals of the aroused emotion (e.g. protection, in the case of fear). Finally, given the expectation that emotional experience directs information processing and information accessibility, the EFM predicts that decision-making and action will be heavily influenced by these emotion-driven processes. In short, the message consumer's emotional state directs message engagement and, in turn, emotion-consistent decision-making and action.

Multiple studies have supported the predictive power of the emotions-as-frames perspective, demonstrating not only that different emotion frames lead to different ways of viewing problems and preferred solutions but also that emotion is an important mediator of that process (e.g. Kühne and Schemer 2013). In fact, a recent meta-analysis on emotions and gain/loss framing effects supports the position that positive emotions mediate the effects of gain-framed messages on persuasive outcomes whereas negative emotions mediate the effects of loss-framed messages (Nabi, Walter, et al. 2019.) It is important to note, however, that other elements of the model (e.g. information accessibility) have rarely been assessed. Further, the EFM has been applied more in the context of news than health persuasion. Still, the EFM has the potential to assist in understanding how emotion-based messages might generate persuasive influence by emphasizing how emotion-relevant information is more likely to be attended to later in the message and how post-message behaviors are likely to be consistent with emotional motivations.

Emotional Flow

A third general model speaking to the persuasive influence of emotions diverges from other perspectives by focusing not on the dominant emotion evoked by a message but rather on the evolution of the emotional experience across message exposure. The recently advanced emotional flow perspective (Nabi 2015; Nabi and Green 2015) asserts that persuasive messages may evoke multiple emotions in sequence as the contents of the messages unfold. It further asserts that the ordering or shifts in emotional states in response to changing message content may be critical to understanding persuasive outcomes. For example, fear appeals begin with threat information followed by efficacy information. The emotional flow perspective suggests that the threat information results in fear arousal, and the efficacy information is associated with feelings of hope. As such, the emotional flow perspective suggests that the emotional shift from fear to hope may help to explain the conditions under which fear appeals are more likely to be effective (see Nabi and Myrick 2018 for supporting evidence for this claim.) Given its recent introduction to the literature, there are few published studies testing the tenets of emotional flow as yet (though see Nabi, Gustafson, and Jensen 2018). However, with its more realistic reflection of the more complex emotional experiences of audiences to messages, particular video-based narrative messages, the emotional flow perspective has strong heuristic value and will likely lead to greater consideration of emotional sequencing in health message design in the coming years.

Conclusion

In sum, a wide range of theoretical perspectives exists to guide health-focused message design, including those focused on motivational drives with emotional underpinnings (e.g. reactance, dissonance), discrete emotions (e.g. fear, hope), and umbrella theories of discrete emotional influence (e.g. CFM, emotional framing). As we look forward to how such theorizing can be improved, each approach has its own possible future paths. Motivational theories, like dissonance, could consider more carefully the role discrete emotions may play in documented effects. Models focused on the persuasive influence of discrete emotions share the idea that appraisals underlying each emotion coupled with efficacy information are both important components. Yet understanding the relative weight of each as well as the conditions under which such information is necessary to include or can be left implicit remain questions open to additional investigation. As well, though general models of emotional influence have been proposed, empirical evidence is sorely needed.

Additional gaps in theorizing also become evident in light of this review. Most notably, the lion's share of attention has been given to the persuasive influence of negative emotional states. As such, there is minimal theorizing regarding the influence of positive emotions on health behavior decision-making. Further, the theories that have been developed reflect processes of mediated, versus interpersonal, influence. Thus, though they may apply to influencing prevention and detection behavioral choices, we do not know whether these theories fully capture the process of influence as it occurs in clinical contexts (e.g. motivating compliance with treatment recommendations). Indeed, the dynamic nature of the provider–patient relationship suggests that variables not typically considered in mediated contexts, such as interpersonal trust, would be of potential value to consider when emotions are harnessed to affect patient behavior.

Finally, it is important to note that extant theorizing has overwhelmingly made two potentially troubling assumptions: first, that audiences will give attention to the message, and second, that messaging is not countered by an environment replete with messages that may support or counter the health message's position. Moving forward, theorizing across this domain would do well to consider the full process of influence from message selection to downstream behavior while also considering the noisy, complicated media environment in which those messages are received.

References

Averill, J. R., Catlin, G., & Chon, K. K. (1990). *Rules of hope*. New York, NY: Springer-Verlag. doi:10.1007/978-1-4613-9674-1

Brehm, J.W. (1966). *A theory of psychological reactance*. New York, NY: Academic Press

Brehm, S.S., & Brehm, J.W. (1981). *Psychological reactance: A theory of freedom and control*. New York, NY: Academic Press.

Burgoon, M., Alvaro, E., Grandpre, J., & Voulodakis, M. (2002). Revisiting the theory of psychological reactance: Communicating threats to attitudinal freedom. In J. P. Dillard & M. Pfau (Eds.), *The persuasion handbook: Developments in theory and practice* (pp. 213–232). Thousand Oaks, CA: Sage. doi:10.4135/9781412976046.n12

Chadwick, A. E. (2015). Toward a theory of persuasive hope: Effects of cognitive appraisals, hope appeals, and hope in the context of climate change. *Health Communication, 30*, 598–611. doi:10.1080/10410236.2014.916777

Cooper, J., Zanna, M. P., & Taves, P. A. (1978). Arousal as a necessary condition for attitude change following induced compliance. *Journal of Personality and Social Psychology, 36*(10), 1101–1106. doi:10.1037/0022-3514.36.10.1101 de Hoog, N., Stroebe, W., & de Wit, J. B. F. (2007). The impact of vulnerability to and severity of a health risk on processing and acceptance of fear-arousing communications: A meta-analysis. *Review of General Psychology, 11,* 258–285.

Dillard, J. P., Li, R., Meczkowski, E., Yang, C., & Shen, L. (2017). Fear responses to threat appeals functional form, methodological considerations, and correspondence between static and dynamic data. *Communication Research, 44,* 997–1018. doi:10.1177/0093650216631097

Dillard, J. P., & Shen, L. (2005). On the nature of reactance and its role in persuasive health communication. *Communication Monographs, 72,* 144– 168. doi:10.1080/03637750500111815

Eisend, M. (2009). A meta-analysis of humor in advertising. *Journal of the Academy of Marketing Science, 37,* 191–203. doi:10.1007/s11747–008–0096-y

Farrelly, M. C., Healton, C. G., Davis, K. C., Messeri, P., Hersey, J. C., & Haviland, M. L. (2002). Getting to the truth: Evaluating national tobacco countermarketing campaigns. *American Journal of Public Health, 92,* 901–907. doi:10.2105/AJPH.92.6.901

Festinger, L. (1957). *A theory of cognitive dissonance.* Palo Alto, CA: Stanford University Press.

Festinger, L., & Carlsmith, J. M. (1959). Cognitive consequences of forced compliance. *Journal of Abnormal and Social Psychology, 58,* 203–210. doi:10.1037/h0041593

Hovland, C. I., Janis, I. L., & Kelley, H. H. (1953). *Communication and persuasion.* New Haven, CT: Yale University Press.

Ilakkuvan, V., Turner, M. M., Cantrell, J., Hair, E., & Vallone, D. (2017). The relationship between advertising-induced anger and self-efficacy on persuasive outcomes: A test of the anger activism model using the truth campaign. *Family&CommunityHealth,40,*72–80. doi:10.1097/FCH.0000000000000126

Janis, I. L. (1967). Effects of fear arousal on attitude change: Recent developments in theory and experimental research. In L. Berkowitz (Ed.), *Advances in experimental social psychology* (Vol. 3, pp. 166–225). New York, NY: Academic Press.

Kühne, R., & Schemer, C. (2013). The emotional effects of news frames on information processing and opinion formation. *Communication Research, 42,* 387–407. doi:10.1177/0093650213514599

Lazarus, R. S. (1991). *Emotion and adaptation.* Oxford, England: Oxford University Press.

Lazarus, R. S. (1999). Hope: An emotion and a vital coping resource against despair. *Social Research, 66,* 653–678.

Leventhal, H. (1970). Findings and theory in the study of fear communications. In L. Berkowitz (Ed.), *Advances in experimental social psychology* (Vol. 5, pp. 119–186). New York, NY: Academic Press. doi:10.1016/s0065-2601(08)60091-x

Miller, C. H., Lane, L. T., Deatrick, L. M., Young, A. M., & Potts, K. A. (2007). Psychological reactance and promotional health messages: The effects of controlling language, lexical concreteness, and the restoration of freedom. *Human Communication Research, 33,* 219–240.

Mongeau, P. A. (2013). Fear appeals. In J. P. Dillard & L. Shen (Eds.), *The Sage handbook of persuasion: Developments in theory and practice* (pp. 184–199). Thousand Oaks, CA: Sage.

Moyer-Gusé, E., & Nabi, R. L. (2010). Explaining the effects of narrative in an entertainment television program: Overcoming resistance to persuasion. *Human Communication Research, 36*, 26–52. doi:10.1111/j.1468-2958.2009 .01367.x

Nabi, R. L. (1999). A cognitive-functional model for the effects of discrete negative emotions on information processing, attitude change, and recall. *Communication Theory, 9*, 292–320. doi:10.1111/j.1468-2885.1999.tb00172.x

Nabi, R. L. (2002). Anger, fear, uncertainty, and attitudes: A test of the cognitive-functional model. *Communication Monographs, 69*, 204–216. doi:10.1080/ 03637750216541

Nabi, R. L. (2003). The framing effects of emotion: Can discrete emotions influence information recall and policy preference? *Communication Research, 30*, 224–247. doi:10.1177/0093650202250881

Nabi, R. L. (2007). Emotion and persuasion: A social cognitive perspective. In D. R. Roskos-Ewoldsen & J. Monahan (Eds.), *Social cognition and communication: Theories and methods* (pp. 377–398). Mahwah, NJ: Erlbaum.

Nabi, R. L. (2015). Emotional flow in persuasive health messages. *Health Communication, 30*, 114–124. doi:10.1080/10410236.2014.974129

Nabi, R. L., & Green, M. C. (2015). The role of a narrative's emotional flow in promoting persuasive outcomes. *Media Psychology, 18*, 137–162. doi:10.10 80/15213269.2014.912585

Nabi, R. L., & Gustafson, A., & Jensen, R. (2018). Framing climate change: Exploring the role of emotion in generating advocacy behavior. *Science Communication, 40*, 442–468. doi:10.1177/1075547018776019

Nabi, R. L., Huskey, R., Nicholls, S. B., Keblusek, L., & Reed, M. (2019). When audiences become advocates: Self-induced behavior change through health message posting in social media. *Computers in Human Behavior, 99*, 260–267.

Nabi, R. L., & Myrick, J. G. (2018). Uplifting fear appeals: Considering the role of hope in fear-based persuasive messages. *Health Communication*, 1–12 (e-print). doi:10.1080/10410236.2017.1422847

Nabi, R. L., Walter, N., Oshidary, N., Endacott, C., Love-Nicols, J., Lew, Z., & Aune, A. (2019). Can emotions capture the elusive gain-loss framing effect? A meta-analysis. *Communication Research*. doi:10.1177/0093650219861256

O'Keefe, D. J. (2000). Guilt and social influence. *Annals of the International Communication Association, 23*, 67–101. doi:10.1080/23808985.2000.11678970

Popova, L. (2012). The extended parallel process model: Illuminating the gaps in research. *Health Education & Behavior, 39*, 455–473. doi:10.1177/1090198111418108

Quick, B. L., Shen, L., & Dillard, J. P. (2013). Reactance theory and persuasion. In J. P. Dillard & L. Shen (Eds.), *The Sage handbook of persuasion: Developments in theory and practice* (2nd ed., pp. 167–183). Thousand Oaks, CA: Sage.

Rains, S. A. (2013). The nature of psychological reactance revisited: A meta-analytic review. *Human Communication Research, 39*, 47–73. doi:10.1111/j.1468-2958.2012.01443.x

Reynolds-Tylus, T., Martinez Gonzalez, A., & Quick, B. L. (2019) The role of choice clustering and descriptive norms in attenuating psychological reactance to water and energy conservation messages, *Environmental Communication*, *13*, 847–863, doi:10.1080/17524032.2018.1461672

Rogers, R. W. (1975). A protection motivation theory of fear appeals and attitude change. *Journal of Psychology*, *91*, 93–114. doi:10.1080/00223980.1975.9915803

Rogers, R. W. (1983). Cognitive and physiological processes in fear appeals and attitude change: A revised theory of protection motivation. In J. T. Cacioppo & R. E. Petty (Eds.), *Social psychophysiology* (pp. 153–176). New York, NY: Guilford.

Rosenberg, B. D., & Siegel, J. T. (2018). A 50-year review of psychological reactance theory: Do not read this article. *Motivation Science*, *4*, 281–300.

Shen, L. (2010). Mitigating psychological reactance: The role of message-induced empathy in persuasion. *Human Communication Research*, *36*, 397– 422. doi:10.1111/j.1468-2958.2010.01381.x

Snyder, C. R. (2000). Hypothesis: There is hope. In C. R. Snyder (Ed.), *Handbook of hope: Theory, measures, and applications* (pp. 3–21). San Diego, CA: Academic Press. doi:10.1016/B978-012654050-5/50003-8

Stice, E., Shaw, H., Becker, C. B., & Rohde, P. (2008). Dissonance-based interventions for the prevention of eating disorders: Using persuasion principles to promote health. *Prevention Science*, *9*, 114–128. doi:10.1007/s11121-008-0093-x

Stone, J., & Fernandez, N. C. (2008). To practice what we preach: The use of hypocrisy and cognitive dissonance to motivate behavior change. *Social and Personality Psychology Compass*, *2*, 1024–1051. doi:10.1111/j.1751-9004.2008.00088.x

Stone, J., & Focella, E. (2011). Hypocrisy, dissonance and the self-regulation processes that improve health. *Self and Identity*, *10*, 295–303. doi:10.1080/152 98868.2010.538550

Stone, J., Wiegand, A. W., Cooper, J., & Aronson, E. (1997). When exemplification fails: Hypocrisy and the motive for self-integrity. *Journal of Personality and Social Psychology*, *72*(1), 54–65. doi:10.1037/0022-3514.72.1.54

Stotland, E. (1969). *The psychology of hope*. San Francisco, CA: Jossey-Bass.

Tannenbaum, M. B., Hepler, J., Zimmerman, R. S., Saul, L., Jacobs, S., Wilson, K., & Albarracin, D. (2015). Appealing to fear: A meta-analysis of fear appeal effectiveness and theories. *Psychological Bulletin*, *141*, 1178–204. doi:10.1037/a0039729

Turner, M. M. (2007). Using emotion in risk communication: The anger activism model. *Public Relations Review*, *33*, 114–119. doi:10.1016/j.pubrev.2006.11.013

Walter, N., Cody, M. J., Xu, L. Z., & Murphy, S. T. (2018). A priest, a rabbi, and a minister walk into a bar: A meta-analysis of humor effects on persuasion. *Human Communication Research*, *44*, 343–373. doi:10.1093/hcr/hqy005

Walter, N., Tukachinsky, R., Pelled, A., & Nabi, R. (2019). Meta-analysis of anger and persuasion: An empirical integration of four models. *Journal of Communication*, *69*(1), 73–93. doi:10.1093/joc/jqy054

Witte, K. (1992). Putting the fear back into fear appeals: The extended parallel process model. *Communication Monographs*, *59*, 329–349. doi:10.1080/03637759209376276

Witte, K., & Allen, M. (2000). A meta-analysis of fear appeals: Implications for effective public health campaigns. *Health Education & Behavior*, *27*, 591–615. doi:10.1177/109019810002700506

Xu, Z., & Guo, H. (2018) A meta-analysis of the effectiveness of guilt on health-related attitudes and intentions, *Health Communication*, *33*, 519–525. doi:10.1080/10410236.2017.1278633

9

Theories of Behavior

Marco Yzer and Rebekah H. Nagler

The theories discussed in this chapter represent a class of theories often referred to as behavioral theory, or, depending on their application, health behavior theory or behavior change theory. There exist a great many theories of behavior. Some of those theories identify a limited set of psychological factors that predict behavior (e.g. the health belief model; see Skinner, Tiro, and Champion 2015), whereas others focus on message and audience features that explain behavior in terms of message rejection or acceptance (e.g. reactance theory; see Quick, Shen, and Dillard 2013) or on factors that can explain a population's adoption of recommended behavior as stages in an adoption life cycle (e.g. diffusion of innovations; Rogers 2003). For the purpose of this chapter, we focus on those theories that "describ[e] rational, emotional, social and personal predictors of healthy and risk behavior" (Cappella 2006, p. S265) and the relations between these predictor variables. Whereas the roots of these theories lie mostly (but certainly not exclusively) in social and cognitive psychology, behavioral theories have demonstrated important potential for informing health communication interventions.

In this chapter, we focus our discussion on three theories – namely, social cognitive theory (Bandura 1986), reasoned action theory (Fishbein and Ajzen 1975, 2010), and the transtheoretical model (Prochaska,

Health Communication Theory, First Edition. Edited by Teresa L. Thompson and Peter J. Schulz.

DiClemente and Norcross 1992). There are three reasons for this selective focus. One, whereas no theory is without limitations, the state of support for the basic premises of social cognitive theory, reasoned action theory, and the transtheoretical model is strong (see, for example, some of the theorists' syntheses of the thousands of studies based on their theories: Bandura 1997, 2005; DiClemente 2018; Fishbein and Ajzen 2010; Prochaska, Redding and Evers 2015). Two, of all possible behavioral theories, social cognitive theory, reasoned action theory, and the transtheoretical model are arguably the most widely used for understanding how health communication interventions can change behavior. And three, the transtheoretical model and in particular social cognitive theory and reasoned action theory have strongly influenced the development of other behavioral theories. See Table 9.1 for a concise description of the three theories.

Before describing each theory in detail, it is useful to consider some broad similarities and differences among behavioral theories. This can help recognize the unique contributions of each theory. The theories discussed here are similar in that they each offer an explanatory account of the process by which particular variables drive health behavior. This marks the relevance of behavioral theory for health communication: the better we understand the factors that underlie a particular behavior, the better able we are to design messages that address those factors and, in turn, influence behavior (Fishbein and Ajzen 2010).

The theories differ in the approach that is taken to behavioral explanation. To begin, we can differentiate between what have been called continuum models and stage models of behavior change (Weinstein, Rothman, and Sutton 1998). Continuum theories of behavior propose a limited number of variables that influence behavior. These variables can be combined in a prediction equation. For example, a theory that proposes that behavior is a function of risk perceptions and control perceptions takes the form of b_1 risk perceptions + b_2 control perceptions = behavior, where b_1 and b_2 are weights that indicate the importance of each variable in predicting behavior. The possible range in scores on risk perceptions and control perceptions create a continuum of behavioral likelihood. For example, consider three people who have low risk and low control perceptions, high risk perceptions and low control perceptions, and high risk and high control perceptions. These three people will be located at the left, midpoint, and right *of the same* risk + control perceptions continuum. Put differently, whereas people can be located at different points on the continuum, there is only one prediction equation, which means that the behavior change process is the same for everyone: behavior change results from a change in risk and control perceptions from negative to positive.

Table 9.1   Summary of social cognitive theory, reasoned action theory, and the transtheoretical model.

	Social cognitive theory	Reasoned action theory	Transtheoretical model
Primary variables	Self-efficacy; outcome expectations; behavior	Beliefs; attitude; perceived norms; perceived control; intention; behavior	Stages of change; self-efficacy; decisional balance; behavior
Central propositions about behavior formation	Among other possibilities, people can learn why (outcome expectations) and how to perform a behavior through observing others. Cognitive capabilities, such as the ability to derive meaning from symbols, aid learning through observation. Other capabilities, such as the ability to use rules of logic and normative rules, help people control whether they should adopt an observed behavior. One's sense of capability (self-efficacy) explains engagement in all aspects of the behavioral process.	Behavior is a function of intention. Intention is shaped by beliefs people hold about the behavior in terms of expectations of outcomes (attitude); support for or pressure against performing the behavior (perceived norms); and capability to perform the behavior (perceived control). Beliefs are formed through learning processes.	Behavior formation is a process in which people move forwards and backwards through stages that differ in how ready one is for behavior change. Whether expected positive outcomes outweigh negative outcomes (decisional balance) determines movement in early stages of readiness. Self-efficacy determines movement through stages where one is preparing for and trying behavior change.

In contrast, stage theories of behavior propose that behavior change reflects an ordered sequence of qualitatively different stages, and that different variables are responsible for moving someone from one state to another. This means that there is not one single prediction equation that explains behavior change, but rather that movement from each set of two adjacent stages has its own prediction equation. Phase transition of water is often used to illustrate a stage approach to change: water exists in three phases, namely solid (i.e. ice), liquid (i.e. water), and gaseous (i.e. steam). Water can be in only one of these phases, and cannot skip from one phase to a non-adjacent phase (i.e. to become steam, ice first needs to transform to water).

It is also useful to consider the nature of the variables that each theory emphasizes as important in explaining behavior. With roots in social and cognitive psychology, it is no surprise that behavioral theories see an important role for individual-level variables, such as attitudinal perceptions, for explaining behavior. Whereas all behavioral theories in principle also accept the idea that non-individual level variables such as social networks or one's media environment importantly contribute to behavior, theories differ in the extent to which they integrate such variables into central behavior change propositions.

Of the theories discussed in this chapter, reasoned action theory is often considered an example of a continuum theory and the transtheoretical model an example of a stage theory, whereas social cognitive theory cannot easily be categorized as either a continuum or stage theory. Further, whereas all three theories agree that both individual and non-individual level variables matter in shaping behavior, social cognitive theory most clearly integrates individual and non-individual levels of influence in its behavior formation propositions.

To explain each theory's central propositions, we will use the example of a hypothetical person who is experiencing depression symptoms. In this example, the behavior to be explained is the person's seeking help from a mental health professional. For presentation purposes we will refer to this person as he, his, and him, yet the points that the examples illustrate are applicable to every gender identity.

Social Cognitive Theory

Albert Bandura's (1986) social cognitive theory is one of the most well-known behavioral theories. Social cognitive theory offers a comprehensive account of behavior formation as a function of the interaction between a person, their behavior, and their environment; learning processes that operate through a number of cognitive capabilities; parameters that delineate the extent to which people learn from external sources; and a set of explanatory and outcome variables, among which outcome expectancies (i.e. expected likelihood that the behavior will result in particular outcomes) and self-efficacy (i.e. perceived capability to successfully perform the behavior) are most prominent.

Origin

In the early twentieth century, behaviorist theory proposed that human behavior is learned through conditioning processes in which some environmental stimulus automatically triggers a response. In contrast, psychodynamic theories, among others, emphasized the idea that behavior is dispositional, driven by impulse or other internal motivational factors. In his social learning theory, Bandura (1977) integrated environmental and dispositional factors. He agreed that behavior can be learned from sources outside a person, yet disagreed with the behaviorist notion that behavior is primarily a reaction to external stimuli. Instead, he argued that people have self-regulatory capacities that allow them to influence their own behavior, within the limits that people's environments impose. Bandura further developed this idea over the next decade. The result, social cognitive theory (Bandura 1986), emphasizes the role of personal agency within a system of constantly interacting social, environmental factors and personal, internal factors. Since its inception, social cognitive theory has put an increasingly important weight on the concept of self-efficacy as central to all processes implied in behavior.

Basic Claims and Notions

The comprehensive nature of social cognitive theory means that it cannot easily be captured in a single diagram. Therefore, in what follows we will unpack the major components of the theory to elucidate how various social cognitive concepts relate to each other.

Human agency and triadic reciprocal causation. First and foremost, social cognitive theory views people as agentic. This means that people can influence their thoughts, feelings, and behaviors. These behaviors, as well as personal factors (such as personality and cognitive skills), are in part shaped by social-environmental factors; at the same time, people's behaviors and personal factors influence the social systems in which they live. Social cognitive theory formalizes this idea in its proposition of triadic reciprocal causation, the idea that personal factors, people's behaviors, and social-environmental factors are both products and determinants of one another.

Information engagement capabilities. One implication of the triadic reciprocal causation model is that the interplay between behavior, personal factors, and the environment results in information that people have about themselves and the world around them. Ultimately, behavior is a transformation of this information into action. People have a number of capabilities that allow this transformation: vicarious learning, symbolizing, self-reflection, and self-regulation. Vicarious learning is learning through observation (rather than through direct experience) how to perform a behavior and what the consequences of that behavior are. For example, while watching a movie a person may observe how a central character struggles with depression, seeks out help, and in time feels better able to cope. Through this experience he learns how to go about seeking help, even if he cannot fall back on his own experience, as in the past he has never done so himself. Symbolization refers to the human capability to use and interpret symbols in order to give meaning to information. In our movie example, non-verbal cues such as brighter colors and the character's improved posture imply that the character's meeting with a mental health professional was beneficial. Self-reflection involves people's determination of the accuracy of their thoughts and the adequacy of their behavior, based on such tools as rules of logic and observation of others. A person may reflect on how few people he knows have sought help, which may lead him to think that he may have been wrong in thinking that most people would support his seeking help for depression. Last, people use their own internal norms and goals to self-regulate – in other words, to maintain or change their thoughts, feelings, and behavior. If a person was raised in an environment where the response to feeling depressed is to buckle up and deal with it, he may have developed a norm of self-sufficiency, which would keep him from seeking help.

Observational learning. Social cognitive theory is perhaps most widely known for its attention to observational learning. In a series of studies in the 1970s, Bandura demonstrated that in contrast to the then prevailing notion that behavior is formed only by learning from the effects of trying the behavior, one can learn a behavior by observing someone else model the behavior (for discussion, see Bandura 2005). Observational learning is a special case of behavior formation, where one learns rules about a behavior (in terms of how, when, why, and to what effect) by observing others perform – or in social cognitive terminology, model – the behavior. The relevance for health communication and more generally for media effects scholarship is that modeled behavior can be observed directly or indirectly, through media representation.

Observational learning involves four subprocesses that can be interpreted as prerequisites for a modeled event to ultimately translate into people modeling their thoughts, feelings, and behavior after what was observed. First, the modeled event needs to be attended to; attention can be driven by such factors as relevance, attractiveness, and so on. Second, the modeled event needs to be remembered. Retention is where we see the importance of symbolization capabilities; retaining information involves extracting meaning from what one observes and transforming the result to memory as symbolic conceptions. Third, reproduction is the retrieval of those symbolic conceptions and translating them into corresponding action. This requires, in part, that people have the necessary physical skills to actually perform a behavior. Last, there must be a motivational reason for people to model observed events. Simply put, motivation is strong if the modeled behavior has more valued outcomes than unwanted outcomes.

Even if people attend to a modeled event, retain it, are able to reproduce the modeled behavior, and are motivated to adopt the modeled behavior, modeling effects will vary in strength. Modeling effects are the strongest when the modeled behavior is rehearsed symbolically and when one identifies with whomever one observes (e.g. because the observed person is perceived to be similar or has an admired status).

Cognitive evaluation processes in observational learning of transgressive behavior. Modeling effects not only vary in strength, but also in nature. For example, modeling effects can be socially inconsequential but personally useful, as when someone learns how to change a flat tire from a YouTube video. Modeling effects also can be socially consequential and positive, as when children learn conversation skills from watching Sesame Street.

Other observed behaviors imply transgression – that is, behaviors that generally are seen as socially unacceptable, such as stealing and aggression towards others. People regulate such behaviors by using social sanctions and self-sanctions. Social sanctions are expectations about social backlash after engagement in the particular behavior. Media play an important role in shaping such social sanction expectations (e.g. by portraying the punishments people receive for engaging in the behavior). Self-sanctions imply interaction with one's personal norms and values. Inhibition occurs when someone does not model an observed behavior because the behavior is inconsistent with one's norms and values, whereas disinhibition occurs when someone adopts the observed behavior. Because engaging in a behavior that is clearly at odds with one's norms and values threatens one's sense of being a decent person, disinhibition requires cognitive reevaluation of the behavior, its effects, and the people who might be affected by it. Reevaluation processes include moral justification, euphemistic labeling, misconstruing consequences, dehumanizing victims, and attribution of blame. These processes have the result that one no longer feels that a behavior is violating rules of conduct. Mass media portrayals have important potential to be a source for these processes (Bandura 2009). For example, entertainment and news media often portray people afflicted with personality disorders as violent (Bowen 2016), which for some may justify discriminatory treatment of those people.

Note that social cognitive theory's propositions about the many factors that need to be in place for someone to adopt an observed behavior, and its emphasis on human agency in regulating these factors, mean that it is unlikely that modeled transgressive behavior will be adopted by most people who observe the behavior. Similarly, the many requirements for observational learning to translate into actual behavior make clear that we cannot expect everyone to respond to health information in the same way.

Self-efficacy and outcome expectations. The concept of self-efficacy plays an important explanatory role in social cognitive theory. Self-efficacy is the extent to which people believe they have the "capabilities to organize and execute the courses of action required to produce given attainments" (Bandura 1997, p. 3). Self-efficacy is contextualized: Given that each behavior poses unique personal and environmental demands, one can feel efficacious with respect to one behavior but not another, or efficacious with respect to a behavior under some but not all circumstances. Because of these reasons, Bandura (1997) recommends measuring self-efficacy as one's perceived capability to execute a behavior under a variety of increasingly challenging circumstances, where one's self-efficacy score indicates confidence in overcoming these challenges. This is consistent with the proposition that people who have strong self-efficacy are resilient in the face of challenges, and do not give up after initial failed behavioral attempts.

Social cognitive theory offers an interesting account of the relation between self-efficacy and outcome expectancies. Self-efficacy is "a judgment of one's capability to accomplish a certain level of performance, whereas an outcome expectation is a judgment of the likely consequence such behavior will produce" (Bandura 1977, p. 391). In social cognitive theory, self-efficacy is a prerequisite for outcome expectancies to matter for behavior. For example, a person may believe that professional help for depression may improve his well-being, but not act on this belief by seeking help because he feels that he is not able to take the step of finding a professional and calling to make an appointment.

Application in Health Communication, Limits, and Merits

Social cognitive theory offers a comprehensive account of behavior. Ironically, this rich, comprehensive account of behavior may have made it difficult for researchers and interventionists to test and use more than one or a few components of social cognitive theory. For example, in a review of the theory, Nabi and Prestin (2017) write: "media scholars find great utility in social cognitive theory as an explanation for . . . effects of media exposure, but the research often falls short of offering rigorous tests of the processes as conceptualized by the theory" (p. 1861). In health communication, social cognitive theory has mostly been used to test modeling as a health message effects mechanism (e.g. Nabi and Clark 2008) and to select self-efficacy as a predictor of behavior (e.g. Stacey et al. 2016). The concept of self-efficacy has been incorporated in numerous other behavioral theories, which is testament to its impact.

Reasoned Action Theory

Reasoned action theory proposes that a small set of psychological variables explains any given behavior. Since its inception in the 1960s (e.g. Fishbein, 1967), the theory has been refined in a sequence of modifications: the theory of reasoned action (Fishbein and Ajzen, 1975), the theory of planned behavior (Ajzen, 1985), the integrative model of behavioral prediction (Fishbein, 2000), and its current formulation, the reasoned action approach to explaining and changing behavior (Fishbein and Ajzen, 2010). The different names assigned to these formulations do not mean that these are fundamentally different theories. They are not. Rather, each represents a next step in the development of what we can refer to in general terms as reasoned action theory. The different formulations build on one another in a developmental fashion and reflect improvements in conceptualization and measurement of the theory's key constructs for the purpose of improving the precision with which behavior can be explained.

Origin

In the first half of the twentieth century, scholarship on the attitude construct evolved from an initial view that attitude is the basis of human behavior to widespread skepticism about the usefulness of the attitude construct for explaining behavior. This skepticism was informed by disappointingly weak research support for the idea that people act on their attitude toward a particular object. Martin Fishbein was among a number of scholars who observed that weak attitude–behavior relations could be explained by the quite heterogeneous conceptual definitions of attitude and the wide array of measures that purportedly all reflected attitude. Building on this observation, Fishbein proposed a "theory of attitude–behavior relationships" that conceptually differentiated between a number of causally related variables: beliefs about a behavior and an evaluation of those beliefs, attitude, intention, and behavior.

Basic Claims and Notions

The theory of reasoned action. Martin Fishbein and Icek Ajzen further developed the "theory of attitude–behavior relationships" into the theory of reasoned action (Fishbein and Ajzen, 1975). According to the theory of reasoned action, behavioral intention is the single best predictor of whether people will or will not perform any given behavior. Intention, or how likely people think it is they will perform a particular behavior at a particular time in the future, is itself a function of attitude and the subjective norm toward performing the behavior. In reasoned action theory, attitude is how one feels about performing the behavior in terms of favorability ratings such as bad or good, negative or positive, unpleasant or pleasant, and so forth. Subjective norm is the extent to which a person feels other people who are important to them will approve or disapprove of the person's performing the behavior.

Attitude and subjective norm are easily accessible evaluative perceptions that are a summary of a potentially large set of highly specific beliefs. These beliefs are thoughts and feelings that represent what people have learned over time about performing a behavior. As in social cognitive theory, beliefs are formed through direct experience with the behavior but can also be learned vicariously or through inference. Attitude is a function of behavioral beliefs. Similar to social cognitive theory's outcome expectancies, behavioral beliefs pertain to the likelihood that performing a behavior will lead to particular outcomes. Behavioral beliefs are weighted by how people evaluate each possible behavioral consequence in terms of desirability. For example, a person may expect that talking to a mental health counselor will allow him to open up about his depression symptoms, but whether this results in feeling favorable toward meeting with a counselor depends on whether opening up is seen as desirable or undesirable.

Subjective norm is a function of normative beliefs, which are beliefs about how likely it is that specific individuals or specific groups of people, such as friends, colleagues, or one's religious community, will approve or disapprove someone's performing a behavior. Normative beliefs are weighted by the extent to which a person is motivated to comply with each normative referent. Thus, for example, a person may expect that his physician will approve of his talking to a counselor about his depression, but also believe that his friends will disapprove. Regardless of whether these beliefs are accurate, if it is more important for him to do what he believes his friends would want him to do than what his physician wants him to do, he will experience an overall sense of normative pressure against talking to a counselor. See Figure 9.1 for a visual representation of the theory of reasoned action.

The theory of planned behavior. To broaden the explanatory scope of the theory to behaviors that are not perceived as under volitional control, Ajzen introduced the theory of planned behavior (1985, 1991), which proposes that in addition to attitude and subjective norm, perceptions of control over performing a particular behavior also shape behavioral intentions. Perceived behavioral control is the extent to which people feel that performing a particular behavior is under their control, or put differently, up to them. To measure perceived behavior control, Ajzen recommended asking how easy or difficult performing a behavior is. Perceived behavioral control strengthens intention to perform the particular behavior and, if perceptions of control match actual control, can even directly drive behavior (see Figure 9.2).

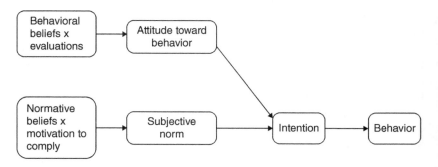

Figure 9.1   The theory of reasoned action.

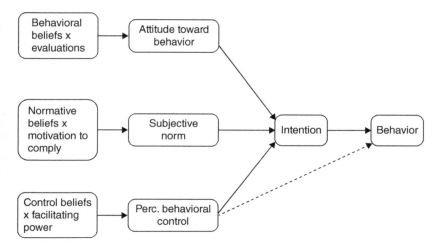

Figure 9.2 The theory of planned behavior.

Perceived behavioral control is a function of control beliefs, which are beliefs about the likelihood of particular resources, opportunities, obstacles, or any other environmental factor that can facilitate or hinder behavioral performance. Control beliefs are weighted by perceptions of how powerful those factors are in facilitating or hindering behavioral performance. For example, someone may believe that his health insurance will not fully cover mental health counseling. When costs are a real issue for him, his perceived behavioral control over meeting with a mental health counselor will be weak.

The integrative model of behavioral prediction. The integrative model of behavioral prediction (Fishbein 2000) builds on work that sought to integrate variables from the leading theories of behavior in order to form the best possible explanation of behavior (Fishbein et al. 1992); it also logically builds on the theory of planned behavior. Similar to the theory of planned behavior, the integrative model proposes that behavioral intention is a function of attitude, perceived normative influence, and control perceptions. In the integrative model, however, perceived norms include both subjective norm – henceforth labeled as injunctive norms – and descriptive norm, which is the extent to which a person believes other people from one's social network engage in the behavior themselves (Cialdini, Reno, and Kallgren, 1990). Fishbein further included Bandura's concept of self-efficacy instead of the theory of planned behavior's perceived behavioral control. He argued that the conceptualization of perceived behavioral control had led to a wide range of measurement approaches, which weakened understanding of how perceptions of one's capacity to perform a behavior shapes behavior change (Yzer, Hennessy, and Fishbein 2004).

The integrative model further emphasizes two propositions that had already been advanced in earlier iterations of reasoned action theory, but that had received little attention from the research community. First, people may not engage in a particular behavior despite their intention to do so when environmental barriers make behavior impossible, or when someone does not have the actual skills needed for performing a behavior. For example, someone may have had the intention to meet with a mental health counselor on a particular day and time, but the bus he depends on for transportation unexpectedly did not run on the day of his appointment. An important implication for health communication interventions is that if people intend to perform a particular health behavior but do not do so, an intervention should address factors – often sociostructural in nature – that impede acting on one's intentions, and thus may not call for message-based strategies (Fishbein and Yzer 2003).

Second, the role of any variable other than those identified as predictors of intention and behavior can best be understood as a possible source of beliefs. These variables have been called external, distal, or, more recently, background factors. These include, among many others, attitudes toward a target (rather than toward a behavior – for example, attitude toward mental healthcare compared to attitude toward my meeting with a counselor to discuss my depression symptoms); individual difference variables; demographic variables; cultural, political, and religious variables; and media messages. Background variables clarify belief-based behavioral processes: exposure to a wide range of variables over time shapes beliefs about a particular behavior through a learning process (see Figure 9.3).

The reasoned action approach to behavioral prediction and change. Based on a review of five decades of reasoned action scholarship, Fishbein and Ajzen (2010) introduced the current formulation of the theory – the reasoned action approach to predicting and changing behavior. The most important modification of the reasoned action approach relative to earlier versions of the theory is the proposition that attitude, perceived normative pressure, and perceived behavioral control each have two aspects. Specifically, attitude comprises instrumental attitude – an evaluation of performing a behavior in terms of positive or negative attributes (e.g. foolish or wise) – and experiential attitude – an evaluation of performing a behavior in terms of positive or negative experiences (e.g. pleasant or unpleasant). Perceived normative

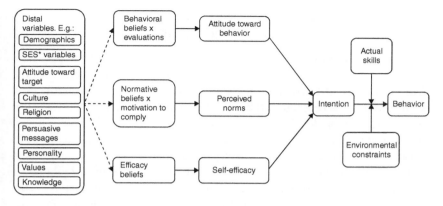

*SES = socioeconomic status

Figure 9.3   The integrative model of behavioral prediction.

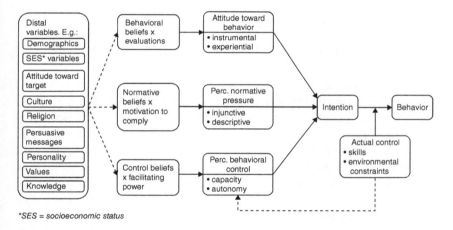

*SES = socioeconomic status

Figure 9.4   The reasoned action model.

pressure comprises injunctive norms and descriptive norms. Perceived behavioral control (which Fishbein and Ajzen argued is conceptually similar to Bandura's notion of self-efficacy, namely the extent to which people believe they are able to successfully perform a behavior) comprises perceived autonomy – the extent to which people perceive that the decision to engage in the behavior is up to them, and perceived capacity – one's perceived ability to perform the behavior (see Figure 9.4).

Application in Health Communication, Limits, and Merits

Reasoned action theory has been widely used to test whether a particular health behavior is under attitudinal, normative, and/or efficacy control, and to identify beliefs that may be most promising to address in health messages (e.g. Dillard 2011). Whereas reasoned action theory is one of the most dominant theories in health behavior research and health communication intervention design, the theory is not without its critics. Some critiques are misconceptions, such as the incorrect contention that reasoned action theory is a theory of rational, deliberative decision-making. Others are justified, such as the concern that the theory does not generate testable hypotheses about when which variable or variables – instrumental attitude, experiential attitude, injunctive norms, descriptive norms, perceived autonomy, and perceived capacity – is most likely to predict a particular behavior.

Transtheoretical Model of Behavior Change

James Prochaska and Carlo DiClemente's (1983, Prochaska and Velicer 1997) transtheoretical model argues that behavior change is a process whereby people progress through different stages of behavioral preparedness that range from unawareness of a health risk (and therefore no intention to change one's behavior) to sustained behavior change. Different cognitions are important in the different stages, which offer interventionists guidance for what to focus on to help people progress from one stage to the next. The model views behavior change as often spiral rather than linear, in the sense that people can move toward behavior change but relapse to previous risk behavior. Because of its emphasis on stages that reflect readiness for change, the transtheoretical model has also been referred to as the stages of change model, at least in some circles.

Origin

To understand the origins of the transtheoretical model, it is useful to point out that both Prochaska and DiClemente were trained as clinical psychologists. Some of their early work focused on clinical therapy approaches to smoking behavior, in which they observed what smokers were experiencing at different points in the process toward quitting (e.g. DiClemente and Prochaska 1982). That work made salient the idea that health behavior change is not an on/off dichotomy, or a matter of now you do, now you don't. For example, smokers may go back and forth between wanting to quit, trying it, relapsing into smoking, and even going back to not wanting to quit. In addition, work on smoking and more generally on addiction reinforced the idea that addiction is caused by a multitude of factors, including genetics, personality, societal variables, and learning processes, among others, and thus no theory that looks at only one of these factors can adequately explain addiction (DiClemente 2018). This led Prochaska and DiClemente to develop a theory that uses insights from multiple theories from multiple disciplines or, in other words, a transtheoretical model. Whereas the origins of the transtheoretical model explain why it has been applied often to addictive behaviors (e.g. smoking), its primary propositions can be applied to non-addictive behaviors as well (e.g. adherence to a mental health counseling and medication regimen).

Basic Claims and Notions

The transtheoretical model focuses on how individual people change. Behavior change is seen as an intentional process, whereby choices at various points in this process are influenced by personal, societal, and biological factors. A primary proposition of the theory is that behavior change is a developmental process, and the essence of such development is captured in the concept of stages of change. The transtheoretical model argues that at different points in time, people are in different stages that vary in readiness for change.

The starting stage in behavior change is the precontemplation stage, where one has no awareness of the need to change one's behavior and therefore no intention to change. Next, contemplation is characterized by an awareness of a problem with one's current behavior, yet no intention to change that behavior. In the preparation stage, an intention to change is formed but no action has been taken yet. In the action stage, some attempts at the new behavior are made, but this new behavior is not yet consistent. In the final stage, maintenance, the new behavior has been sustained into a behavioral pattern that has endured for some time. Table 9.2 presents commonly used operational definitions of the stages of change.

People can be in any of these stages for shorter or longer periods. They can move forward to sustained behavior change (e.g. someone affected by depression may consistently meet with a counselor and adhere to a recommended medication regimen), and then relapse or move backward (e.g. stop seeing a counselor and stop taking medication).

Table 9.2   Operational definitions of stages of change.

Stage of change	Operational definition
precontemplation	no intention to change
contemplation	some intention to change, no behavior
preparation	intention to change, inconsistent behavior
action	consistent behavior but for less than 6* months
maintenance	consistent behavior for more than 6* months

Note. * To stage people in action and maintenance stages, 3 and 12 months also have been used to quantify duration of behavior.

The transtheoretical model proposes a number of stage-specific processes that are needed to move from one particular stage to a next. These processes include cognitive mechanisms, such as consciousness raising and reevaluation of the behavior, and action mechanisms, such as self-liberation (i.e. making the personal choice to commit to a new behavior) and reinforcement management (i.e. making changes in those environmental factors that may hamper or facilitate the new behavior). These processes originate in a wide array of theories across multiple fields or, put differently, reflect a transtheoretical approach to behavior change. The transtheoretical model proposes that cognitive mechanisms are more important to move people through the early stages of behavior change – precontemplation and contemplation – whereas the action mechanisms are more important to move people through the later stages – preparation, action, and maintenance. This is consistent with the operational stage definitions in Table 9.2: preparation, action, and maintenance have action or behavior components, whereas precontemplation and contemplation do not, focusing more on cognitions (e.g. awareness and intention).

The transtheoretical model proposes that two concepts, decisional balance and self-efficacy, further describe movement through stages. Decisional balance is the relative superiority of perceptions of costs and benefits of a particular behavior. (These perceptions are conceptually similar to social cognitive theory's outcome expectancies and reasoned action theory's behavioral beliefs.) Decisional balance changes when one moves through early stages. For example, in precontemplation, someone may feel that the costs of seeking help for depression (e.g. feeling embarrassed, the potential of stigma, possibly being misunderstood by a counselor) outweigh the benefits (e.g. feeling relief, have someone to confide in). In contemplation, these benefits outweigh costs. The transtheoretical model adopts Bandura's (1997) concept of self-efficacy as a marker of movement through later stages of change. Whereas self-efficacy is accepted as potentially playing a role in movement through all stages, it is particularly relevant for movement through preparation, action, and maintenance. This is consistent with Bandura's work on self-efficacy, which showed that people are more likely to try a new behavior and persist in their attempts when they have strong self-efficacy (Bandura 1997).

Application in Health Communication, Limits, and Merits

The cyclical description of behavior change with likely relapses maps well onto addiction recovery pathways, and the transtheoretical model therefore is widely used in recovery treatment programs. An often-used description of addiction recovery in this regard is that "the journey of recovery is a process, not a destination." This is a useful reminder to those working in health communication that behavior change is not a matter of moving people from non-action to action – it requires understanding of the predictors of relapse as well as of behavioral maintenance (e.g. Rothman et al. 2011).

Most health interventions that use the transtheoretical model appear to focus primarily on using an intention-behavior algorithm to determine in which stage of change people reside. Less attention has been given to the use of stage-specific progression processes, the role of decisional balance, self-efficacy, and other transtheoretical model constructs (e.g. Hutchison, Breckon, and Johnston 2008). Those interventions that do include transtheoretical constructs beyond stages of change have been found to be more effective (Romain et al. 2018).

The primary limitations of the transtheoretical model have to do with the conceptualization of stages of change and stage progression processes. The transtheoretical model operationalizes stages of change in terms of behavioral intention (i.e. no intention versus intention to change) and behavior (i.e. how long someone has performed the behavior). This essentially makes stages of change identical to reasoned action theory's differentiation between predictors of intention and predictors of behavior given intention. Perhaps part of the issue with the stages of change construct is the transtheoretical model's seemingly arbitrary algorithm to determine stage membership – is someone who has engaged in a behavior for five and a half months really different from someone who has done so for six months? Relatedly, there is limited support for the variables and processes that the transtheoretical model argues explain progress from one stage to another. These observations have led some to argue that the five stages of change are not discrete stages, where moving from one to another is accompanied by a qualitative transformation (Bandura 1997).

Conclusions

In this chapter we discussed social cognitive theory, reasoned action theory, and the transtheoretical model as three leading theories of behavioral prediction – that is, theories that describe the processes by which particular predictor variables explain behavior. Decades after their introduction, these theories continue to be important for the health communication field. In recognition of their usefulness for explaining current health behavior problems, these theories are still widely used in research and form the foundation of many health communication interventions across a range of health issues.

In addition, social cognitive theory, reasoned action theory, and the transtheoretical model have been advantageous to the development of new behavioral theories. In the health communication field, for example, the theory of social normative behavior (Rimal 2008; Rimal and Real 2005) and the societal risk reduction motivation model (Cho and Kuang 2014) build in part on concepts developed in social cognitive theory and reasoned action theory, thus offering important new areas of attention. The theory of social normative behavior emphasizes the role of descriptive norms in shaping health behavior and argues that effects of descriptive norms on intention and behavior are moderated by injunctive norms, outcome expectancies, and group identity. The societal risk reduction motivation model emphasizes the role of societal risk perceptions – or the extent to which one believes a particular health issue is a risk for society at large – in shaping those behaviors that in turn can "influence political, economic, and sociocultural contexts of risk" (Cho and Kuang, 2014, p. 126), such as voting for a particular policy. Efficacy beliefs, including self-efficacy, are argued to moderate effects of societal risk perceptions on behavior.

These examples highlight the broad influence of social cognitive theory, reasoned action theory, and the transtheoretical model on health communication research, theory, and intervention. All three theories share the objective of maximizing the precision with which health behavior can be explained, and in looking across them we can identify a finite set of key factors or determinants of behavior change, including beliefs, attitudes, perceived normative pressure, self-efficacy, and behavioral intention. Ultimately, understanding the factors that explain behavior is a prerequisite for changing behavior through health communication, and appreciating the synergies across these theories may enable us to better intervene, and, in turn, improve public health.

References

Ajzen, I. (1985). From intentions to actions: A theory of planned behavior. In J. Kuhl & J. Beckman (Eds.), *Action-control: From cognition to behavior* (pp. 11–39). Heidelberg, Germany: Springer.

Ajzen, I. (1991). The theory of planned behavior. *Organizational Behavior and Human Decision Processes, 50*, 179–211.

Bandura, A. (1977). *Social learning theory.* Englewood Cliffs, NJ: Prentice Hall.

Bandura, A. (1986). *Social foundations of thought and action: A social-cognitive theory.* Englewood Cliffs, NJ: Prentice Hall.

Bandura, A. (1997). *Self-efficacy: The exercise of control.* New York, NY: Freeman.

Bandura A. (2005). The evolution of social cognitive theory. In K. G. Smith & M. A. Hitt (Eds.), *Great minds in management* (pp. 9–35). Oxford: Oxford University Press.

Bandura, A. (2009). Social cognitive theory of mass communication. In J. Bryant & M. B. Oliver (Eds.), *Media effects: Advances in theory and research* (2nd ed., pp. 99–124.) Mahwah, NJ: Erlbaum.

Bowen, M. L. (2016). Stigma: Content analysis of the representation of people with personality disorder in the UK popular press, 2001–2012. *International Journal of Mental Health Nursing, 25*, 598–605.

Cappella, J. N. (2006). Integrating message effects and behavior change theories: Organizing comments and unanswered questions. *Journal of Communication, 56*, S265–S279.

Cho, H., & Kuang, K. (2014). The societal risk reduction motivation model. In H. Cho, T.O. Reimer, & K. A. McComas (Eds.), *The Sage handbook of risk communication* (pp. 117–131). Thousand Oaks, CA: Sage.

Cialdini, R. B., Reno, R. R., & Kallgren, C. A. (1990). A focus theory of normative conduct: Recycling the concept of norms to reduce littering in public places. *Journal of Personality and Social Psychology, 58*, 1015–1026.

DiClemente, C. C. (2018). *Addiction and change: How addictions develop and addicted people recover.* New York, NY: Guilford Press.

DiClemente, C. C., & Prochaska, J. O. (1982). Self-change and therapy change of smoking behavior: A comparison of processes of change of cessation and maintenance. *Addictive Behaviors, 7*, 133–142.

Dillard, J. P. (2011). An application of the integrative model to women's intention to be vaccinated against HPV: Implications for message design. *Health Communication, 26,* 479–486.

Fishbein, M. (1967). Attitude and the prediction of behavior. In M. Fishbein (Ed.), *Readings in attitude theory and measurement* (pp. 477–492). New York, NY: Wiley.

Fishbein, M. (2000). The role of theory in HIV prevention. *AIDS Care, 12,* 273–278.

Fishbein, M., & Ajzen, I. (1975). *Belief, attitude, intention, and behavior: An introduction to theory and research.* Reading, MA: Addison-Wesley.

Fishbein, M., & Ajzen, I. (2010). *Predicting and changing behavior: The reasoned action approach.* New York, NY: Psychology Press.

Fishbein, M., Bandura, A., Triandis, H. C., Kanfer, F. H., Becker, M., & Middlestadt, S. E. (1992). Factors influencing behavior and behavior change. (Report prepared for the National Institute of Mental Health). Bethesda, MD: National Institute of Mental Health.

Fishbein, M., & Yzer, M. C. (2003). Using theory to design effective health behavior interventions. *Communication Theory, 13,* 164–183.

Hutchison, A. J., Breckon, J. D., & Johnston, L. H. (2008). Physical activity behavior change interventions based on the transtheoretical model: A systematic review. *Health Education and Behavior, 36,* 829–845.

Nabi, R. L., & Clark, S. (2008). Exploring the limits of social cognitive theory: Why negatively reinforced behaviors on TV may be modeled anyway. *Journal of Communication, 3,* 407–427.

Nabi, R. L., & Prestin, A. (2017). Social learning theory and social cognitive theory. In P. Rossler, C. Hoffner, & L. van Zoonen (Eds.), *International encyclopedia of media effects* (pp. 1855–1867). Hoboken, NJ: Wiley Blackwell.

Prochaska, J. O., & DiClemente, C. C. (1983). Stages and processes of self-change of smoking: Toward an integrative model of change. *Journal of Consulting and Clinical Psychology, 51,* 390–395.

Prochaska, J. O., DiClemente, C. C., & Norcross, J. C. (1992). In search of how people change: Applications to the addictive behaviors. *American Psychologist, 47,* 1102–1114.

Prochaska, J. O., Redding, C. A., & Evers, K. E. (2015). The transtheoretical model and stages of change. In K. Glanz, B. K. Rimer & K. Viswanath (Eds.), *Health behavior: Theory, research, and practice* (5th ed., pp. 125–148). San Francisco, CA: Jossey-Bass.

Prochaska, J. O., & Velicer, W. F. (1997). The transtheoretical model of health behavior change. *American Journal of Health Promotion, 12,* 38–48.

Quick, B. L., Shen, L. J., & Dillard, J. P. (2013). Reactance theory and persuasion. In J. P. Dillard & L. J. Shen (Eds.), *The persuasion handbook: Developments in theory and practice* (2nd ed., pp. 167–183). Los Angeles, CA: Sage.

Rimal, R. (2008). Modeling the relationship between descriptive norms and behaviors: A test and extension of the theory of normative social behavior (TNSB). *Health Communication, 23,* 103–116.

Rimal, R. N., & Real, K. (2005). How behaviors are influenced by perceived norms: A test of the theory of normative social behavior. *Communication Research, 32,* 389–414.

Rogers, E. M. (2003). *Diffusion of innovations.* New York, NY: Simon and Schuster.

Romain, A. J., Bortolon, C., Gourlan, M., Carayol, M., Lareyre, O., Ninot, G., . . . Bernard, P. (2018). Matched or nonmatched interventions based on the transtheoretical model to promote physical activity. A meta-analysis of randomized controlled trials. *Journal of Sport and Health Science, 7,* 50–57.

Rothman, A. J., Baldwin, A. S., Hertel, A. W., & Fuglestad, P. T. (2011). Self-regulation and behavior change: Disentangling behavioral initiation and behavioral maintenance. In K. D. Vohs & R. F. Baumeister (Eds.), *Handbook of self-regulation: Research, theory, and applications* (p. 106–122). New York, NY: Guilford Press.

Skinner, C. S., Tiro, J., & Champion, V. L. (2015). The health belief model. In K. Glanz, B. K. Rimer & K. Viswanath (Eds.), *Health behavior: Theory, research, and practice* (5th ed., pp. 75–94). San Francisco, CA: Jossey-Bass.

Stacey, F. G., James, E. L., Chapman, K., & Lubans, D. R. (2016). Social cognitive theory mediators of physical activity in a lifestyle program for cancer survivors and carers: Findings from the ENRICH randomized controlled trial. *International Journal of Behavioral Nutrition and Physical Activity, 13,* 1–13.

Weinstein, N. D., Rothman, A. J., & Sutton, S. (1998). Stage theories of health behavior: Conceptual and methodological issues. *Health Psychology, 17,* 290–299.

Yzer, M. C., Hennessy, M., & Fishbein, M. (2004). The usefulness of perceived difficulty for health research. *Psychology, Health and Medicine, 9,* 149–162.

10

Theories of Message Effects

James D. Robinson, Yan Tian, and Jeanine W. Turner

Health communication scholars and researchers have long been interested in the impact of health information on audience members. Whether the information comes from a reliable source or is simply part of entertainment programming, there is little doubt that attitudes and beliefs are influenced by such messages. In 2012, 72% of all internet users reported that they had looked online for health information within the previous year (Fox and Duggan 2013). The number of adults with a smartphone has increased from 35% in 2011 to 81% (Pew Research Center 2019).

A quick examination of other technologies suggests there are 78.9 million desktop computers, 231.67 million laptop computers, and 180.57 million tablet computers in the US (Statista 2020) and even with the precipitous decrease in households with at least one television, more than 95% of all homes still have one or more television set (Statista 2019). Coupled with the fact that 90% of US adults are using the internet (Anderson et al. 2019), it is safe to say that the vast majority of adults are exposed to health messages by choice or by chance.

This chapter examines how theories of message effects have been used by health communication scholars to better understand the impact

Health Communication Theory, First Edition. Edited by Teresa L. Thompson and Peter J. Schulz.
© 2021 John Wiley & Sons, Inc. Published 2021 by John Wiley & Sons, Inc.

of health messages in both the face-to-face and mediated contexts. While these theories were not originally developed for the use in health communication, they have been adopted because of the importance of the mass and social media as a tool for public health.

Agenda Setting

Agenda setting was first proposed by McCombs and Shaw (1972) to explain why audience members believe one issue is more important than another issue. Originally focused on political communication, McCombs and Shaw found that voter perception of issue salience was nearly identical to the prominence the issue received in the media. Experiments by Iyengar, Peters, and Kinder (1982) demonstrated that voter evaluations of the president's performance changed with issue prominence – putting to rest concerns that audience perceptions of salience actually lead to issue prominence in the media.

Studying the underlying mechanism of agenda setting, Weaver (1977) found audience members with high uncertainty about an issue and high levels of personal relevance were more likely to have their agenda set by the media than audience members who perceive low personal relevance and high certainty. Takeshita's (2006) work suggests the careful weighing of information motivated by uncertainty and relevance can result in the relationship between prominence in the media and issue salience we typically call agenda setting. Takeshita (2006) also found evidence that cognitive priming produces agenda setting effects. In the case of cognitive priming, exposure to information primes the proverbial cognitive pump or brain. Thus, repeated exposure to an issue and effortful thinking about an issue can produce agenda setting-like effects.

In health communication, agenda setting has been used to examine the role the media play in beliefs about obesity (Campo and Mastin 2007; Len-Rios and Qiu 2007), cancer (Cohen et al. 2008), HIV/AIDS (Caburnay et al. 2008), and organ donation (Feeley, O'Mally, and Covert 2016). Agenda setting has also been used to frame studies focusing on doctor – patient interactions. Heritage et al. (2007) found that 40% of all patients have more than one agenda and physicians usually focus on the first concern mentioned. Similarly, in follow-up visits physicians tend to bring their own agenda and do not ask questions designed to identify new health problems or issues (Beckman and Frankel 1984; Rey-Bellet, et al. 2017). Finally, physicians have less understanding of a patient's problem when they do not solicit the patient's agenda (Dyche and Swiderski 2005). More research on agenda setting in the healthcare context is sorely needed.

Cultivation Theory

Similar to the agenda-setting theory, cultivation theory also focuses on powerful effects of media.

Proponents of cultivation theory believe television viewing influences perceptions of reality. Like other institutions, television demonstrates standardized roles and behaviors in our society, and plays an important role in shaping our judgements, attitudes, values, and behaviors (Gerbner and Gross 1976). Heavy television viewers are more likely than light reviewers to believe in the norms and realties that are consistent with what is shown on television (Gerbner et al. 2002).

Cultivation research investigates the relationship between frequency of television viewing and perceptions of the real world (Shanahan et al. 2004). Research based on the original theory focused on the myths and themes that ran throughout television. Using content analysis and survey methods Gerbner and colleagues found that heavy television viewers are more likely to choose answers that were close to what is portrayed in the television world than were light viewers (Gerbner et al. 2002).

More recently, cultivation theory has begun to focus on specific television genres or even programs (Morgan and Shannahan 2010). Instead of treating the television message as a coherent system, researchers suspected that genre-specific television viewing could provide more robust support for the cultivation theory than overall television viewing (Chory-Assad and Tamborini 2003). For example, Holbert et al. (2003) found no relationship between overall viewing and pro-environmental behaviors, while the pro-environmental behaviors were predicted by viewing public affairs and nature documentaries. Studies also indicate the shift of cultivation research from focusing on long-term effects to focusing on short-term effects, and the shift of locus of meaning from messages to receivers (Potter 2014). These shifts help provide new insights into understanding how media affect audience's attitudes and behaviors. It may well be that measurement issues or factors that have been shown to impact the relationship between attitudes and behavior also impact cultivation effects. Certainly more research on this idea is needed.

Cultivation theory has been applied in health communication contexts to understand the relationship between television exposure and audience perceptions of health-related topics, including audience perceptions of physicians (Tian and Yoo 2018). Other genre-specific cultivation research suggested that viewing local television news predicts increased fatalistic beliefs in cancer prevention (Lee and Niederdeppe 2011), and a similar conclusion was drawn for the relationship between medical drama viewing and beliefs about cancer (Chung 2014). A cultivation hypothesis on the negative relationship between television exposure and estimates of smoking in the real world, based on the decreased smoking rate on television, however, was not supported (Shanahan et al. 2004).

Researchers have also tested the relationship between television viewing and health outcome measures with cultivation theory. Survey studies suggested that television viewing is associated with negative psychosocial profiles of a female audience (Hammermeister et al. 2005) and early onset of smoking behaviors among adolescents (Gutschoven and Van den Bulck 2005). Research also suggests TV viewing is associated with the discrepancy between the real and ideal self – a discrepancy that might be related to behaviors such as going to a gym, for instance (Eisend and Möller 2007).

Cultivation theory may also be used in health education campaigns (Brodie et al. 2001). Sherry (2002) argued that entertainment education interventions will be most effective when they reach high levels of theme saturation. Saturation occurs when a storyline is shared across multiple dramas or extended across other show genres. An empirical study adopted this approach, having two storylines on breast cancer genetics featured in two popular medical dramas. and the results suggested that exposure to both storylines is more effective than exposure to each individual storyline alone in changing attitudinal and behavioral outcomes (Hether et al. 2008). While frequency of exposure or amount of media use is a key component in cultivation theory, message characteristics and audience engagement are essential in the next theory, narrative engagement theory.

Narrative Engagement Framework

In some ways, narrative engagement (NE) can be viewed as the vehicle used by storytellers to get information across to their audiences without directly addressing an issue. Supporters of NE believe message effectiveness can be increased by grounding health messages within stories that are relevant to and/or about the audience (Miller-Day and

Hecht 2013). Narrative then is messaging that focuses on important events and experiences and narrative is believed to be effective because it requires the audience to create a mental model of meaning to understand the story. During the development of the mental model, the audience may incorporate their own experience into the storyline (Graesser, Olde, and Klettke 2002).

While narratives need not be true, they should capture audience interest and provide insight into a particular health issue or behavior. This means the narrative should include a plot line with an identifiable beginning and end, the story should occur within a context that is relevant and similar to the audience's situation, and the narrative should incorporate characters that behave in an understandable and identifiable manner.

Typically, health information campaigns focusing on the use of factual information to raise audience awareness, salience, response efficacy, and self-efficacy are augmented by a story that is intended to help the audience to better understand the health information being provided. The NE typically employs a similar strategy but incorporates that information within a story in an effort to engage the audience and motivate them to change their beliefs, attitudes, intentions, and behavior. Several researchers have successfully measured engagement (e.g. Busselle and Bilandzic 2009; Beentjes et al. 2009) in an effort to discover the characteristics that enhance the persuasiveness of narratives.

Hecht, Miller-Day and colleagues used NE as they developed and deployed their *keepin' it REAL* curriculum to reduce drug abuse in young people. They employ the personal narratives of young people who are similar to the kids participating in their drug prevention program. Using real drug story experiences allows message developers an opportunity to discover how young people see drugs and create more effective anti-drug messages (Hecht and Miller-Day 2009; Pettigrew et al. Hecht, 2011).

The narrative approach assumes people are storytelling beasts and that stories are how we understand ourselves and our experiences. Using NE, audience members can gain symbolic experience of the front, back, and middle stage views of the health issue. These insights can serve to motivate further thinking about the issue, motivate health information seeking, and illustrate how others – real or fictional – respond (Green 2006; Kreuter et al. 2007).

Research suggests vivid, concrete, and personalized elements increase the effectiveness of stories as persuasive tools (Nisbett and Ross 1980; Zillmann 2000). In addition, personalized stories promote narrative engagement, increase personal relevance, help overcome resistance to anti-drug messaging, and increase identification with the program and program content (Hecht and Miller-Day 2010; Miller et al. 2000).

However, in a study focused on health policy, Zhou and Niederdeppe (2017) found that message personalization was less effective than depersonalization in generating public support for policies regarding food deserts. They argue that personalization or depersonalization needs to be consistent with the goals of the campaign. Unidentifiable collectives or groups are more influential in policy messages than identifiable individuals. Similarly, providing the inner states or feelings of the identifiable individuals is a good strategy for personal health behavior messages but not for developing health policy support. These findings are consistent with research suggesting personal narratives may undermine public support for health policies (Barry, Brescoll, and Gollust 2013) because the inclusion of personal narratives increases counterarguing (Niederdeppe, Roh, and Dreisbach 2016) and diverts attention from societal causes of health problems (Iyengar 1991). With mixed findings on the effects of personal narratives, it is important to review other theories that also focus on messages and effects, among which framing theory is an important one.

Framing Theory

Bateson (1972) suggested message frames function as meta-communication, providing contextual information that shapes what people think about and how they think about a particular issue or topic. Using prospect theory (Kahneman and Tversky 1979) as the basis for framing, researchers have argued that individuals are more likely to take risks when information is presented in a negative frame (a frame based on potential losses for the individual) and less likely to occur when the message is framed positively or as an opportunity for gain (Loroz 2007; Tversky and Kahneman 1986). This is interesting because gain frames (40% of the people will be cured) and loss frames (60% of the people will die) produce the same conclusion or outcome. While prospect theory is clear about how people should respond, a significant meta-analysis suggests the research is not so clear (O'Keefe and Jensen 2006).

For example, sometimes positively framed messages are more effective (Jeong, Zhao, and Khouja 2012) and sometimes negatively framed messages are more effective (Chang 2007). Regulatory focus theory (Crowe and Higgins 1997) has been used to help clarify these by suggesting that people use different strategies in making decisions to attain a goal. In short, people can focus on their desired outcomes (a promotion focus) or they can focus on the avoidance of undesirable outcomes (an avoidance focus). Higgins (2000) argued that the fit between regulatory focus of the individual and the framing strategy used in the message increases the likelihood of message influence. In short, it may not be simply the positive or negative framing of a message that matters as much as that the framing of the message is consistent with the focus of the receiver. This idea that a message will be more effective if the receiver has a promotion focus and the message is framed positively or if the receiver has an avoidance focus and the message is framed negatively has received some support (Lee and Aaker 2004).

Other scholars have employed construal-level theory (CLT; Liberman and Trope 1998) in an attempt to explain the incongruity in framing studies. Proponents of CLT believe that psychological closeness determines how people think about distal objects, persons, places, or events. So people considering an immediate health behavior change such as exercise will produce construals that are concrete – they will focus on things like the types of exercises they will perform. People who are not considering exercise will produce more abstract construals.

This difference is important because messages framed positively or as an opportunity for personal gain will be more influential when a person feels psychologically close to the issue addressed in the message. Similarly, a person who feels psychologically distant from the activity will be more likely to be influenced if the message is loss framed or framed negatively. The increase in message effectiveness occurs because of the enhanced fluency or ease of understanding and processing meanings (Lee and Aaker 2004; Lee and Labroo 2004).

Ahn (2015) recently examined message personalization and immersive virtual environments (IVE) in a test of CLT. Arguing that messages tailored to the self should produce feelings of relevance, Ahn (2015) found that personalized messages reduce social distance or make the individual feel like they are more susceptibile to the health issue. In addition, individuals exposed to personalized messages reduced their sugar-sweetened beverage (SSB) consumption for one week. After one week, however, intentions to drink SSBs decreased. This suggests the impact of reduced social distance was relatively short-lived. Participants exposed to the messages in an IVE reported reduced temporal distance and a decrease in soft drink consumption one week following exposure. This reduction in temporal distance means that the individuals felt that their behavior was a more proximate cause of a health problem when the message was presented in the IVE. Ahn suggests social distance influences behavioral intentions immediately following an experiment but temporal distance influences actual behavior after the effects of social distance have dissipated. It appears that motivating individuals to think of themselves in a negative light may result in an effort to psychologically distance themselves from their past (Ahn 2015).

Other factors that influence the effectiveness of message framing include risk perception (Meyers-Levy and Maheswaran 2004), issue involvement (Meyers-Levy and Maheswaran 1990), and processing depth (Block and Keller 1995). The subjective ease of processing information can also lead to increased feelings of efficacy and more positive behavioral intentions (Lee and Aaker 2004; Lee and Labroo 2004). Lower-level construals promote self-control (independently from reflective cognitive processing) across various behavioral domains, including health (Fujita 2008).

Inoculation Theory

Inoculation theory focuses on how people can be prepared to defend themselves against the persuasive efforts of others. McGuire (1964) suggested people were susceptible to persuasion if they did not have sufficient information, motivation, or practice in defending their beliefs. Inoculation messages forewarn the individual that an attack against their attitude is imminent, point out their attitude is vulnerable to an attack, and include refutational preemption. Refutational preemption is threat-specific information that individuals can use to defend themselves against the persuasive efforts of others.

So if a child holds a negative attitude toward recreational drug use and a parent believes peers will pressure their child to smoke marijuana – or like the kids say "flammicate some dank" – forewarning their child and providing them with arguments for and counterarguments against smoking marijuana should help them defend themselves.

Researchers have successfully used inoculation theory as a vehicle for developing more effective health messages (Godbold and Pfau 2000). This is an excellent use for the theory since audiences are exposed to health messages in the traditional media, social media, and their interpersonal interactions and more importantly many of the messages to which they are exposed are not consistent with healthy behavior (e.g. Comasco et al. 2010; Prinstein and Dodge 2008). A meta-analysis suggests that both refutationally different (an argument combined with an unrelated counterargument) and refutationally same messages (a message that contains an argument and a counterargument) are effective (Banas and Rains 2010). Similarly, both active refutational messages (counterarguments developed by the receiver) and passive refutational messages (counterarguments provided by a speaker) are effective (Banas and Rains 2010). Further, both messages delivered interpersonally and messages delivered through the mass media are effective (Compton, Jackson, and Dimmock 2016), which is important for health campaigns.

Pfau and Van Brokern (1994) demonstrated inoculation effects can last as long as 84 weeks, and inoculation effects have been shown to help individuals retain anti-alcohol beliefs (Cornelis, Cauberghe, and De Pelsmacker 2013), marijuana use (Parker, Ivanov, and Compton J. 2012), condom use (Parker et al. 2012), attitudes toward vaccines (Wong and Harrison 2014), and resistance to food advertisements (Mason and Miller 2013).

Compton and Pfau (2009) have argued that word-of-mouth communication may serve to increase the effectiveness of inoculation messages. Previous research suggests the conversations elicited by the inoculation may be as influential as the original message (Robinson and Levy 1986) and may motivate further conversation – including participation in public policy discussions (McLeod, Scheufele, and Moy 1999). The argument that inoculation motivates future talk is compelling and suggests inoculation may be a more effective strategy than was initially thought.

Uses and Gratifications Theory

Herzog's (1944) investigation into why women listened to daytime serial radio programs is now recognized as a pioneering uses and gratifications (UG) study. She found they listened as an outlet for emotional release, a method of escaping their boredom, and as a source for identifying solutions to their problems. Katz, Blumler, and Gurevitch (1974) then identified five ontological assumptions about audiences: (i) The audience is actively involved in the selection of media channels and media content, (ii) people use the media based on their beliefs about the effectiveness of the media as a source of gratification, (iii) the media is one source of need satisfaction among others (e.g. interpersonal interaction or hobbies), (iv) the audience knows what their needs are and why they are using the media to meet those needs, and (v) researchers need to recognize that the individual uses of the mass media are idiosyncratic and best understood from the perspective of the individual – and not from a societal or cultural perspective. Katz et al. (1974) identified four categories of audience media uses that are consistent with other such typologies (McQuail, Blumler, and Brown 1972). The needs are: (i) cognitive, (ii) affective, (iii) social integrative, and (iv) tension release. Finally, the motives for media use vary for a variety of reasons including age (Greenberg 1974), education level (Rubin 1984), and social class (Greenberg and Dominick 1969) among others.

UG is increasingly being used by scholars in the context of health communication. For example, research suggests that patients use websites, blogs, and online social support groups (Cotton and Gupta 2004; Rice 2006; Warner and Procaccino 2007; Ybarra and Suman 2006) when they seek additional health information (Brashers, Haas, and Neidig 1999). Lee, Hwang, and Hawkins (2006) reported patients uncertain about their cancer diagnosis spent more time searching for health information than their better-informed counterparts. Similarly, those patients diagnosed with cancer who reported receiving insufficient emotional support from traditional sources spent more time in online support groups (Tustin 2010) and patients unsatisfied with their medical care are more likely to seek additional information from the internet (Sen 2008).

Other researchers have used UG to understand use of diet/fitness apps. It turns out people use their smartphone for a variety of different reasons including: tracking (recording diet and/or fitness efforts); interacting (receiving feedback about diet and/or fitness); information acquisition (learning about health and exercise from the app); networkability (social interaction with other users via the app); and gamification of health behavior tracking to increase interest and their level of motivation; normative/fad/image management (everybody's doing it).

Lee and Cho (2017) found that tracking and networkability predicted intentions to continue use of their smartphone for health. In addition, the quality of information the user gains from the app – particularly the credibility of the information and their ability to comprehend that information – also enhances prediction of intention to continue use. Interestingly enough, image management/trendiness of the app but not entertainment also increased the likelihood of intention to continue (Lee and Cho 2017). While these findings support the UG model, they are also important because interest in preventative healthcare has been shown to be related to desired lifetime (Deeks et al. 2009). It may well be that increasing expectations about longevity will motivate positive health behaviors.

Media Complementarity Theory

Communication scholars have always been interested in media usage and proponents of the time displacement hypothesis believe time spent with new media displaces older media use and even interpersonal activities (Putnam 2000). While time displacement hypothesis looks at media use as a zero-sum game (Dutta-Bergman 2004a), media complementarity theory suggests that consumers may use different media channels in a complementary way for their own needs and gratifications (Dutta-Bergman 2004a, 2004b). Instead of displacement, people interested in a particular topic will use a combination of media channels to satisfy their individual needs in this topic and continue to use them as long as the channels fulfill their informational needs.

Dutta-Bergman (2004a) conducted a secondary analysis of the Pew Research Center data to test media complementarity. He found positive relationships between consumers' uses of online and traditional media channels for specific news content domains (e.g. political news, entertainment news). Similarly, individuals were found to use the internet and telephone complementarily to communicate with families and friends right after a crisis (Dutta-Bergman 2004b). Consumers' interest and/or need in a topic or domain, together with channels' effectiveness in gratifying the consumers' needs, could affect media usage process more than the simple availability of the channels (Dutta-Bergman 2004a, 2004b).

Using the Health Information National Trends Survey (HINTS) data, Tian and Robinson (2008a) found that the degree to which consumers pay attention to health information in traditional mass media (i.e. newspapers, magazines, radio, television) is positively associated with the attention they pay to health information on the internet and both are positively associated with visits to their healthcare provider. Similar media complementarity patterns were revealed between active health information seeking online and incidental health information use online, as well as between incidental information use online and incidental health information use from traditional media (Tian and Robinson 2009). These complementary relationships were also observed in people from India (Lin and Dutta 2017).

Scholars have also examined characteristics of information sources. Ruppel and Rains (2012) conceptualized source characteristics with four items relevant to health information searching: access to medical expertise, tailorability, anonymity, and convenience. Also using the HINTS data, they found that individuals use sources complementarily based on tailorability and anonymity. In addition, they found that the use of source pairs with high tailorability and convenience increases during the health information search process. A second study suggested individuals use sources complementarily based on all four source characteristics, while an experimental study indicated that health threat can affect individuals' use of sources pairs that are high in access to medical expertise and anonymity (Rains and Ruppel 2016). While the severity of a threat seems likely to impact media complementarity, more research in this area is needed.

Another line of research applying the media complementarity theory investigates predicting and moderating variables that affect media complementarity. Tian and Robinson (2008b) found a complementary relationship between incidental health information use from traditional media (newspapers and magazines) and from the internet for non-senior but not senior cancer survivors. Lin and Dutta (2017) reported that younger people in India use greater numbers of media channels in a complementary fashion than older users. Analysis of HINTS Puerto Rico data suggested that education and gender are positively related to individual-level media complementarity of health information seeking among respondents from Puerto Rico (Tian and Robinson 2013). Finally, Ruppel and Burke (2014) found that social competence moderates the complementarity between telephone and text message, since individuals with high social competence use telephone and text messaging complementarily, while individuals with low social competence use email and text messaging complementarily.

Media complementarity scholarship in health communication has investigated the relationship among different communication channels including face-to-face and mediated channels, traditional mass media, and new media channels. Studies involve participants with various demographic backgrounds and sociopsychological characteristics including younger and older adults, cancer survivors and cancer-free adults, individuals living in the US, in Puerto Rico, and in India, and individuals with different levels of social competence. Nonetheless, more research into media complementarity is needed

Conclusion

The theories discussed in this chapter focus on media use and message effects. While they provide important understandings of how audiences use media for health information and communication, and how messages affect audience health attitudes and behaviors, the theories are gaining new life with the changes of media technologies. As many aspects of communication are being redefined, it is important to revisit and refine the theories, and to conduct health campaigns and health education informed by theories relevant to today's media consumers.

References

Ahn, S. J. (2015). Incorporating immersive virtual environments in health promotion campaigns: A construal-level theory approach. *Health Communication, 30*, 545–556. doi:10.1080/10410236.2013.869650

Anderson, M., Perrin, A. Jiang, J., & Kumar M. (2019). 10% of Americans don't use the internet. Who are they? Retrieved January 28, 2020, from https://www.pewresearch.org/fact-tank/2019/04/22/some-americans-dont-use-the-internet-who-are-they/

Banas J., & Rains S. (2010). A meta-analysis of research on inoculation theory. *Communication Monographs, 77*, 281–331. doi:10.1080/03637751003758193

Barry, C. L., Brescoll, V. L., & Gollust, S. E. (2013). Framing childhood obesity: How individualizing the problem affects public support for prevention. *Political Psychology, 34*, 327–349.

Bateson, G. (1972). *Steps to an ecology of mind: A theory of play and fantasy.* Chicago, IL: University of Chicago Press.

Beckman, H. B., & Frankel, R. M. (1984). The effect of physician behavior on the collection of data. *Annals of Internal Medicine, 101*, 692–696. doi:10.7326/0003-4819-101-5-692.

Beentjes, J., de Graaf, A., Hoeken, H., & Sanders, J. (2009). Do American television stories influence Dutch people's opinions about society? In R. P. Konig & F. J. M. Huysmans (Eds.). *Meaningful media: Communication research on the social construction of reality* (pp. 245–254). Nijmegen, Netherlands: Tandem Felix.

Block, L. G., & Keller, P. A. (1995). When to accentuate the negative: The effects of perceived efficacy and message framing on intentions to perform a health-related behavior. *Journal of Marketing Research, 32*, 192–203.

Brashers, D. E., Haas, S. M., & Neidig, J. L. (1999). The patient self-advocacy scale: Measuring patient involvement in health care decision-making interaction. *Health Communication, 11*, 97–12.

Brodie, M., Foehr, U., Rideout, V., Baer, N., Miller, C., Flournoy, R., & Altman, D. (2001). Communicating health information through the entertainment media. *Health Affairs, 20*, 192–199. doi:10.1377/hlthaff.20.1.192

Busselle R., & Bilandzic, H. (2009). Measuring narrative engagement. *Media Psychology, 12*, 321–347. doi:10.1080/15213260903287259.

Caburnay, C. A., Kreuter, M. W., Cameron, G. T., Luke, D. A., Cohen, E., McDaniels, L., . . . Atkins, P. (2008). Black newspapers as a tool for cancer education in African Americancommunities. *Ethnicity & Disease, 18*, 488–495.

Campo, S., & Mastin, T. (2007). Placing the burden on the individual: Overweight and obesity in African American and mainstream women's magazines. *Health Communication, 22*, 229–240.

Chang, C.T. (2007). Health-care product advertising: The influences of message framing and perceived product characteristics. *Psychology & Marketing, 24*, 143–169.

Chory-Assad, R. M., & Tamborini, R. (2003). Television exposure and the public's perceptions of physicians. *Journal of Broadcasting & Electronic Media, 47*, 197–215.

Chung, J. E. (2014). Medical dramas and viewer perception of health: Testing cultivation effects. *Human Communication Research, 40*, 333–349.

Cohen, E. L., Caburnay, C. A., Luke, D. A., Rodgers, S., Cameron, G. T., & Kreuter, M. W. (2008). Cancer coverage in general-audience and Black newspapers. *Health Communication, 23*, 427–435.

Comasco E., Berglund K., Oreland L., & Nilsson K. W. (2010). Why do adolescents drink? Motivational patterns related to alcohol consumption and alcohol related problems. *Substance Use & Misuse, 45*, 1589–1604. doi:10.3109/10826081003690159

Compton, J., Jackson, B., & Dimmock, J. (2016). Persuading others to avoid persuasion: Inoculation theory and resistant health attitudes. *Frontiers in Psychology, 7*, 122. doi:10.3389/fpsyg.2016.00122

Compton, J., & Pfau, M. (2009). Spreading inoculation: Inoculation, resistance to influence, and word-of-mouth communication. *Communication Theory, 19*, 9–28.

Cornelis, E., Cauberghe, V., & De Pelsmacker, P. (2013). Two-sided messages for health risk prevention: The role of argument type, refutation, and issue ambivalence. *Substance Use & Misuse, 48*, 719–730.

Cotton, S. R., & Gupta, S. S. (2004). Characteristics of online and offline health information seekers and factors that discriminate between them. *Social Science & Medicine, 59*, 1795–1806.

Crowe, E., & Higgins, E.T. (1997). Regulatory focus and strategic inclinations: Promotion and prevention in decision-making. *Organizational Behavior and Human Decision Processes, 69*, 117–132.

Deeks, A., Lombardo, C., Michelmore, J., & Teede, H. (2009). The effects of gender and age on health related behaviors. *BMC Public Health, 9*, 213. doi:10.1186/1471-2458-9-213.

Dutta-Bergman, M. J. (2004a). Complementarity in consumption of news types across traditionaland new media. *Journal of Broadcasting & Electronic Media, 48*, 41–60.

Dutta-Bergman, M. J. (2004b). Interpersonal communication after 9/11 via telephone and internet: A theory of channel complementarity. *New Media & Society, 6*, 659–673.

Dyche, L., & Swiderski, D. (2005). The effect of physician solicitation approaches on ability to identify patient concerns. *Journal of General Internal Medicine, 20*, 267–270. doi:10.1111/j.1525-1497.2005.40266.x

Eisend, M., & Möller, J. (2007). The influence of TV viewing on consumers' body images and related consumption behavior. *Marketing Letters, 18*, 101–116.

Feeley, T. H., O'Mally, A. K., & Covert, J. M. (2016). A content analysis of organ donation stories printed in U.S. newspapers: Application of newsworthiness. *Health Communication, 31*, 495–503. doi:10.1080/10410236.2014.973549

Fox, S., & Duggan, M. (2013). Health online 2013. Retrieved January 28, 2020 from https://www.pewresearch.org/internet/2013/01/15/health-online-2013/

Fujita, K. (2008). Seeing the forest beyond the trees: A construal-level approach to self-control. *Social and Personality Psychology Compass, 2*, 1475–1496.

Gerbner, G., & Gross, L. (1976). Living with television. The violence profile. *Journal of Communication, 26*, 182–190.

Gerbner, G., Gross, L., Morgan, M., Signorielli, N., & Shanahan, J. (2002). Growing up with television: Cultivation processes. In J. Bryant & D. Zillmann (Eds.), *Media effects: Advances in theory and research* (2nd ed., pp. 43–67). Mahwah, NJ: Erlbaum.

Godbold, L. C., & Pfau, M. (2000). Conferring resistance to peer pressure among adolescents. *Communication Research, 27*, 411–437.

Graesser, A. C., Olde, B., & Klettke, B. (2002). How does the mind construct and represent stories? In M. C. Green, J. J. Strange, & T. C. Brock (Eds.), *Narrative impact: Social and cognitive foundations* (p. 229–262). Mahwah, NJ: Erlbaum.

Green, M. C. (2006). Narratives and cancer communication. *Journal of Communication, 56*, 163–183. doi:10.1111/j.1460-2466.2006.00288.x

Greenberg, B.S. (1974). Gratifications of television viewing and their correlates for British children. In J. G. Blumler and E. Katz (Eds.) *The uses of mass communications: Current perspectives on gratifications research.* Beverly Hills, CA: Sage.

Greenberg, B., & Dominick, J. (1969). Racial and social class differences in teenagers use of television. *Journal of Broadcasting, 13*, 331–334.

Gutschoven, K., & Van den Bulck, J. (2005). Television viewing and age at smoking initiation: Does a relationship exist between higher levels of television viewing and earlier onset of smoking? *Nicotine & Tobacco Research, 7*, 381–385.

Hammermeister, J., Brock, B., Winterstein, D., & Page, R. (2005). Life without TV? Cultivation theory and psychosocial health characteristics of television-free individuals and their television-viewing counterparts. *Health Communication, 17*, 253–264.

Hecht, M. L., & Miller-Day, M. (2009). The drug resistance strategies project: Using narrative theory to enhance adolescents' communication competence. In L. Frey and K. Cissna (Eds). *Routledge handbook of applied communication* (pp. 535–557). New York, NY: Routledge.

Hecht, M. L., & Miller-Day, M. (2010). "Applied" aspects of the drug resistance strategies project, *Special Issue of the Journal of Applied Communication Research, 38*, 215–229. doi:10.1080/00909882.2010.490848

Heritage, J., Robinson, J. D., Elliott, M. N., Beckett, M., & Wilkes, M. (2007). Reducing patients' unmet concerns in primary care: The difference one word can make. *Journal of General Internal Medicine, 22*, 1429–1433. doi:10.1007/s11606-007-0279-0

Herzog, H. (1944). What do we really know about daytime serial listeners? In P. F. Lazarsfeld and F. N. Stanton (Eds.), *Radio Research 1942–43* (pp. 3–33). New York, NY: Duell, Solan & Pearce.

Hether, H. J., Huang, G. C., Beck, V., Murphy, S. T., & Valente, T. W. (2008). Entertainment-education in a media-saturated environment: Examining the impact of single and multiple exposures to breast cancer storylines on two popular medical dramas. *Journal of Health Communication, 13*, 808–823, doi:10.1080/10810730802487471

Higgins, E. T. (2000). Making a good decision: Value from fit. *American Psychologist, 55*, 1217–1230.

Holbert, R. L., Kwak, N., & Shah, D. (2003). Environmental concern, patterns of television viewing, and pro-environmental behaviors: Integrating models of media consumption and effects. *Journal of Broadcasting & Electronic Media, 47*, 177–196.

Iyengar S. (1991). *Is anyone responsible?* Chicago, IL: University of Chicago Press.

Iyengar, S., Peters, M. D., & Kinder. D. R. (1982). Experimental demonstration of the "not-so-minimal" consequences of television news programs. *American Political Science Review, 76*, 848–858.

Jeong, B., Zhao, K., & Khouja, M. (2012). Consumer piracy risk: Conceptualization and measurement in music sharing. *International Journal of Electronic Commerce, 16*, 89–118.

Kahneman, D., & Tversky, A. (1979). Prospect theory: An analysis of decision under risk. *Econometrica, 47*, 263–291.

Katz, E., Blumler, J. G., & Gurevitch, M. (1974). Utilization of mass communication by the individual. In J. G. Blumler & E. Katz (Eds.), *The uses of mass communications: Current perspectives on gratifications research* (pp. 19–34). Beverly Hills, CA: Sage.

Kreuter, M. W., Green, M. C., Cappella, J. N., Slater, M. D., Wise, M. E., Storey, D., Woolley, S. (2007). Narrative communication in cancer prevention and control: A framework to guide research and application. *Annals of Behavioral Medicine, 33*, 221–235. doi:10.1007/BF02879904

Lee, A. Y., & Aaker, J. L. (2004). Bringing the frame into focus: The influence of regulatory fit on processing fluency and persuasion. *Journal of Personality and Social Psychology, 86*, 205–218. doi:10.1037/0022-3514.86.2.205

Lee A. Y., & Labroo, A. A. (2004). The effect of conceptual and perceptual fluency on brand evaluation. *Journal of Marketing Research, 41*, 151–165.

Lee, C., & Niederdeppe, J. (2011). Genre-specific cultivation effects: Lagged associations between overall TV viewing, local TV news viewing, and fatalistic beliefs about cancer prevention. *Communication Research, 38*, 731–753.

Lee, H. E., & Cho, J. (2017). What motivates users to continue using diet and fitness apps: Application of the uses and gratifications approach. *Health Communication, 32*, 1445–1453. doi:10.1080/10410236.2016.1167998

Lee, S., Hwang, H., & Hawkins, R. (2006, June). Why do patients use the internet? The effects of insufficiency on patients' health-related internet use. Paper presented at the annual meeting of the International Communication Association, Dresden, Germany.

Len-Ríos, M. E., & Qiu, Q. (2007). Negative articles predict clinical trial reluctance. *Newspaper Research Journal, 28*, 24–39.

Liberman, N., & Trope, Y. (1998). The role of feasibility and desirability considerations in near and distant future decisions: A test of temporal construal theory. *Journal of Personality and Social Psychology, 75*, 5–18. doi:10.1037/0022-3514.75.1.5

Lin, J., & Dutta, M. (2017). A replication of channel complementarity theory among internet users in India. *Health Communication, 32*, 483–492.

Loroz, P. S. (2007). The interaction of message frames and reference points in prosocial persuasive appeals. *Psychology & Marketing, 24*, 1001–1023.

Mason A. M., & Miller C. H. (2013). Inoculation message treatments for curbing noncommunicable disease development. *Revista Panamericana de Salud Pubublica, 34*, 29–35.

McLeod, J. M., Scheufele, D. A., & Moy, P. (1999). Community, communication, and participation: The role of mass media and interpersonal discussion in local political participation. *Political Communication, 16*, 315–336.

McCombs, M. E., & Shaw, D. L. (1972). The agenda-setting function of the mass media. *Public Opinion Quarterly, 36*, 176–187.

McGuire, W. J. (1964). Inducing resistance to persuasion: Some contemporary approaches. In L. Berkowitz (Ed.), *Advances in experimental social psychology* (Vol. 1; pp. 191–220). New York, NY: Academic Press.

McQuail, D., Blumler, J. G., & Brown, J. (1972). The television audience: A revised perspective. In D. McQuail (Ed.), *Sociology of mass communication* (pp. 135–65). Middlesex, England: Penguin.

Meyers-Levy, J., & Maheswaran, D. (1990). Message framing effects on product judgments. In M. E. Goldberg, G. Gorn, & Pollay, R. W. (Eds.), *NA advances in consumer research*, (Vol. 17; pp. 531–534). Provo, UT: Association for Consumer Research.

Meyers-Levy, J., & Maheswaran, D. (2004). Exploring message framing outcomes when systematic, heuristic, or both types of processing occur. *Journal of Consumer Psychology, 14*, 159–167.

Miller, M., Alberts, J., Hecht, M. Trost, M., & Krizek, R. (2000). *Adolescent relationships and drug use.* Mahwah, NJ: Erlbaum.

Miller-Day, M., & Hecht, M. L. (2013). Narrative means to preventative ends: A narrative engagement framework for designing prevention interventions. *Health Communication, 28*, 657–670. doi:10.1080/10410236.2012.762861

Morgan, M., & Shanahan, J. (2010). The state of cultivation. *Journal of Broadcasting & Electronic Media, 54*, 337–355.

Niederdeppe, J., Roh, S., & Dreisbach, C. (2016). How narrative focus and a statistical map shape health policy support among state legislators. *Health Communication, 31*, 242–255.

Nisbett, R., & Ross, L. (1980). *Human inference: Strategies and shortcomings of social judgment.* Englewood Cliffs: Prentice Hall.

O'Keefe, D. J., & Jensen, J. D. (2006). The advantages of compliance or the disadvantages Of noncompliance? A meta-analytic review of the relative persuasive effectiveness of gain-framed and loss-framed messages. *Communication Yearbook, 30*, 1–43.

Parker K. A., Ivanov B., & Compton J. (2012). Inoculation's efficacy with young adults' risky behaviors: Can inoculation confer cross-protection over related but untreated issues? *Health Communication, 27*, 223–233.

Pettigrew, J., Miller-Day, M., Krieger, J. L., & Hecht ML. (2011). Alcohol and other drug resistance strategies employed by rural adolescents. *Journal of Applied Communication Research, 39*, 103–122. doi:10.1080/00909882.2011.556139

Pew Research Center (2019). Mobile fact sheet. Retrieved January 28, 2020, from https://www.pewresearch.org/internet/fact-sheet/mobile/

Pfau M., & Van Bockern S. (1994). The persistence of inoculation in conferring resistance to smoking initiation among adolescents: The second year. *Human Communication Research, 20*, 413–430.

Potter, W. J. (2014). A critical analysis of cultivation theory. *Journal of Communication, 64*, 1015–1036.

Prinstein M. J., & Dodge K. A. (2008). *Understanding peer influence in children and adolescents*. New York, NY: Guilford.

Putnam, R. D. (2000). *Bowling alone: The collapse and revival of American community*. New York, NY: Simon & Schuster.

Rains, S. A., & Ruppel, E. K. (2016). Channel complementarity theory and the health information-seeking process: Further investigating the implications of source characteristic complementarity. *Communication Research, 43*, 232–252.

Rey-Bellet, S., Dubois, J., Vannottic, M., Zuercher, M., Faouzi, M., Devaud, K., . . ., Rodondi, P. (2017). Agenda setting during follow-up encounters in a university primary care outpatient clinic. *Health Communication, 32*, 714–720. doi:10.1080/10410236.2016.1168003

Rice, R. E. (2006). Influences, usages, and outcomes of internet health information searching: Multivariate results from the Pew surveys. *International Journal of Medical Informatics, 75*, 8–28.

Robinson, J. P., & Levy, M. R. (1986). *The main source: Learning from television news*. Beverly Hills, CA: Sage.

Rubin, A. M. (1984). Ritualized and instrumental television viewing. *Journal of Communication, 34*, 67–77.

Ruppel, E. K., & Burke, T. J. (2014). Complementary channel use and the role of social competence. *Journal of Computer-Mediated Communication, 20*, 37–51. doi:10.1111/jcc4.12091

Ruppel, E. K., & Rains, S.A. (2012) Information sources and the health information-seeking process: An application and extension of channel complementarity theory. *Communication Monographs, 79*, 385–405. doi:10.1080/03637751.2012.697627

Sen, N. (2008, November). Patient dissatisfaction as a motivating factor in online health seeking. A paper presented at the annual meeting of the National Communication Association's annual conference, San Diego, CA.

Shanahan, J., Scheufele, D., Yang, F., & Hizi, S. (2004). Cultivation and spiral of silence effects: The case of smoking. *Mass Communication & Society, 7*, 413–428. doi:10.1207/s15327825mcs0704_3

Sherry, J. L. (2002). Media saturation and entertainment education. *Communication Theory, 12*, 206–224.

Statista (2019). Number of TV households in the U.S. 2000–2020. Retrieved January 28, 2020, from https://www-statista-com.libproxy.udayton.edu/statistics/243789/number-of-tv-households-in-the-us/

Statista (2020). Installed base of personal computing devices (desktops, tablets, and laptops) in the United States from 2017 to 2022, by device type (in millions). Retrieved January 28, 2020, from https://www.statista.com/statistics/670172/united-states-installed-base-desktops-laptops-tablets/

Takeshita, T. (2006). Current critical problems in agenda-setting research. *International Journal of Public Opinion Research, 18*, 275–296.

Tian, Y., & Robinson, J. D. (2008a). Media use and health information seeking: An empirical test of complementarity theory. *Health Communication, 23,* 184–190.

Tian, Y., & Robinson, J. D. (2008b). Incidental health information use and media complementarity: A comparison of senior and non-senior cancer patients. *Patient Education and Counseling, 71,* 340–344.

Tian, Y., & Robinson, J. D. (2009). Incidental health information use on the internet. *Health Communication, 24,* 41–49.

Tian, Y., & Robinson, J. D. (2013). Media complementarity and health information seeking in Puerto Rico. *Journal of Health Communication, 19,* 710–720. doi:10.1080/10810730.2013.821558

Tian, Y., & Yoo, J. (2018). Medical drama viewing and medical trust: A moderated mediation approach. *Health Communication, 35*(1), 46–55. doi:10.1080/10 410236.2018.1536959

Tustin, N. (2010). The role of patient satisfaction in online health information seeking. *Journal of Health Communication, 15,* 3–17.

Tversky, A., & Kahneman, D. (1986). The behavioral foundations of economic theory. *The Journal of Business, 59,* s251–s278.

Warner, D., & Procaccino, J. D. (2007). Women seeking health information: Distinguishing the web users. *Journal of Health Communication, 12,* 787–814.

Weaver, D. H. (1977). Political issues and voter need for orientation. In D. L. Shaw & M. E. McCombs (Eds.), *The emergence of American political issues* (pp. 107–119). St. Paul, MN: West.

Wong N., Harrison K. J. (2014). Nuances in inoculation: Protecting positive attitudes toward the HPV vaccine and the practice of vaccinating children. *Journal of Women's Health, Issues & Care, 3*(6). doi:10.4172/2325-9795. 1000170

Ybarra, M. L., & Suman, M. (2006). Help seeking behavior and the internet: A national survey. *International Journal of Medical Information, 75,* 29–41.

Zhou, S., & Niederdeppe, J. (2017). The promises and pitfalls of personalization in narratives to promote social change. *Communication Monographs, 84,* 319–342.

Zillmann, D. (2000). Mood management in the context of selective exposure theory. In M. F. Roloff (Ed.), *Communication yearbook 23* (pp. 103–123). Thousand Oaks, CA: Sage.

PART IV

Perspectives on Organizations and Society

11

Social Psychological Influences on Health Communication: An Examination of Four Theories

Yanqin Liu and Anthony J. Roberto

Generally speaking, *social psychology* seeks to explain and predict how our beliefs, attitudes, and behavior influence – and are influenced by – our social environment. Here, the social environment is defined broadly to include a variety of relationship factors (e.g. family, friends, classmates, and co-workers), community factors (e.g. school, work, faith-based, healthcare, and other organizations), and societal factors (e.g. culturally shared beliefs and traditions, social norms, cultural values, and the mass media). The fields of social psychology and communication share much in common in that they both seek to answer basic questions about human behavior (Greenaway, Gallois, and Haslam 2017). A key difference between these approaches is that the former focuses

Health Communication Theory, First Edition. Edited by Teresa L. Thompson and Peter J. Schulz.
© 2021 John Wiley & Sons, Inc. Published 2021 by John Wiley & Sons, Inc.

on social behavior in general, while the latter focuses on communicative behaviors in particular (Hornsey, Gallois, and Duck 2008). Nonetheless, "the two disciplines have the same background, heritage, and interests" and "they have the capacity to support, complement, and extend each other" (Hornsey et al., p. 764). Perhaps most importantly from the perspective of this book, both approaches focus on how to influence others. To illustrate, you have already read (or will read) about many different social psychology theories in just about every other chapter in this book. This chapter will focus on four additional social psychological theories that did not fall neatly into one of these other chapters, but that are also an important part of the health communication discipline: (i) diffusion of innovation, (ii) social judgment theory, (iii) self-determination theory, and (iv) social comparison theory.

Diffusion of Innovation

Diffusion of innovation (DOI) is a theoretical framework that emphasizes how, why, and at what rate a new idea, practice, or product is spread widely among individuals (Rogers 2003). In this section, we will provide a brief overview of the four main elements of diffusion of innovation. Next, we will review the innovation-decision process. Third, we will talk about five main attributes of innovations that help explain the rate of adoption. Lastly, we will identify five adopter categories regarding innovativeness.

Four Main Elements in the Diffusion of Innovations

Rogers (2003) defined diffusion as the process by which (i) an *innovation* (ii) is *communicated* through certain *channels* (iii) over *time* (iv) among members of a *social system*. These four elements work together to impact how quickly a new health promotion and disease prevention practice will spread. Each of them will be discussed briefly here.

Innovation. An innovation is an idea, practice, or product that is new or perceived as new to an individual or organization of adoption. For example, palliative care (i.e. care focused on providing relief from the symptoms and stress of an illness; also called comfort care and supportive care) has been frequently applied to improve a patient's quality of life when this person has a life-threatening disease. The first US palliative medicine program was launched in 1987 at the Cleveland Clinic Cancer Center in Ohio (Walsh 2001). However, many lay people and health professionals are not aware of palliative care. That means, palliative care is still new to them.

Communication channels. Communication channels refer to the means of transmitting messages from one person to another (Rogers 2003). Traditionally, there are two primary communication channels in our society. The first one encompasses mass communication channels, which refer to media that transmit messages to large audiences quickly, such as television, newspaper, and radio. The second one includes interpersonal communication channels involving face-to-face interaction between two or more individuals. While interpersonal communication may not be as fast as mass communication, it can be quite effective in persuading individuals to accept a new idea, practice, or product. Although social media as a communication channel was not included in the DOI originally, the development of new technologies has guided researchers to expand the scope of channels. As well as mass and interpersonal communication, social media has become another influential platform to spread new ideas, practices, or products.

Time. Time is closely related to the DOI in three different aspects. First, the innovation-decision process consists of five steps (i.e. knowledge, persuasion, decision, implementation, and confirmation) that include the time when a person passes from first knowing about an innovation to adopting or rejecting an innovation. Second, individuals are classified into five adopter categories based on when they adopt an innovation (i.e. innovators, early adopters, early majority, late majority, and laggards). Third, the rate of adoption (i.e. the relative speed at which an innovation is adopted) is measured as the number of members of the system that adopt the innovation in a given time period.

Social system. A social system is defined as a set of interrelated individuals, groups, and organizations that are engaged in solving a common problem or achieve a common task (Rogers 2003). Sharing a joint goal can connect different members of a social system together. Palliative care is again a good example. At the individual level are the patients diagnosed with life-threatening diseases. At the group level are the palliative care doctors, primary care doctors, nurses, social workers, pharmacists, chaplains, physical therapists, dieticians, and volunteers collaborating to help patients. At the organizational level are the palliative medicine programs, research institutions, and national organizations that provide necessary support.

The Innovation-Decision Process

A person's decision to use an innovation does not happen immediately. It involves multiple information-seeking and information-processing activities over time. The *innovation-decision process* refers to the way a person moves from first knowing about an innovation to strengthening the decision to adopt or reject an innovation (Rogers 2003). This process consists of five stages, which will be reviewed briefly below.

The first stage is *knowledge*, which occurs when a person becomes aware of an innovation and builds some understanding of how and why the innovation works. An individual cannot adopt an innovation without knowing about it. We can gain knowledge of an innovation in different manners (e.g. watching others use it, reading news articles, and receiving a flyer in public occasions). There are three important types of knowledge at this stage: (i) learning that an innovation exists, (ii) learning how to use an innovation properly, and (iii) learning how and why an innovation works.

The second stage is *persuasion*, which occurs when a person forms a favorable or unfavorable attitude toward an innovation. At this stage individuals become engaged in the innovation. They seek, obtain, and interpret information about the innovation. This process will guide their feelings about the innovation (do you believe it is good or bad, pleasant or unpleasant, beneficial or harmful, etc.?).

The third stage is *decision*, which occurs when a person chooses to adopt or reject the innovation. This stage does not focus on the actual use of an innovation. Rather, it involves actively seeking further information (e.g. strengths and weaknesses) to evaluate the innovation and other activities that lead to the adoption or rejection of an innovation. The goal is to decide whether people should adopt the innovation.

The fourth stage is *implementation*, which refers to the time when a person starts to adopt the innovation. As Rogers (2003) discusses, "until the implementation stage, the innovation-decision process has been a strictly mental exercise of thinking and deciding. But implementation involves overt behavior change as the new idea is actually put into practice" (p. 179). In other words, at this stage individuals put an innovation into use and can find out whether an innovation meets their expectations.

The last stage is *confirmation*, which refers to the time when a person seeks reinforcement and supports their choice to adopt or reject the innovation. In some circumstances, implementation means the completion of the innovation-decision process. However, this is not always the case. Individuals may continue exploring the innovation and further assess the outcomes of their decision to adopt or reject an innovation. Given that people change their minds all the time, it is important to spend time considering the decisions they have already made.

Attributes of Innovations that Influence Diffusion

It is not surprising that innovations may diffuse at different rates based upon different reasons. There are five perceptual attributes related to the innovation-decision process: relative advantage, compatibility, complexity, trialability, and observability. *Relative advantage* refers to the perceived benefits of adopting an innovation. *Compatibility* refers to the degree to which an innovation is perceived as consistent with the existing values and beliefs, lifestyles, and needs of potential adopters. *Complexity* refers to the degree to which an innovation is perceived as difficult to understand and use. *Trialability* refers to the degree to which an innovation can be experimented with on a limited basis. *Observability* refers to the degree to which benefits of an innovation are visible to others. And it is worth noting that relative advantage, compatibility, trialability, and observability are all positively related to an innovation's rate of adoption, while complexity is negatively related to an innovation's rate of adoption.

Adapter Categories

Obviously, not all people accept an innovation at the same time. At first, only a few people show interest in it. Later, more and more individuals adopt the innovation. Based on the findings of previous empirical studies, Rogers (2003) used a measure of "innovativeness" (i.e. the degree to which an individual is relatively earlier in adopting new ideas than other members of a social system) to distinguish five categories of adopters that will be discussed below. In most cases, the distributions of adaptor categories follow a bell-shaped normal curve.

Innovators are made up of the first 2.5% of people in a social system to use an innovation. They seek information actively about new ideas, have a considerable amount of media exposure and strong interpersonal networks, and show willingness to cope with high-level uncertainty about an innovation and accept occasional failure. *Early adopters* include the next 13.5% of people to adopt an innovation. Because early adopters are not too far ahead of the average member of a social system, they are considered as role models to adopt an innovation and frequently offer guidance and advice for potential adopters. The *early majority* adopt an innovation just *before* the average member of a social system and make up the next 34% of individuals who adopt an innovation. They interact a lot with their peers, but seldom serve as leaders for providing advice and guidance. The *late majority* adopt an innovation just *after* the average member of a social system and make up the next 34% of individuals. They are skeptical and cautious about an innovation and may not accept an innovation until most members in the social system have done so or a lot of support is available before the adoption. Finally, *laggards* are the slowest to adopt an innovation and comprise the last 16% of individuals. They are quite traditional, socially isolated, suspicious of innovations, and resistant to changes. They may not want to adopt an innovation unless using the traditional way is not working any more working or the innovation has been working for others.

In sum, DOI provides a conceptual lens to explore how members of a social system make the decision to accept an innovation. This theory contributes to the adoption of important health promotion programs and serves as a powerful tool to facilitate both planned and spontaneous spread of a new idea, practice, or product. For instance, Lin and Bautista (2017) found that high observability of mHealth app usage drives young users to try innovative mHealth technologies, which can help app development companies create marketing strategies for the target audience. DOI is a macro-level theory as it focuses on how social factors influence behavior change. Other social psychological theories focus on how individual factors such as beliefs, attitudes, and intentions impact behavior change. The balance of this chapter will focus on three individual approaches, beginning with social judgment theory, which is discussed next.

Social Judgment Theory

The main premise of social judgment theory (SJT) is that the effects of a health communication message depend on how the receiver evaluates the position it advocates compared to their current point of view (Sherif, Sherif, and Nebergall 1965; Sherif and Hovland 1961). To illustrate, Smith et al. (2006) used SJT to better understand students' perceptions of alcohol consumption as part of a social norms campaign. By way of introduction, take a moment to read the question and response options in Figure 11.1 (which were adapted from the Smith et al. study):

After the respondent has read through the entire list, they are asked to please place a *star* (★) next to the *one* position that is found most acceptable or likely. Next, the respondent should place a *plus sign* (+) next to any other positions that seem acceptable or likely to this respondent. Finally, they should put a *minus sign* (–) next to any positions that are unacceptable or unlikely to them. They are instructed to keep in mind that it is not necessary to place a mark next to all 11 positions, and that positions on which the respondent has no opinion, about which they do not feel strongly, or have not fully decided should be left blank.

What percentage of students at your university typically drink five or fewer drinks when they party?

_____ 0%

_____ 10%

_____ 20%

_____ 30%

_____ 40%

_____ 50%

_____ 60%

_____ 70%

_____ 80%

_____ 90%

_____ 100%

Figure 11.1 Ordered alternatives questionnaire about students' perceptions of alcohol consumption.

Ordered Alternatives Questionnaire

As you probably noticed, these 11 response options were not presented in a random order. Instead, the alternatives were presented in a specific order ranging from one extreme to the other (thus the name "ordered alternatives questionnaire"). In other words, the *ordered alternatives questionnaire* presents a set of options designed to represent various positions on the issue being studied, ranging from the extreme view on one side to the extreme view on the other side. This allows a health communicator to identify participants' most preferred positions, as well as other positions they find agreeable, disagreeable, or about which they have no opinion.

Anchor, Latitude of Acceptance, Latitude of Rejection, and Latitude of Noncommitment

The *anchor* is the position a person finds most acceptable (i.e. the one marked with a star). According to SJT, the anchor serves as a point of reference for judging the discrepancy between the position advocated by a health communication message and the receiver's own position on the issue. For our running example for this theory, imagine a hypothetical student who selected 70% as his or her most preferred position.

The *latitude of acceptance* includes a person's anchor *and* any other positions he or she finds acceptable (i.e. the one marked with a star *and* any marked with a plus sign). These are the positions that may be a little more or less extreme than one's preferred position, but that a person still finds tolerable. For example, while our hypothetical student selected 70% as his or her most preferred position, he or she might still see the 50% and 60% options to be acceptable or reasonable.

The *latitude of rejection* includes any positions a person finds unacceptable (i.e. those marked with a minus sign). These are the positions a person disagrees with or views as unreasonable. For example, our hypothetical student might find the extremes at both ends of the continuum to be unacceptable or unreasonable, in which case he or she would put a minus sign next to the 0%, 10% 20%, 80%, 90%, and 100% options.

Finally, the *latitude of noncommitment* includes any positions on which a person has no opinion, about which he or she does not feel strongly, or has not fully decided (i.e. any positions not marked). In our running example, 30% and 40% were not marked and therefore make up the hypothetical student's latitude of noncommitment.

Of course, the hypothetical example represents just one of many possible options. Different people may have different anchors and latitude structures. And, people with the same anchor might have different latitudes of acceptance, rejection, and noncommitment. Perhaps most importantly, SJT posits that a person's reaction to a health message will depend on his or her (i) anchor – i.e. most preferred position, (i) judgment of various alternatives – i.e. latitudes of acceptance, rejection, and noncommitment, and (iii) level of ego involvement with the issue – which is discussed next.

The Effects of Ego-Involvement and the Latitudes

Ego-involvement concerns the extent to which an issue is personally relevant or meaningful to an individual, or how important it is to his or her self-concept or self-esteem. For example, is the issue central to one's sense of self or well-being, is the person strongly committed to it, does he or she think about it a lot, etc. (Griffin 2012; O'Keefe 2016)? As the following sections will illustrate, ego-involvement is a central concept in SJT as it has a strong impact on (i) our judgments on an issue – whether a given statement falls into one's latitude of acceptance, rejection, or noncommitment, (ii) how much one distorts incoming information to fit these judgments, and ultimately (iii) the effectiveness of health communication messages.

Assimilation effect. Assimilate means to make similar, so the *assimilation effect* involves interpreting a message that falls within people's latitude of acceptance as closer, or more similar, to their position than it actually is. To return to our hypothetical example, consider the student who selected 70% as his or her most preferred position. Now suppose he or she was exposed to a social norms campaign telling him or her that 50% was actually the correct number. An assimilation effect would occur if the receiver interpreted the message as *more similar* to his or her own than it actually is (e.g. perhaps as 60%). So, instead of moving this person from 70% to 50% as hoped, the assimilation effect would cause him or her to move only slightly toward the advocated position (i.e. perhaps to 60%).

Contrast effect. To contrast means to focus on differences, so the *contrast effect* involves interpreting a message that falls within people's latitude of rejection as farther away, or more different, from their own position than it actually is. Returning to our running example, suppose the social norms campaign tries to convince our hypothetical student that 20% is the correct number (which falls at the edge of his or her latitude of rejection). A contrast effect would occur if the receiver interpreted the message as *more different* from this student's position than it actually is (e.g. perhaps as 10%). Given how far the position is perceived to be from the student's anchor of 70%, coupled with the fact that it is perceived as falling further into his or her latitude of rejection than it actually does, means this student will likely not change his or her position at all.

Boomerang effect. In this context, boomerang means to have a negative effect, or to backfire. So, a *boomerang effect* would cause a person to become more committed to his or her current position or to do the opposite of what was requested. To conclude our example, imagine a social norms campaign trying to convince our hypothetical student that only about 10% of students at their university typically drink five or fewer drinks when they party (which is very far away from his or her anchor and well into his or her latitude of rejection). Instead of moving toward accepting the advocated position, this individual might become even more committed to their current position (i.e. go all in on position 70%) or move in the opposite direction (i.e. move *away* from the advocated position toward 80%).

In sum, SJT suggests that an individual's opinion on a topic cannot be adequately represented by a single point along a continuum and is better represented by the person's latitudes of acceptance, noncommitment, and rejection. It also posits that health communication messages will be most effective when they target the edge of the audience's latitude of acceptance and noncommitment. Additionally, SJT highlights that ego involvement can impact health communication in at least three ways. First, ego-involvement affects the structure of an individual's latitudes (i.e. highly involved individuals tend to have larger latitudes of rejection). Second, ego-involvement impacts judgments made about a message, or whether a message is perceived as more similar to (assimilation) or different from (contrast) one's anchor than it actually is. Finally, ego-involvement influences the potential effectiveness of a health communication message (i.e. assimilated messages will not cause as much change, and contrasted messages are more likely to cause boomerang effects than they otherwise might). Readers interested in another good example of SJT in action are referred to Salazar (2017), who developed an insightful activity to help individuals construct persuasive arguments guided by this theory.

Next, we discuss self-determination theory, which focuses on how individual motivations impact behavior change.

Self-Determination Theory

Self-determination theory (SDT) is an empirically derived theory designed to explain human motivation in various social circumstances (Ryan and Deci 2017). The researchers who study SDT address how people can create the conditions to motivate *themselves* – as opposed to being motivated by others (Deci and Flaste 1995). SDT posits that: (i) motivation is an important predictor of behavioral outcomes; and (ii) satisfaction of the three basic psychological needs (i.e. competence, autonomy, and relatedness) influences motivation. In this section we will first review three basic psychological needs. Second, we will review two primary types of motivation. Third, we will examine the reconceptualization of motivation. Fourth, we will discuss how people feel motivated to take an action.

Basic Psychological Needs

SDT states that humans have three basic psychological needs: a need to feel competent, a need to feel autonomous, and a need to feel related (Ryan and Deci 2017). SDT illustrates that *intrinsic motivation* (i.e. feeling motivated by our internal desire to do something for its own sake) flourishes in a wide variety of social contexts that satisfy these three universal psychological human needs. Having social environments that satisfies these three fundamental needs will support people's personal growth and well-being.

Competence refers to the need to feel a sense of confidence and capacity to act. Feeling sufficiently competent at the task is important to make people motivated to perform a role. For example, when patients feel confident that they understand the benefits of following physicians' suggestions on their health, they are more likely to take their opinions seriously. This is closely related to the concept of self-efficacy which was introduced in Chapters 8 and 9.

Autonomy refers to the need to feel that the choice is up to you. When autonomous, behavior is a manifestation of one's true self. Autonomy is often confused with the concept of independence. Independence means not relying on external resources and doing for yourself, while autonomy refers to acting freely with a sense of choice, flexibility, and personal freedom (Ryan and Deci 2017). For example, people will feel autonomous about taking a workout class when they believe it is their choice to do so. This is closely related to the concept of perceived behavioral control which was introduced in Chapter 9 of this book.

Relatedness refers to the need to feel connected to others, to care for and be cared for by others, to have meaningful relationships with others, and to have a sense of belonging to a community. For example, when romantic partners express more affection through cuddling and kissing, they are more likely to experience satisfaction of the need for relatedness than others without affectionate behaviors.

To summarize, SDT postulates that intrinsic motivation is sustained by satisfaction of the three fundamental psychological needs: competence, autonomy, and relatedness. These three psychological needs work together to energize intrinsically motivated behaviors and improve the quality of life of individuals. Failing to satisfy these needs may undermine intrinsic motivation and lead people to display poor health as well as social malfunctioning (Ryan and Deci 2017).

Extrinsic and Intrinsic Motivations

There are two primary types of motivation, extrinsic motivation and intrinsic motivation, which shape who we are and how we behave (Deci and Ryan 2008). *Extrinsic motivation* means that people's energies for taking an action come from external sources and rewards such as grading systems and evaluations, while *intrinsic motivation* refers to doing something for the enjoyment of the activity itself (Ryan and Deci 2017). The interplay between extrinsic and intrinsic motivations is the territory of SDT (Ryan and Deci 2017).

Intrinsic motivation is characterized by the experience of interest and pleasure (e.g. playing a video game with friends for fun). The reward for intrinsic motivation is in the doing of the activity rather than the final outcome. Intrinsic motivation is typically associated with richer experience, better understanding, higher quality of performance, greater creativity, and improved problem-solving. For example, when people are intrinsically motivated to exercise, they actively engage in physical activities for internal satisfaction. The rewards linked to intrinsic motivation are the feelings of interest and enjoyment of freely engaging in the behavior. What Ryan and Deci's (2017) work has indicated is that intrinsic motivation is essential for people's creativity, responsibility, problem-solving, and psychological and physical wellness.

Extrinsic motivations, on the other hand, are those that are external or outside an individual's control. The reward for extrinisic motivation is in the desirable outcome (e.g. scholarships). Extrinsic motivation is typically negatively related to intrinsic motivation – more extrinsic motivation is associated with less intrinsic motivation, and vice versa. However, recent studies have provided a more complicated picture beyond the classic distinction between extrinsic and intrinsic motivations (Ryan and Deci 2017). For example, individuals are likely to feel autonomously extrinsically motivated. This means that people can internalize external prompts and accept them as their own. With this in mind, the most important distinction within SDT is not intrinsic versus extrinsic motivation, but autonomous versus controlled motivation. Next, we will talk about the reconceptualization of motivation.

Autonomous Motivation and Controlled Motivation

Central to the SDT is whether a behavior is autonomous or controlled (Deci and Ryan 2000). To be *autonomous* means to feel free in one's actions and choices. Autonomous people are fully willing to do what they do as it is in line with their interests and values. Their behaviors originate from their true sense of self. Autonomously motivated behaviors allow people to feel satisfaction of the three basic psychological needs. Research indicates a positive relationship between autonomous motivation and people's health (Deci and Ryan 2008; Teixeira, Patrick, and Mata 2011; Williams et al. 2002).

To the contrary, to be *controlled* means to feel pressured to act. When controlled, people may still feel competent or connected to others, but their need for autonomy will not be satisfied. This may undermine their intrinsic motivation. Think about a man who maintains a healthy diet not because he wants to but because his wife asks him to eat healthy and keeps telling him the negative consequences of eating his favorite junk food. This person is eating healthily but in a way that is controlled by someone else; he will not feel he has the freedom to choose what he wants. SDT suggests that people tend to be more autonomous when the three basic psychological needs described above are being met (Ryan and Deci 2002).

More recently, SDT researchers and theorists have switched from using intrinsic versus extrinsic motivations to autonomous versus controlled motivations. Autonomous motivation includes *intrinsic motivation* and *internalized extrinsic motivation* (i.e. being willing to accept and endorse the value of a behavior as one's own). With this new conceptualization, people can be autonomously motivated when they have extrinsically motivated behaviors. For example, a personal trainer may have asked a bride-to-be to exercise three times per week to look and feel her best on her big day. The bride-to-be was initially motivated to exercise to get in shape by her wedding day. However, during this process she gradually internalized the importance of regular exercise, and in doing so became more autonomously motivated. Through internalization, people become willing to accept responsibility for behaviors that are important but not quite enjoyable (Deci and Flaste 1995).

In contrast with autonomous motivation, controlled motivation encompasses *external regulation* (i.e. being motivated by external rewards or punishments) and *introjected regulation* (i.e. starting to internalize the value of a behavior but having not truly accepted it as one's own). External regulation is the least autonomous form of extrinsic motivation and has been contrasted with intrinsic motivation in the earlier stage of SDT research (Ryan and Deci 2002). As a more autonomous form of extrinsic motivation, introjected regulation involves trying to accept the value of a behavior but it is still controlling. For example, imagine a medical school student whose parents are doctors. They encouraged her to go to medical school. She tried hard to do so to make her parents happy until she realized health communication is what she would like to study.

Autonomy Support

According to SDT, in order to make people feel autonomously motivated, we should create an autonomy-supportive environment (Ryan and Deci 2017). *Autonomy support* describes an interpersonal or a group environment in which authority figures (e.g. doctors or parents) take the perspective of individuals under the authority (e.g. patients or children) into account and encourage them to accept more responsibility for their behaviors (Deci and Flaste 1995). The concept of autonomy support involves minimizing pressure by avoiding controlling language, acknowledging others' perspectives and feelings, providing choices, and giving a meaningful rationale for recommended behaviors. Research indicates that autonomy support is positively related to people's satisfaction of the needs for autonomy, competence, and relatedness in health behavior (Ng et al. 2012). For example, when physicians are autonomy supportive, they are more likely to understand such high-risk behaviors on the part of patients as overeating, substance abuse, and unprotected sex, and will work with patients to develop personalized treatment plans (Deci and Flaste 1995; Ryan and Deci 2017).

Autonomy support is hard work. It requires being clear, being consistent in managing consequences, and setting limits empathetically. Pressuring people to act in a certain way may weaken their feelings of self-determination. In contrast, providing them with choices regarding how to do something can help them engage more in the activities. As an important feature to support autonomy, providing choices engenders willingness and personal freedom and may lead to better solutions. Setting effective limits is another central feature to embrace autonomy. Making the limits as wide as possible and allowing choices within them can help keep people from feeling restricted. Setting limits is not about control but about helping people recognize the consequences of choices and behave responsibly. In these ways, autonomous motivation can be facilitated, and people's basic psychological needs can be satisfied.

In sum, SDT contributes to the development of the concept of motivation. This theory presents strong empirical evidence that satisfaction of the three universal psychological needs and being motivated autonomously are positively associated with both physical and mental health. SDT also suggests that we provide autonomy-supportive environments to help people become motivated to take an action. By focusing on human motivation and personality, SDT has been widely applied in many health communication contexts (e.g. message design for promoting physical activity and healthy eating, patient-centered communication, and health information seeking). For instance, Hull et al. (2016) found that competence, autonomy, and relatedness have deeply interconnected effects on the use of an online health support system among breast cancer patients. SDT is not the only theoretical framework addressing the importance of motivational factors on individuals' health and well-being. Next, we will talk about social comparison theory.

Social Comparison Theory

People often compare themselves with others for different purposes such as assessing themselves (e.g. how healthy my diet is), learning from others (e.g. my sister did a better job in staying in shape, because she eats healthier and exercises more than me), and feeling better about their own situations (e.g. I suffered from one concussion, but I am luckier than my teammate who suffered from three concussions). *Social comparison* refers to the process in which people determine their social and personal worth (e.g. attractiveness, personality, and intelligence) based on how they stack up against others. Social comparison theory (SCT) is an important social psychological framework emphasizing people's judgments, experiences, and behavior (Corcoran, Crusius, and Mussweiler 2011). This section will review main hypotheses in SCT and talk about why people engage in social comparisons, to whom people compare themselves, and how social comparisons influence the self.

Festinger's Theory of Social Comparison Processes

Initially proposed by Leon Festinger (1954), SCT highlights that individuals have a fundamental need to maintain a stable and accurate self-view. This theoretical framework addresses how people use others to fulfill their own needs to gather and interpret knowledge about themselves. Festinger (1954) advanced several hypotheses to explain why people engage in social comparisons, with whom people will compare, and the consequences of social comparisons. The main hypotheses include:

1. Humans are driven to evaluate their opinions and abilities.
2. When objective and nonsocial means are not available, people will evaluate their opinions and abilities by comparing them to the opinions and abilities of others.
3. There is a unidirectional drive upward for the comparison of abilities but not for opinions.
4. Individuals do not tend to evaluate their abilities or opinions by comparison with others who are very divergent from themselves.
5. Social comparison leads to pressures toward uniformity.

The major processes of social comparison include acquiring social information, thinking about social information in relation to the self, and reacting to social comparisons (Wood 1996).

Motives for Social Comparison

Some of Festinger's hypotheses focus on people's motives (i.e. why people engage in social comparisons). Social comparisons are commonly viewed as strategic processes to satisfy goals of self-evaluation, self-enhancement, and self-improvement (Corcoran, Crusius, and Mussweiler 2011). *Self-evaluation* refers to the process of determining where people stand relative to others in terms of attributes, skills, and social expectations (Krayer, Ingledew, and Iphofen 2008). When people engage in subjective judgments of their self-concepts (e.g. how does my physical attractiveness compare to my best friend's?), they are involved in the process of self-evaluation. Comparing with similar others provides people diagnostic information for an accurate self-evaluation. When we know that we are similar to the standard, we are likely to assimilate our self-evaluations toward the target. When we know that we are not similar to the target, we are likely to contrast our self-evaluations away from the target. For example, a high school student would be more likely to compare with her classmate (rather than an elementary school student) in terms of athletic ability.

However, sometimes people do not seek accurate feedback about themselves but select dissimilar others whom they expect to be superior or inferior for the purposes of self-enhancement and self-improvement. *Self-enhancement* refers to the process of comparing in a way that produces a positive evaluation of the self (Wills 1981). For self-enhancement, people compare themselves to others who are worse off. People seek an inferior target to protect their self-esteem and boost their self-view with a favorable comparison (e.g. I have a better personality than my brother). *Self-improvement* helps people learn how to better the self (e.g. how can I learn from my peers to be more physically active?). Different from self-evaluation, both self-enhancement and self-improvement are helpful for people to look for differences from the comparison target on certain dimensions.

Types of Social Comparison

Another important question related to social comparison is, "With whom do people decide to compare themselves?" To evaluate their physical attractiveness, for instance, a girl could compare herself with her sister, friend, co-worker, a movie star, or any other real or imaginary person she knows from her social networks or mass media. How does she select her comparison target to satisfy her need for self-evaluation, self-enhancement, or self-improvement? In the following we will review three types of social comparison.

Lateral comparison occurs when people seek comparisons with others who are similar to them on important characteristics (e.g. age, gender, or school performance) that help them accurately evaluate themselves on the focal attribute. For example, college male students compare their physical fitness levels with other male students' in the same college.

Downward comparison occurs when people seek comparisons with lower standards (i.e. others who are worse than themselves) for the need to maintain a positive self-view. The major benefit of downward comparison is an improvement in people's well-being and satisfaction. Comparison with a less-fortunate other enables people to feel better about their own situations. Affleck and Tennen (1991) studied a group of infertile women and found they used downward comparison as a coping strategy, "I think I'm fortunate compared to other people. I could have worse problems than infertility."

Finally, *upward comparison* occurs when people seek comparisons with higher standards (i.e. others who are better than themselves) for the need to improve themselves. Research illustrates an overall preference for upward comparison rather than downward or lateral comparison (Gerber, Wheeler, and Suls 2017). Upward comparisons motivate people to make a change. For example, Lockwood and Kunda (1997) showed that role models who exceeded a person's own ability triggered inspiration when it was possible for this person to be as successful as role models. However, upward comparisons can have negative impacts on people's health. Several studies showed that upward comparison on social networking sites was significantly associated with higher ratings of depressive symptoms (Seabrook, Kern, and Rickard 2016). Comparing female college students' behaviors through social media, traditional media, and in person, Fardouly, Pinkus, and Vartanian (2017) found that upward appearance comparisons were associated with less positive moods and appearance satisfaction than when no comparisons were made across these three contexts.

Consequences of Social Comparison

Social comparison has been linked to various consequences. In the original formulation of SCT, Festinger (1954) predicted a pressure toward uniformity, which will result in assimilation. For example, when a woman is not satisfied with her physical attractiveness and would like to learn from her favorite Instagram model to improve makeup skills, she may choose the same products which the model uses rather than those appropriate for her skin type. In this case, social comparison may cause a change in a person's characteristics and produce a similarity between the person and the standard.

Although Festinger did not emphasize the contrastive consequences during the initial development of SCT, later studies have indicated that people are likely to feel better or worse after a downward or an upward comparison (Corcoran, Crusius, and Mussweiler 2011). For example, having the best performance can help a trainee boost self-confidence in a CrossFit training. Meanwhile, being not as successful as others can make a trainee feel very frustrated or encourage harder working to achieve the level of the upward target. The whole process may lead to a positive or negative contrast.

In sum, social comparison arises when people are not able to evaluate themselves by objective standards and have a fundamental desire to gain informative feedback about their opinions and abilities through comparisons with others. Although Festinger's classical SCT (1954) mainly focuses on humans' needs to have accurate self-evaluations, more researchers have successfully expanded the scope of SCT and examined the dynamics of lateral, upward, and downward comparisons in a wide range of health communication domains (e.g. body satisfaction, eating behaviors, stress management, and acute and chronic illness). For example, Myers and Crowther's meta-analysis (2009) indicated that more use of social comparison was positively related to higher level of body dissatisfaction. The effect for social comparison and body dissatisfaction was stronger for women than men. In another study, Umstead et al. (2018) illustrated that downward comparison can help restore one's sense of well-being after a health threat. These findings have guided health communication researchers' efforts to understand how we use social information to evaluate our skills and abilities.

Conclusion

This chapter reviewed four different social psychological theories that are used by health communication researchers and practitioners to better understand and more effectively influence our health and well-being. The chapter began by examining DOI, which focuses on how, why, and at what rate a new health idea, practice, or product will spread among individuals. Second, it summarized SJT, which suggests that the effectiveness of a health message depends on how the receiver evaluates the position it advocates compared to their current point of view. Third, it reviewed SDT, which highlights how satisfaction of the three basic psychological needs and motivation impact health behavior. Finally, it described SCT, which focuses on how individuals tend to compare themselves to others, and how these comparisons can positively or negatively impact our self-image and sense of well-being.

All four of the theories discussed in this chapter provide helpful insights regarding how to get people to engage in healthy behaviors. They suggest that behavior change is a complicated process that involves effortful engagement at different stages. When researchers and practitioners develop health communication interventions, they should have a deep understanding of what motivates people. Luckily, the theories reviewed in this chapter highlight how we can offer supportive social environments to encourage behavior change. Such insights provide a valuable tool to those seeking to design, implement, and evaluate effective health communication interventions.

References

Affleck, G., & Tennen, H. (1991). Social comparison and coping with major medical problems. In J. Suls & T. A. Wills (Eds.), *Social comparison: Contemporary theory and research* (pp. 369–393). Hillsdale, NJ: Erlbaum.

Corcoran, K., Crusius, J., & Mussweiler, T. (2011). Social comparison: Motives, standards, and mechanisms. In D. Chadee (Ed.), *Theories in social psychology* (pp. 119–139). Oxford, UK: Wiley Blackwell.

Deci, E. L., & Flaste, R. (1995). *Why we do what we do: The dynamics of personal autonomy.* New York, NY: G. P. Putnam's Sons.

Deci, E. L., & Ryan, R. M. (2000). The "what" and "why" of goal pursuits: Human needs and the self-determination of behavior. *Psychological Inquiry, 11,* 227–268. doi:10.1207/S15327965PLI1104_01

Deci, E. L., & Ryan, R. M. (2008) Facilitating optimal motivation and psychological well-being across life's domains. *Canadian Psychology, 49,* 14–23. doi:10.1037/0708-5591.49.1.14

Fardouly, J., Pinkus, R. T., & Vartanian, L. R. (2017). The impact of appearance comparisons made through social media, traditional media, and in person in women's everyday lives. *Body Image, 20,* 31–39. doi:10.1016/j.bodyim.2016.11.002

Festinger, L. (1954). A theory of social comparison processes. *Human Relations, 7,* 117–140. doi:10.1177/001872675400700202

Gerber, J. P., Wheeler, L., & Suls, J. (2017). A social comparison theory meta-analysis 60+ years on. *Psychological Bulletin, 144,* 177–197. doi:10.1037/bul0000127

Greenaway, K., Gallois, C., & Haslam, S. (2017). Social psychological approaches to intergroup communication. *Oxford research encyclopedia of communication.* Retrieved from https://oxfordre.com/communication/view/10.1093/acrefore/9780190228613.001.0001/acrefore-9780190228613-e-483

Griffin, E. (2012). *A first look at communication theory* (8th ed.). New York, NY: McGraw Hill.

Hornsey, M. J., Gallois, C., & Duck, J. M. (2008). The intersection of communication and social psychology: Points of contact and points of difference. *Journal of Communication, 58,* 749–766. doi:10.1111/j.1460-2466.2008. 00412.x

Hull, S. J., Abril, E. P., Shah, D. V., Choi, M., Chih, M. Y., Kim, S. C., . . . Gustafson, D. H. (2016). Self-determination theory and computer-mediated support: Modeling effects on breast cancer patient's quality-of-life. *Health Communication, 31,* 1205–1214. doi:10.1080/10410236.2015.1048422

Krayer, A., Ingledew, D. K., & Iphofen, R. (2008). Social comparison and body image in adolescence: A grounded theory approach. *Health Education Research, 23,* 892–903. doi:10.1093/her/cym076

Lin, T. T., & Bautista, J. R. (2017). Understanding the relationships between mHealth apps' characteristics, trialability, and mHealth literacy. *Journal of Health Communication, 22,* 346–354. doi:10.1080/10810730.2017.1296508

Lockwood, P., & Kunda, Z. (1997). Superstars and me: Predicting the impact of role models on the self. *Journal of Personality and Social Psychology, 73,* 91–103. doi:10.1037/0022-3514.73.1.91

Myers, T. A., & Crowther, J. H. (2009). Social comparison as a predictor of body dissatisfaction: A meta-analytic review. *Journal of Abnormal Psychology, 118,* 683–698. doi:10.1037/a0016763

Ng, J. Y., Ntoumanis, N., Thøgersen-Ntoumani, C., Deci, E. L., Ryan, R. M., Duda, J. L., & Williams, G. C. (2012). Self-determination theory applied to health contexts: A meta-analysis. *Perspectives on Psychological Science, 7,* 325–340. doi:10.1177/1745691612447309

O'Keefe, D. J. (2016). *Persuasion: Theory and research* (3rd ed.). Thousand Oaks, CA: Sage.

Rogers, E. M. (2003). *Diffusion of innovation* (5th ed.). New York, NY: Free Press.

Ryan, R. M., & Deci, E. L. (2002). An overview of self-determination theory: An organismic-dialectical perspective. In E. L. Deci & R. M. Ryan (Eds.), *Handbook of self-determination research* (pp. 3–33). Rochester, NY: University of Rochester Press.

Ryan, R. M., & Deci, E. L. (2017). *Self-determination theory: Basic psychological needs in motivation, development, and wellness.* New York, NY: Guilford.

Salazar, L. R. (2017). Changing resistant audience attitudes using social judgment theory's anchor point perspectives. *Communication Teacher, 31,* 90–93. doi:10.1080/17404622.2017.1285412

Seabrook, E. M., Kern, M. L., & Rickard, N. S. (2016). Social networking sites, depression, and anxiety: A systematic review. *JMIR Mental Health, 3,* e50. doi:10.2196/mental.5842

Sherif, M., & Hovland, C. I. (1961). *Social judgment: Assimilation and contrast effects in communication and attitude change.* Westport, CT: Greenwood Press.

Sherif, C. W., Sherif, M., & Nebergall, R. E. (1965). *Attitude and attitude change: The social judgment-involvement approach.* Westport, CT: Greenwood Press.

Smith, S. W., Atkin, C. K., Martell, D., Allen, R., & Hembroff, L. (2006). A social judgment theory approach to conducting formative research in a social norms campaign. *Communication Theory, 16,* 141–152. doi:10.1111/j.1468-2885. 2006.00009.x

Teixeira, P. J., Patrick, H., & Mata, J. (2011). Why we eat what we eat: The role of autonomous motivation in eating behaviour regulation. *Nutrition Bulletin, 36,* 102–107. doi:10.1111/j.1467-3010.2010.01876.x

Umstead, K. L., Kalia, S. S., Madeo, A. C., Erby, L. H., Blank, T. O., Visvanathan, K., & Roter, D. L. (2018). Social comparisons and quality of life following a prostate cancer diagnosis. *Journal of Psychosocial Oncology, 36,* 350–363. doi:10.1080/07347332.2017.1417950

Walsh, D. (2001). The Harry R. Horvitz Center for Palliative Medicine (1987–1999): Development of a novel comprehensive integrated program. *American Journal of Hospice and Palliative Medicine, 18,* 239–250. doi:10.1177/104990910101800408

Williams, G. G., Gagné, M., Ryan, R. M., & Deci, E. L. (2002). Facilitating autonomous motivation for smoking cessation. *Health Psychology, 21,* 40–50. doi:10.1037/0278-6133.21.1.40

Wills, T. A. (1981). Downward comparison principles in social psychology. *Psychological Bulletin, 90,* 245–271. doi:10.1037/0033-2909.90.2.245

Wood, J. V. (1996). What is social comparison and how should we study it? *Personality and Social Psychology Bulletin, 22,* 520–537. doi:10.1177/0146167296225009

12

Theories of Public Relations

Arunima Krishna

One of the central foci of public relations theory building in the last few decades has been the concept of publics. Ever since Grunig (1968) advanced the situational theory of publics, much public relations literature has been dedicated to understanding the nature (e.g. Hallahan 2000), types (e.g. Ni and Kim 2009), characteristics (e.g. Krishna 2018), and behaviors (e.g. Chen, Hung-Baesecke, and Kim 2017) of publics. Several of the investigations on publics have been centered on health-related issues, including anti-vaccine activism (e.g. Krishna 2017), organ donation (e.g. J.-N. Kim, Shen and Morgan 2011), food safety (e.g. J.-N. Kim et al. 2012; Vardeman and Aldoory 2008), and HIV/AIDS (e.g. Chay-Nemeth 2001) among many others. The present chapter focuses on two public-centered theories that have emerged from the discipline of public relations, collectively referred to as the situational theories, to help explicate cognitive processes and behaviors of health-related publics.

This chapter begins with a review of the parent situational theory, i.e. the situational theory of publics (STP; Grunig 1997), tracing its theoretical origins and assumptions with a brief summary of the applications of the theory in health contexts. The STP will be followed by the situational

Health Communication Theory, First Edition. Edited by Teresa L. Thompson and Peter J. Schulz.

theory of problem-solving (STOPS; J.-N. Kim and Grunig 2011; J.-N. Kim and Krishna 2014), the theoretical successor to the STP. Along with a summary of the theory, this section will also review the shared and distinct theoretical assumptions underpinning both theories, and conclude with a discussion of the application of the STOPS in health contexts.

The Situational Theory of Publics

The situational theory of publics (STP; Grunig 1968, 1997) is a theory of public relations that explains individuals' communicative behaviors in the process of making a decision. The central postulate of the STP is that when faced with a decision, individuals tend to seek further information about the issue at hand to make the best possible decision. However, the degree to which individuals seek and attend to information depends on the extent to which the individual stops to think about the issue, i.e. problem recognition; how involved they are in the issue, i.e. involvement recognition; and the barriers they perceive in their path toward making a decision, i.e. constraint recognition (Grunig 1997).

Theoretical Origins of the Situational Theory of Publics

In the 1960s, when Grunig (1968) posited the STP, communication theory development was characterized by a focus on understanding the ways to best influence the public's attitudes. What situational theorists refer to as the "symbolic, interpretive paradigm" (J.-N. Kim et al. 2013, p. 201), considers persuasion as the primary focus of communication, and assumes that communication is what a message sender does to affect the attitudes and behaviors of an audience. Grunig (1968, 1997) challenged this paradigm as limiting, asymmetric, and biased toward the sender, and contended instead that any behavioral or attitudinal effects that emerge from communication efforts are not just the result of effective messaging, but also a function of the receivers' interpretation and epistemic motivations resulting from the message. Advocating for an audience autonomy (vs. audience control; McQuail 1997) paradigm, Grunig (1968) was one of the first to in public relations view communication as a "*purposive* and *situational* human action" (J.-N. Kim and Krishna 2014, p. 72), rather than merely a message that a sender transmits to a receiver.

In addition to critiquing the audience control paradigm of extant communication theory building, Grunig (1968) also criticized existing microeconomic decision-making theories for treating communication as a constant in the decision-making process. The supposition of perfect information in economic theory assumes that a rational decision-maker has complete information regarding choices, alternatives, prices, availability, and other factors when making an economic decision. However, as situational theorists note, "knowledge or information is neither free nor given in decision situations" (J.-N. Kim and Krishna 2014, p. 72). The assumption of perfect knowledge is particularly problematic in health-related decision-making, as health-related knowledge can vary across age, education, income, and context. The STP therefore posits that individuals faced with a decision, economic or otherwise, engage communicative behaviors to obtain the information required for them to make said decision. In so doing, rather than treating information as a constant, the STP positions information acquisition behaviors as the dependent variable, conceptualized to be a function of their situational perceptions (Grunig 1997). Additionally, the STP posits that individuals' information behaviors vary across different situations and problems.

Furthermore, Grunig (1968) in his articulation of the STP interrogated the existing notions of what constitutes a public. Rejecting notions of a "general public," or a static, amorphous body of individuals, Grunig (1968) drew upon Lippmann (1925) and Dewey's (1927) arguments to posit a situation-specific conceptualization of a "public." Rather than viewing a public as a fixed entity who serve as audiences in the political sphere, Grunig (1968, 1997) advanced the notion that "publics begin as disconnected systems of individuals experiencing common problems, but they can evolve into organized and powerful activist groups" (p. 9). In other words, the general population consists of individuals at different levels of engagement over a variety of issues or problems, and individuals connected by situation-specific perceptions constitute an issue-specific public. In so doing, Grunig (1968, 1997) articulated what is arguably the first publics-centered theory of public relations.

Central Constructs of the Situational Theory of Publics

As noted earlier, the STP posits that individuals' issue-specific information acquisition behaviors are dependent on their activeness about the issue. The STP operationalizes issue activeness through three variables. The first variable of the STP framework is problem recognition, which is defined as a state in which "people detect that something should be done about a situation and stop to think about what to do" (Grunig 1997, p. 10). Inspired by Dewey's (1938) concept of a problematic situation, Grunig (1997) asserted that when individuals come across a situation that they deem problematic they are likely to engage in communicative behaviors. Importantly, the theory posits that it is an individual's perception of a situation being problematic that triggers communicative behaviors.

Constraint recognition, the second variable in the STP framework, refers to when "people perceive that there are obstacles in a situation that limit their ability to do anything about the situation" (Grunig 1997, p. 10). Constraint recognition lowers individuals' likelihood of engaging in communicative behaviors, as people may have less need to communicate when obstacles prevent them from making decisions. For example, when deciding whether to socially distance or quarantine oneself during the Covid-19 pandemic, individuals who work in essential businesses (e.g. first responders, sanitation workers, healthcare professionals, etc.) would experience high levels of constraint recognition since their ability to stay home and work is limited. Such individuals would be unlikely to search for information regarding social distancing. The final independent variable in the framework, level of involvement, is defined as "the extent to which people connect themselves with a situation" (Grunig 1997, p. 10). That is, when people are involved in a problem they are likely to want to communicate about it.

In addition to these three variables, early versions of the STP also included a fourth variable called the referent criterion, which Grunig (1997) conceptualized to be "a solution carried from previous situations to a new situation" (p. 11). The presence of a previous solution would lower an individual's need for additional information and therefore lower communicative behavior. However, several tests of this hypothesis failed to confirm it (e.g. Grunig and Disbrow 1977), and the variable was subsequently dropped from the theoretical framework.

The final two components of the STP framework are information seeking and information processing, the two dependent variables of the model. The STP posited communicative behaviors to consist of information acquisition behaviors, consistent with the prevalent trend in communication research at the time (Ni and Kim 2009). Drawing on Clarke and Kline's (1974) concepts, Grunig (1997) argued for information acquisition to be a two-dimensional construct, consisting of an active and a passive dimension of information acquisition. Accordingly, information seeking refers to an active, premeditated search for issue-specific information (e.g. a Google search), whereas information processing is conceptualized to be the unintentional discovery of issue-related information (Grunig 1997). Information seeking and information processing form the two dependent variables of the STP.

Identifying Publics using the Situational Theory of Publics

As one of the first publics-centered theories of public relations, the STP explicates the conditions under which individuals seek information about problematic situations. One of the key theoretical advancements offered by the STP is the notion of the public sphere consisting of multiple publics about a number of different issues rather than a single, fixed entity serving as an audience for message senders. Accordingly, one of the key applications of the STP is the ability to identify and segment issue-specific publics based on the framework and subsequently predict their information behaviors. Grunig (1997) posited that based on individuals' reported problem recognition, constraint recognition, and level of involvement about an issue it is possible to classify them into four categories of issue-specific publics. The first of these publics are active/ activist publics, or those who report high levels of problem recognition and involvement, and very low levels of constraint recognition (Grunig and Hunt 1984). Individuals who volunteer and fundraise for organizations like the American Cancer Society would constitute activist/active publics about cancer awareness and advocacy as they have recognized cancer as a social problem, feel involved in it, and feel like they can do something about it. Active/activist publics are therefore conceptualized to display the highest level of communicative behaviors about an issue.

The second category of publics is aware publics. Aware publics consist of individuals who display either high problem recognition, low constraint recognition and level of involvement, or high levels of all three variables. Given their high levels of problem recognition about the issue at hand, these publics may be the most receptive to communication campaigns designed to influence their communicative and behavioral actions. Smokers who want to quit may be considered aware publics, as they recognize that smoking is a problem and have a personal connection to it, but feel constrained against actually quitting due to their dependence on cigarettes.

The third type of public proposed by Grunig and Hunt (1984) is latent publics. Latent publics include those who display either high problem and constraint recognition and low involvement, or low problem recognition and high constraint recognition involvement, or low levels of all three. These publics are those who may be affected by the problem but have not perceived the situation as being problematic or have not yet felt the effects of the problem even though they recognize its existence. Consider the initial reaction to the Covid-19 pandemic especially in the United States, when the virus was dismissed by many as "just a flu" (De Giorgio 2020, p. 1).

Such individuals would be classified as latent publics about Covid-19 because although they may be affected by the problem, they had not yet understood the risk or recognized their connection to it. Latent publics therefore may represent the most challenging subset of the population, at least from a health communication perspective, given that although they are affected by the problem they do not believe it to be an issue. The challenge for health communicators, then, is to devise campaigns, messages, and tools to help impact their perceptions of a problematic health-related situation. Finally, nonpublics are those who are neither affected by the problem, nor do they hold any perceptions about the issue at all.

Application

Although the STP was originally developed as a theory of public relations, the concepts explicated within the framework as well as the ability to segment publics into active/activist, aware, latent, and nonpublics has led to the application of the theory to several health-related contexts. A key variable of interest among health and risk communication scholars has been the idea of level of involvement. For example, Avery (2010) examined the role of publics' involvement in health issues on their preferences for accessing health information and found that those reporting high involvement in health issues reported higher engagement with newspaper articles, magazines, and federal health agencies for health related information.

Similarly, Aldoory (2001) demonstrated the importance of involvement or issue relevance in determining the extent to which women paid attention to messages about health issues. She identified a set of factors affecting women's involvement with health messages. Tindall and Vardeman-Winter (2011), in their investigation of how women of color made sense of a heart disease campaign targeted at them, found that lack of cultural meaning-making factors contributed to a perceived lack of relevance, and a corresponding lack of involvement from women in the issue, thus reducing the efficacy of the campaign. Furthermore, Grunig and Ipes (1983) in examining the effectiveness of campaigns against drunk driving noted that such messages needed to go beyond merely providing publics with information about the problem; the campaigns also serve to establish relevance and reduce constraints in publics' pathways to solving the problem.

Appraisal

As one of the first publics-centered theories of public relations, the situational theory of publics has been a foundation on which much public relations theory building and scholarship has been built. However, the theory is not without limitations. First, the STP adopts a limited view of communicative behaviors as encompassing merely information seeking and processing (J.-N. Kim and Grunig 2011). For health contexts in particular, where publics' physical actions are considered most important, a clearer and more comprehensive conceptualization of communicative behavior is warranted (Aldoory and Sha 2007). Second, although the concept of the referent criterion was dropped from the theory, scholars have called for its reconceptualization and reintegration into the theory (e.g. J.-N. Kim, Ni and Sha 2008). Scholars have also noted the limits to the explanatory power of the STP due to its theoretical origins in economic decision-making and information use (J.-N. Kim and Grunig 2011). Such an assumption limits the scope of the kinds of communicative behaviors that may be explained using the theory. These and other limitations of the STP inspired the development of its successor, the situational theory of problem-solving.

The Situational Theory of Problem-Solving

The limitations of the situational theory of publics, as outlined above, prompted the rethinking and refining of the theory. Although several scholars over the years have contributed to the STP framework to increase its explanatory power (e.g. Aldoory 2001), it was not until J.-N. Kim and Grunig (2011) that a comprehensive successor to the STP, the situational theory of problem-solving (STOPS) was proposed. Like the STP, the STOPS, too, is a theory that explains how and why individuals communicate about problematic life situations. However, rather than being a theory of public relations, the STOPS is a more general theory of communication that explains a variety of different behaviors that individuals can engage in in the process of problem-solving. The central postulate of the STOPS is as follows: individuals who recognize a gap between their expected and experienced state, i.e. a problem, see few constraints in their path toward addressing said problem, and feel connected to the problem are motivated to do something about the problem, and engage in a variety of active and passive communicative behaviors in trying to address the problem. The section that follows articulates the theoretical origins of the STOPS, focusing particularly on the theoretical departures from the STP that the STOPS made in the articulation of this theory of communication.

Theoretical Origins of the Situational Theory of Problem-Solving

The STOPS in many ways adopts the theoretical underpinnings of its parent theory, the STP. Like the STP, the STOPS rejects the audience control paradigm of communication research and instead focuses on audience autonomy, viewing audiences as active communicators in their own right (J.-N. Kim and Krishna 2014). Furthermore, like the STP, the STOPS, too, considers communication as a variable rather a constant, as was the assumption of much economic theory building. Communication instead is a purposeful activity that one undertakes when faced with a problematic life situation (J.-N. Kim and Krishna 2014). The most significant departure between the STP and the STOPS is in the conceptual frame adopted by each of the two theories. While the STP was articulated as a theory of decision-making, the STOPS considers the focus of the theory as problem-solving (J.-N. Kim and Grunig 2011).

This conceptual shift from decision-making to problem-solving has important implications for the development of the theory. Envisaging individuals as problem-solvers rather than decision-makers broadens the scope of the communicative behaviors in which they may engage (J.-N. Kim and Grunig 2011). For decision-makers faced with choices, communicative behaviors would logically be limited to seeking out information about the various choices and make the best possible decision for themselves. However, rethinking the purpose of communication as coping with and solving a problem expands the horizons of what communicative behaviors could be explained as part of the theoretical framework. As social actors (vs. an economic actor making a decision), problem-solvers may not only seek information but also share such information with others and evaluate and select certain information over others as they try to cope with the problematic situation. Thus, this theoretical shift enables the explication of communicative behaviors beyond information seeking and attending as part of the situational theory.

Central Constructs of the Situational Theory of Problem-Solving

The shift in the theoretical focus of the situational theory from being one of economic decision-making to problem-solving warranted the redefinition of the existing concepts of the STP as well as the articulation of additional constructs to better explain the problem-solving process. In the sections that follow, the key changes in conceptualization advanced by the STOPS are articulated.

Communicative Action in Problem-Solving

The first key change to the parent theory advanced by the STOPS is the expansion of the communicative behaviors explained by the theory. Whereas decision-makers' communicative behaviors are limited to information seeking, problem-solvers' communicative behaviors are more varied. Not only do problem-solvers seek information, they also transmit information to others and select information from among a metaphorical sea of data to parse information they deem relevant and accurate (J.-N. Kim and Krishna 2014). Accordingly, as a complementary model to the STOPS framework, J.-N. Kim, Grunig, and Ni (2010) proposed communicative action in problem-solving (CAPS) to represent a range of communicative behaviors in which individuals may engage during the problem-solving process. The CAPS model comprises three information behaviors, i.e. information acquisition, information transmission, and information selection. Each of these three information behaviors consists of two dimensions, an active and a passive dimension, following Lippmann's (1925) view of publics as consisting of actors and spectators. Thus, the CAPS model includes six communicative actions that individuals engage in during the problem-solving process and serves as the dependent variable of the STOPS framework. Each of these communicative behaviors is discussed next.

The first set of behaviors captured by the CAPS is information acquisition, borrowing from Grunig's (1997) original conceptualization. Problem-solvers are likely to turn to external sources of information to better understand their problem and find applicable solutions, and engage in information acquisition. Information acquisition may manifest in the form of active information seeking, where problem-solvers actively look for issue-related information, or passive information attending, which refers to individuals' serendipitous acquisition of information without actually making an effort to do so. It is important to note that information seeking and attending, indeed all active and passive behaviors discussed herein, are not mutually exclusive. In fact, the presence of active information behaviors presumes the presence of passive behaviors, but not vice versa.

The second set of information behaviors that make up the CAPS is information selection, which consists of active information forefending and passive information permitting. Information forefending refers to problem-solvers' active acceptance or rejection of certain types of sources of information. For example, a parent searching for information regarding childhood vaccines may come across a variety of different data from different sources trying to persuade them to either vaccinate or not vaccinate their children. The individual's acceptance of certain data and sources, say the CDC's recommendation of appropriate vaccine schedules over a "natural health" website's call to limit vaccines, would be an example of active information forefending. Passive information permitting represents individuals' acceptance of any and all information regarding the problem, as long as the individual deems them relevant to the problem at hand.

The third and final set of information behaviors captured by the CAPS is information transmission, which consists of active information forwarding and passive information sharing. A powerful addition to the situational theory, information transmission helps increase the ecological functionality of the conceptualization of communicative behaviors by presuming individuals not just as information consumers but also information providers (J.-N. Kim and Krishna 2014). As social actors, individuals are situated among other social actors to whom they may be motivated to transmit information that they have come across for a variety of reasons (see Krishna and Kim 2020). Such communicative actions are accounted for in the CAPS in the form of active information forwarding, where individuals communicate their findings in the problem-solving process to others unprompted, and passive information sharing, wherein problem-solvers provide information to others when asked to do so.

Antecedents of CAPS

In addition to expanding the scope of communicative behaviors explained by the theory, the STOPS also served to refine, redefine, and revisit the antecedents of the CAPS. Specifically, whereas constraint recognition was retained as defined by the STP, J.-N. Kim and Grunig (2011) proposed a redefinition of problem recognition and a reconceptualization of level of involvement to involvement recognition. The STOPS also reintroduced the referent criterion as a predictor of CAPS, and introduced a motivational mediator between the three perceptual variables and CAPS. All of these constructs are explicated next.

First, the STOPS proposed a redefinition of Grunig's (1997) original conceptualization of problem recognition. While problem recognition was originally defined as a state in which "people detect that something should be done about a situation and stop to think about what to do"

(Grunig 1997, p. 10), the STOPS defines problem recognition as "one's perception that something is missing and that there is no immediately applicable solution to it" (J.-N. Kim and Grunig 2011, p. 11). Problem recognition, then, is a perceptual problem that follows an individual's realization of a gap between expected and experienced states. For example, upon learning of a family member's cancer diagnosis one may want to know about treatment options but may not have the requisite medical knowledge to gain access to these options. Such a gap will trigger problem recognition about cancer treatment options, and if the other perceptual conditions are met, further lead to motivation and communicative action about cancer treatment options. This new definition omits the "stop to think about it" aspect of Grunig's (1997) original definition, because situational theorists posit that the extent to which one is motivated about a problem is influenced by more perceptual factors than just problem recognition (see J.-N. Kim and Krishna 2014).

Next, J.-N. Kim and Grunig (2011) reconceptualized Grunig's (1997) level of involvement, or "the extent to which people connect themselves with a situation" (p. 10), as involvement recognition, an individual's perceived involvement or closeness to the problem rather than an actual connection. The reconceptualization of involvement as a perception may help explain the varied responses from governments around the world during the initial stages of the Covid-19 pandemic. Whereas some governments were quick to adopt mitigation plans such as social distancing and lockdowns, others, including the United States, did not mandate such measures perhaps due to a lack of perceived involvement in the problem. Such a reconceptualization not only parallels the definitional structure of the other two antecedents, i.e. problem recognition and constraint recognition, but also shifts focus to the importance of individuals' perceptions of closeness rather than actual closeness, which may be harder to operationalize.

The next change between the STP and the STOPS is the reintroduction of the referent criterion. Although early tests of the STP failed to establish significant relationships between the referent criterion and communicative behaviors, leading to its elimination from the STP framework, the expansion of the scope of communicative behaviors captured in the STOPS warranted a revisiting of the potential role of the referent criterion. Referent criterion refers to existing frames of knowledge that an individual can draw upon based on previous problem-solving experiences. These existing frames form the cognitive lens through which an individual may seek, select, and transmit information they collect during the problem-solving process (J.-N. Kim and Krishna 2014). For example, an individual's bad physiological reaction to the influenza vaccine may translate to a knowledge frame that they may carry forward when seeking, evaluating, and transmitting about childhood vaccines, even though the scientific connection between the influenza vaccine and childhood vaccines may be tenuous at best.

Finally, the STOPS introduced a motivational mediator between the three perceptual variables, i.e. problem, constraint, and involvement recognition, and the CAPS. This mediator, which J.-N. Kim and Grunig (2011) called situational motivation in problem-solving, sums up and carries forward the effects of the three perceptual variables on to the CAPS. Situational motivation in problem-solving is defined as "the extent to which a person stops to think about, is curious about, or wants more understanding of a problem" (J.-N. Kim and Grunig 2011, p. 16). As is evident from this conceptual definition, situational motivation in problem-solving represents the "stop to think about it" part of the original definition of problem recognition, and is predicted not just by problem recognition, but also constraint and involvement recognition. The introduction of situational motivation in problem-solving has important implications for research and practice thanks to its role as a mediator between perceptions and behaviors. Indeed, scholars have used situational motivation as a proxy for the three perceptual predictors to segment publics (e.g. J.-N. Kim, Shen and Morgan 2011; Krishna 2017), identified situational and cross-situational antecedents to situational motivation (e.g. S. Kim, Krishna, and Dhanesh 2019), and noted behavioral outcomes of such motivation (Krishna 2018).

Application

As with the STP, the STOPS, too, has been applied and tested using a variety of different health contexts. Scholars have used the STOPS framework to better understand communicative behaviors about health issues such as organ donation (e.g. J.-N. Kim, Shen, and Morgan 2011), food safety (e.g. J.-N. Kim et al. 2012), anti-vaccine activism (McKeever et al. 2016; Krishna 2017), cervical cancer prevention (e.g. Yoo, Kim, and Lee, 2018), and coping with chronic diseases (e.g. J.-N. Kim and S. Lee 2014) among many others. These investigations have taken several different paths to utilizing the theory to advance knowledge about health issues. Some scholars have replicated and expanded the STOPS model to incorporate other situational and cross-situational explanations for communicative action in problem-solving. For example, McKeever et al. (2016) found mothers' opposition for childhood vaccinations to be associated with communicative action in problem-solving. Similarly, Krishna (2018) found that anti-vaccine attitudes positively predicted situational motivation in problem-solving, active communicative behaviors, and intention not to vaccinate. Shen, Xu and Wang (2019) also demonstrated the utility of the STOPS in understanding health-related issues by modeling individuals' online information acquisition behaviors about cancer. Furthermore, Yan et al. (2018) examined people's perceptions of diet and nutrition, and integrated affective risk perception with the perceptual predictors of the STOPS to predict situational motivation and behavioral health outcomes.

Other scholars have made use of the STOPS framework to segment individuals into active, aware, latent, and nonpublics to understand the similarities and differences between subgroups. J.-N. Kim et al. (2011), for example, segmented publics about organ donation into subgroups and found active publics to be the most active communicators about the issue. They also found that those highly motivated about organ donation were also motivated about other health-related issues, coining the term problem-chain recognition effect (J.-N. Kim et al. 2011). Krishna (2017) provided further insight into active/activist publics by identifying misinformed, vocal subsets of activist publics about childhood vaccines termed lacuna publics. Using situational motivation as a proxy for perceptual predictors, Krishna (2017) identified lacuna publics as those with extreme anti-vaccine attitudes, low factual knowledge, and high motivation. Such individuals were found to be more vocal than nonlacuna publics, echoing McKeever et al.'s (2016) study.

Conclusion

As arguably one of the first publics-centered theories of public relations, the situational theory of publics has enjoyed a long history of testing, expansion, critique, and criticism. Its value in providing theoretically grounded explanations for a variety of different social issues, including health-related issues, has been demonstrated by numerous scholars over the years. Its successor, the situational theory of problem-solving, too, has found application in explicating several health-related issues as described in this chapter. However, a good theory never stagnates, and as the nature of publics and communication evolve, so too must the situational theories. As they stand now, the situational theories provide a powerful theoretically grounded mechanism to examine the nature, perceptions, motivations and behaviors of publics, particularly as related to health issues.

References

Aldoory, L. (2001). Making health communications meaningful for women: Factors that influence involvement. *Journal of Public Relations Research*, *13*, 163–185. doi:10.1207/S1532754XJPRR1302_3

Aldoory, L., & Sha, B. L. (2007). The situational theory of publics: Practical applications, methodological challenges, and theoretical horizons. In E. L. Toth (Ed.), *The future of excellence in public relations and communication management: Challenges for the next generation*, (pp. 339–355). Mahwah, NJ: Erlbaum.

Avery, E. (2010). Contextual and audience moderators of channel selection and message reception of public health information in routine and crisis situations. *Journal of Public Relations Research*, *22*, 378–403. doi:10.1080/10627261003801404

Chay-Nemeth, C. (2001). Revisiting publics: A critical archaeology of publics in the Thai HIV/AIDS issue. *Journal of Public Relations Research*, *13*, 127–161. doi:10.1207/S1532754XJPRR1302_2

Chen, Y. R. R., Hung-Baesecke, C. J. F., & Kim, J.-N. (2017). Identifying active hot-issue communicators and subgroup identifiers: Examining the situational theory of problem solving. *Journalism & Mass Communication Quarterly*, *94*, 124–147. doi:10.1177/1077699016629371

Clarke, P., & Kline, F. G. (1974). Media effects reconsidered: Some new strategies for communication research. *Communication Research*, *1*, 224–270. doi:10.1177/009365027400100205

De Giorgio, A. (2020). COVID-19 is not just a flu. Learn from Italy and act now. *Travel Medicine and Infectious Disease*, 1–4. doi:10.1016/j.tmaid.2020.101655

Dewey, J. (1927). *The public and its problems*. Chicago, IL: Swallow.

Dewey, J. (1938). *Experience and education*. New York, NY: Macmillan.

Grunig, J. E. (1968). *Information, entrepreneurship, and economic development: A study of the decision making processes of Colombian Latifundistas (Unpublished doctoral dissertation)*. University of Wisconsin, Madison.

Grunig, J. E. (1997). A situational theory of publics: Conceptual history, recent challenges and new research. In D. Moss, T. MacManus, & D. Verčič (Eds.), *Public relations research: An international perspective* (pp. 3–46). London, England: International Thompson Business Press.

Grunig, J. E., & Disbrow, J. A. (1977). Developing a probabilistic model for communications decision making. *Communication Research*, *4*, 145–168. doi:10.1177/009365027700400202

Grunig, J. E., & Hunt, T. (1984). *Managing public relations*. New York, NY: Holt, Rinehart and Winston.

Grunig, J. E., & Ipes, D. A. (1983). The anatomy of a campaign against drunk driving. *Public Relations Review*, *9*, 36–52. doi:10.1016/S0363-8111(83)80004-6

Hallahan, K. (2000). Inactive publics: The forgotten publics in public relations. *Public Relations Review*, *26*, 499–515. doi:10.1016/S0363-8111(00)00061-8

Kim, J.-N., & Grunig, J. E. (2011). Problem solving and communicative action: A situational theory of problem solving. *Journal of Communication, 61*, 120–149. doi:10.1111/j.1460-2466.2010.01529.x

Kim, J.-N., Grunig, J. E., & Ni, L. (2010). Reconceptualizing the communicative action of publics: Acquisition, selection, and transmission of information in problematic situations. *International Journal of Strategic Communication, 4*, 126–154. doi:10.1080/15531181003701913

Kim, J.-N., Hung-Baesecke, C.-J., Yang, S-U., & Grunig, J. E. (2013). A strategic management approach to reputation, relationships, and publics: The research heritage of the Excellence Theory. In C. Carroll (Ed.), *Handbook of communication and corporate reputation* (pp. 197–212). New York: Wiley Blackwell.

Kim, J.-N., & Krishna, A. (2014). Publics and lay informatics: A review of the situational theory of problem solving. *Annals of the International Communication Association, 38*, 71–105. doi:10.1080/23808985.2014.11679159

Kim, J. N., & Lee, S. (2014). Communication and cybercoping: Coping with chronic illness through communicative action in online support networks. *Journal of Health Communication, 19*, 775–794. doi:10.1080/10810730.2013.864724

Kim, J.-N., Ni, L., Kim, S. H., & Kim, J. R. (2012). What makes people hot? Applying the situational theory of problem solving to hot-issue publics. *Journal of Public Relations Research, 24*, 144–164. doi:10.1080/1062726X.2012.626133

Kim, J.-N., Ni, L., & Sha, B. L. (2008). Breaking down the stakeholder environment: Explicating approaches to the segmentation of publics for public relations research. *Journalism & Mass Communication Quarterly, 85*, 751–768. doi:10.1177/107769900808500403

Kim, J.-N., Shen, H., & Morgan, S. E. (2011). Information behaviors and problem chain recognition effect: Applying situational theory of problem solving in organ donation issues. *Health Communication, 26*, 171–184. doi:10.1080/10410236.2010.544282

Kim, S., Krishna, A., & Dhanesh, G. (2019). Economics or ethics? Exploring the role of CSR expectations in explaining consumers' perceptions, motivations, and communication behaviors about corporate misconduct. *Public Relations Review, 45*, 76–87. doi:10.1016/j.pubrev.2018.10.011

Krishna, A. (2017). Motivation with misinformation: Conceptualizing lacuna individuals and publics as knowledge-deficient, issue-negative activists. *Journal of Public Relations Research, 29*, 176–193. doi:10.1080/1062726X.2017.1363047

Krishna, A. (2018). Poison or prevention? Understanding the linkages between vaccine-negative individuals' knowledge deficiency, motivations, and active communication behaviors. *Health Communication, 33*, 1088–1096. doi:10.1080/10410236.2017.1331307

Krishna, A., & Kim, S. (2020). Exploring customers' situational and word-of-mouth motivations in corporate misconduct. *Public Relations Review, 46*, 1–8. doi:10.1016/j.pubrev.2020.101892

Lippmann, W. (1925). *The phantom public*. New York: Harcourt Brace Jovanovich.

McKeever, B. W., McKeever, R., Holton, A. E., & Li, J. Y. (2016). Silent majority: Childhood vaccinations and antecedents to communicative action. *Mass Communication and Society, 19*, 476–498. doi:10.1080/15205436.2016.1148172

McQuail, D. (1997). *Audience analysis*. Thousand Oaks, CA: Sage.

Ni, L., & Kim, J.-N. (2009). Classifying publics: Communication behaviors and problem-solving characteristics in controversial issues. *International Journal of Strategic Communication, 3*, 217–241. doi:10.1080/15531180903221261

Shen, H., Xu, J., & Wang, Y. (2019). Applying situational theory of problem solving in cancer information seeking: A cross-sectional analysis of 2014 HINTS survey. *Journal of Health Communication, 24*, 165–173. doi:10.1080/10810 730.2019.1587111

Tindall, N. T., & Vardeman-Winter, J. (2011). Complications in segmenting campaign publics: Women of color explain their problems, involvement, and constraints in reading heart disease communication. *Howard Journal of Communications, 22*, 280–301. doi:10.1080/10646175.2011.590407

Vardeman, J. E., & Aldoory, L. (2008). A qualitative study of how women make meaning of contradictory media messages about the risks of eating fish. *Health Communication, 23*, 282–291. doi:10.1080/10410230802056396

Yan, J., Wei, J., Zhao, D., Vinnikova, A., Li, L., & Wang, S. (2018). Communicating online diet-nutrition information and influencing health behavioral intention: The role of risk perceptions, problem recognition, and situational motivation. *Journal of Health Communication, 23*, 624–633. doi:10.1080/1 0810730.2018.1500657

Yoo, S. W., Kim, J., & Lee, Y. (2018). The effect of health beliefs, media perceptions, and communicative behaviors on health behavioral intention: An integrated health campaign model on social media. *Health Communication, 33*, 32–40. doi:10.1080/10410236.2016.1242033

13

Theories of Uncertainty

Austin S. Babrow, Marianne S. Matthias, Sarah M. Parsloe, and Anne M. Stone

For over 2500 years, commentators have observed that uncertainty constitutes a substantial challenge in communication about health and illness. Hippocrates' first aphorism characterized the problem and offered a solution: "Life is short, and Art long; the crisis fleeting; experience perilous, and decision difficult. The physician must not only be prepared to do what is right himself (sic), but also to make the patient, the attendants, and externals cooperate" (Hippocrates," n.d.). As Babrow (2020) commented:

> This marvel of brevity has taught physicians three vital lessons. First, it emphasized the treacherous uncertainties of healthcare. Second, it recognized that communication is essential in dealing with these perils. Third, it encoded paternal control in the genetics of the communicative response to uncertainty and in the doctor–patient relationship borne out of these interactions. (p. 827)

Medical practice has undergone revolutionary change in the ensuing millennia, but the challenge of communication and uncertainty has persisted and even grown (Babrow 2020). Moreover, we have come to

Health Communication Theory, First Edition. Edited by Teresa L. Thompson and Peter J. Schulz.
© 2021 John Wiley & Sons, Inc. Published 2021 by John Wiley & Sons, Inc.

understand that uncertainties pervade not only illness and healthcare, but important areas of health, as well (e.g. Matthias and Babrow 2007; Vos, Anthony, and O'Hair 2014).

Despite this long history, systematic studies of uncertainty and health communication are a recent development. Mishel's (1988, 1990) uncertainty in illness model crystalized awareness of the challenges of uncertainty in nursing practice, but it emphasized psychological processes and considered communication only tangentially. In 1984, Katz published an exceptionally insightful book that encapsulated physician communication about uncertainty in *The Silent World of Doctor and Patient*. Still, work on communication and uncertainty was relatively rare (Babrow 2020, figs. 2–4).

Albrecht and Adelmans's (1987) provocative argument that social support is fundamentally a matter of uncertainty reduction stimulated interest in the relationship between communication and uncertainty in the context of health. Since that work appeared, research on uncertainty and health communication has flourished. Four models, in particular, have come to prominence in the health communication literature: harm reduction, uncertainty management theory, the theory of motivated information management, and problematic integration theory. This chapter reviews these four theories.

Harm Reduction

Origins and Central Concepts

Much of the earliest work on communication and uncertainty was based on the idea that uncertainty must be reduced or eliminated (e.g. Albrecht and Adelman 1987; Berger and Calabrese 1975). Insistence on certainty is perhaps nowhere more evident than in abstinence-only approaches to risky behavior. These approaches are predicated on an extreme intolerance of uncertainty in at least two senses. First, they assume that absolute certainty, in the form of complete cessation of harmful behavior, is both possible and desirable. Second, when it comes to risky behavior, they assume that promotion of anything short of complete abstinence is both pragmatically and morally suspect. In short, when it comes to patently risky behavior, absolutism is the only acceptable policy in this school of thinking.

In contrast, the harm reduction (HR) framework deals with uncertainty by reframing risky behaviors as potentially beneficial, or at least less harmful. HR emerged when, beginning in the 1920s, healthcare workers and researchers began to recognize that many unhealthy behaviors (alcohol and drug abuse) were not only recalcitrant, but that discouraging these behaviors could increase harm (Hilton et al. 2001). HR neither condones nor condemns harmful behaviors, but respects the individual's capacity to make rational, informed choices (Hilton et al. 2001). This approach even acknowledges that harmful behaviors such as illicit drug use can potentially be beneficial and appropriate (Marlatt 1998). For these reasons, in 1987 the Canadian government officially adopted harm reduction as the framework for Canada's National Drug Strategy, and Vancouver opened the country's first official needle exchange (Hilton et al. 2001). The first International Conference on the Reduction of Drug-Related Harm, held in 1990, and the establishment of Harm Reduction International in 1996 helped to solidify the HR movement (Hilton et al 2001).

HR is rooted in principles of social justice and addresses discrimination by seeking to remove judgment and stigma and to ensure that no one is excluded from services because of drug use, race, gender, gender identity, sexual orientation, choice of work, or economic status (Harm Reduction International 2017). The HR approach deliberately avoids stigmatizing language (e.g. "drug abusers," "addicts"; Harm Reduction International). Moreover, HR stands in direct contrast with abstinence views of drug use and other harmful behaviors. Abstinence models favor maintaining illicit drug laws and treatment programs and increasing law enforcement to combat drug use (Hilton et al. 2001). Proponents of the abstinence model cite the dramatic decrease of illegal drug use in the US after tougher drug laws were passed in the early twentieth century (Hilton et al. 2001). In contrast to the view of drug dependence as harmful, HR advocates accept that some harm is inevitable, and they argue that employing harsh, prohibitionist approaches undermines individual agency and autonomy, ultimately leading to failure to manage risky behavior (Hilton et al. 2001).

HR is thus a perspective which argues that efforts to achieve absolute certainty in the form of complete cessation of harmful behavior are unlikely to be successful and, particularly when combined with moralistic judgments, may exacerbate risky behavior. As an alternative, the HR perspective accepts the irreducible uncertainty of risky behavior. HR advocates contend that this acceptance is key to strategies that can reduce harm. In turn, these advocates claim that harm is reduced beyond anything attainable by abstinence only programs by instead creating and promoting an infrastructure that facilitates less risky behavior (e.g. needle exchanges, methadone maintenance). To bolster these communication and policy strategies, HR practitioners advocate for and promote easy access to services and treatments consistent with the ideal of reducing harm.

Applications

Evidence from a variety of contexts supports the effectiveness of HR approaches. HR has been shown to reduce HIV infection among intravenous drug users, as well as to decrease incidence of other drug-related problems, including crime, diseases (viral hepatitis, tuberculosis), and accidental death (Hilton et al. 2001). Needle exchange programs and safe drug injection sites consistently lead to significant reductions in needle sharing and reuse, overdose, improper disposal of used needles, and death, and to increases in participation in addiction treatment programs (Logan and Marlatt 2010). HR approaches have been used for individuals with opioid use disorder (OUD); medication assisted therapy, in which an "opioid substitute" such as buprenorphine or methadone is prescribed to patients with OUD, has been shown to be effective in reducing illicit opioid use, HIV risk behaviors, criminal activity, and opioid-related death (Logan and Marlatt 2010; Sordo et al. 2017). In the context of teen alcohol consumption, HR programs have led to significant short-term, but not long-term, reductions in alcohol use, in contrast to abstinence-based programs such as DARE (Drug Abuse Resistance Education), which have led to either no change or potentially harmful effects (Logan and Marlatt 2010).

From a health communication perspective, HR involves understanding why individuals engage in risky behaviors, and constructing messages that help them to reduce health risks associated with these behaviors (Haas and Mattson 2014). Communication-oriented HR approaches include providing information about risks and effects of controlled and illegal substances in a neutral, nonjudgmental manner (Abelman 2017; Geist-Martin, Ray, and Sharf 2003); tailoring health promotion efforts about alcohol use in college students toward reducing excessive drinking of hard liquor and participation in drinking games (Eversman 2015); and encouraging someone who uses drugs to consult mental health services, not to prevent further drug use, but in an effort to facilitate safer use (Abelman 2017). HR health communication approaches can include providing advice on reducing dangers of drug use during pregnancy or breastfeeding (Geist-Martin et al. 2003), and HR approaches have been advocated as a means to improve the effectiveness of HIV test counseling (Mattson 2000).

Appraisal

In sum, HR is a pragmatic, non-judgmental approach toward risky behaviors aimed at reducing potential harm of these behaviors in a manner that respects individual agency and autonomy. Evidence indicates that this framework can be effective, particularly in contrast to abstinence messages. However, HR applications have limitations and criticisms. The approach has been criticized for its use in tobacco consumption, given questions about whether there is a "safe" level of tobacco use (Eversman 2015). In addition, HR has come under scrutiny because, for drug use, it does not address the underlying problem of addiction. With increasing recognition of addiction as a legitimate disease rather than a moral failing, this criticism may gain ground, as many (but not all) HR approaches do not attempt to treat addiction. HR has also been criticized for ignoring moral imperatives altogether while permitting and even facilitating immoral behaviors (Hathaway 2001; Keane 2003). In addition, rather than being a fully specified theory espousing ideas of autonomy and respect, HR has been criticized for being simply a grouping of various practices and goals with disparate outcomes (Keane 2003). Finally, whereas HR implicitly accepts the uncertainty that arises when interventions let go of the unrealistic and potentially counterproductive goal of complete abstinence, three prominent frameworks explicitly theorize about uncertainty: uncertainty management theory, the theory of motivated information management, and problematic integration theory. These are reviewed in what follows.

Uncertainty Management Theory

Origins and Central Concepts

Drawing on concepts elaborated in Mishel's (1988, 1990) uncertainty in illness theory (UIT), Dale Brashers developed his uncertainty management theory (UMT) to acknowledge that uncertainty is not always undesirable in health-related contexts. Rather, UMT posits that, depending on a person's emotional response to and appraisal of uncertainty, he or she may be motivated to reduce, maintain, or increase their uncertainty (Brashers 2001, 2007). In some cases, an individual might perceive uncertainty as undesirable or threatening. For example, a patient might seek to reduce her uncertainty about whether a particular treatment is likely to be successful so that she might be more confident about her treatment decision. Alternatively, an individual might view uncertainty as an opportunity – a way to avoid confronting the idea that unpleasant, painful, and/or life-threatening experiences are imminent. Thus, according to UMT, individuals may elect to maintain or increase their sense of uncertainty when doing so allows the person to experience hope in an otherwise hopeless situation (Ford, Babrow, and Stohl 1996).

As the above examples suggest, UMT has frequently been conceptualized in terms of information seeking and avoiding (Hogan and Brashers 2009). Indeed, individuals may seek or avoid interactions with particular others (e.g. friends, family members, other patients, health-care providers) – as well as gather information from websites, pamplets, newspapers, and other sources – in an attempt to reduce, preserve, or maintain their uncertainty (Brasher set al.2002). For instance, a patient who appraises cancer-related uncertainty negatively might seek interactions with health experts who can provide statistical information about chances for survival. In contrast, a patient who appraises cancer-related uncertainty positively might seek support from friends and family members who participate in framing cancer as inherently unpredictable and, thus, potentially "beatable."

However, work with UMT has revealed that individuals may face dilemmas in managing uncertainty through information seeking and avoidance, particularly when they encounter new, conflicting information as they draw on multiple sources of information over time (e.g. Rains 2014). Additional dilemmas arise from the collaborative nature of information management, especially when individuals struggle to coordinate their goals (Brashers, Goldsmith, and Hsieh 2002).

Applications

UMT has been applied in a variety of health-related contexts and has recently been used as a foundation for scale development (e.g. Carcioppolo, Yang, and Yang 2016). This is not surprising given that much of the work using UMT has been qualitative, focused on articulating experiences of uncertainty in health contexts including HIV/AIDS (e.g. Brashers et al. 2000), cancer (e.g. Miller 2014; Donovan et al. 2015), organ transplantation (e.g. Martin et al. 2010), and Alzheimer's disease (e.g. Stone and Jones 2009). Carcioppolo and colleagues (2016) drew from qualitative interview data from previous studies (e.g. Brashers et al. 2000; Miller 2014), as well as content analysis work focused on uncertainty management (e.g. Barbour et al. 2012), to develop and validate four scales to measure uncertainty. Specifically, these scales measure "the desire to (1) seek information to reduce uncertainty, (2) seek information to increase uncertainty, (3) avoid information to maintain uncertainty, and (4) avoid information perceived as insufficient" (p. 979). These validated measures of uncertainty preferences allow researchers to measure the complex experiences of uncertainty and provide an important opportunity for future research using UMT.

Appraisal

Clearly, UMT has been applied to a variety of contexts, facilitating cross-context theorizing about sources of uncertainty and the strategies that individuals use in response to uncertainty. UMT allows researchers to explore the factors that shape responses to experiencing uncertainty. UMT also formed the foundation for a recent articulation of a peer-led uncertainty management intervention for people recently diagnosed with HIV (Brashers et al. 2017). This educational intervention focused on helping people newly infected with HIV learn about HIV, treatments, and resources. The intervention also focused on developing communication skills to use when working with healthcare providers and coordinating care with members of their social network. Study results suggest that those who participated in the intervention (versus those in the control group) reported better outcomes related to illness uncertainty, depression, and satisfaction with social support. Although the spirit of health communication is often driven by praxis, the results are largely descriptive and not always easily applied. Brashers et al. (2017) give applied researchers an excellent example of a theory-driven intervention that produced positive results for the target population.

UMT also opens avenues for researching the dilemmas that arise in cases where interactants appraise and respond to uncertainty differently, employing potentially incompatible uncertainty management strategies. As such, UMT might serve as a useful framework for exploring experiences of conflict that emerge as dyads (e.g. doctors and their patients) and groups (e.g. families, friend groups) attempt to manage uncertainty collaboratively.

As noted above, applications of UMT have mostly focused on information seeking and avoidance behaviors as the primary means through which individuals reduce, maintain, or increase uncertainty. Such a focus may overlook additional strategies – particularly strategies that involve altering a person's initial appraisal of uncertainty. Additionally, the concept of "management" in UMT suggests that responses to uncertainty are purposeful, logical, and within a persons' control. As such, applications of UMT may not attend to the ways in which attempts to manage uncertainty are shaped – and sometimes undermined – by unsolicited information and unexpected encounters with others. In other words, while UMT theorizes about how individuals attempt to exert a sense of control during experiences of uncertainty, it does not explore how they respond when these attempts at control are disrupted. This critique points to the importance of considering the ways that making sense of and responding to uncertainty is a collaborative – often reactive and improvisational – process.

Moreover, it is tempting for scholars working with UMT to think about uncertainty as a singular experience, rather than thinking in terms of uncertain*ies*. While some applications of UMT have sought to enumerate the multiple sources of uncertainty that individuals attempt to manage in a given health context, few have considered the ways in which these sources of uncertainty are overlapping and interwoven, complicating efforts to "manage" a coherent response. In the following model, the authors attempted not so much to explicate the interweaving of multiple uncertainties and the resulting challenges to their management. Rather the next theory focuses on the concept of information management as a means of uncertainty management.

The Theory of Motivated Information Management

Origins and Central Concepts

Afifi and Weiner published the first statement of the theory of motivated information management (TMIM) in 2004. Since then the model has enjoyed significant attention, application, and further development. The TMIM is rooted in the post-positivist tradition of "bounded rationality." In this perspective, human decision and action are guided by the human motivation to maximize subjectively expected utility within constraints such as available information, time, and motivational influences. Afifi (2015) has written that the theory was intended to extend Brashers's UMT and problematic integration theory (discussed below) by specifying the cognitive processes that occur when an individual experiences uncertainty about an important issue and considers seeking information from another person. Collectively, these cognitive processes constitute information management (IM).

IM is a potentially recursive three-stage process that begins with an interpretive phase. In it, the individual recognizes that their level of experienced uncertainty differs from their desired level of uncertainty.

Any perceived uncertainty discrepancy in turn gives rise to anxiety proportional to the magnitude of the discrepancy (Afifi and Weiner 2004), and to other emotional reactions, particularly "fear, disgust, jealousy, envy, and hope" (Afifi and Morse 2009, p. 94).[1] The greater the magnitude of anxiety and other emotional reactions, the greater the likelihood that IM will move to a second phase: evaluation.

In the evaluation stage, the individual appraises potential information seeking behavior in terms of perceived outcomes and efficacy (Afifi 2015). Reflecting its roots in rational choice theory, both informational outcomes and other outcomes of the process of seeking information (e.g. effects on seeker-source relationship) are judged for their likelihood of occurrence and their positive or negative utility. In turn, these outcome expectancies (OE) shape the individual's efficacy expectations (EE). More specifically, OE are hypothesized to influence one or more of four particular efficacy judgments: the individual appraises (i) their ability to complete the necessary information seeking communication tasks, (ii) the potential source's ability to provide the desired information, (iii) source honesty, and (iv) the seeker's ability to cope with information they might receive. The theory predicts that individuals are motivated to seek information to the extent that (i) they expect positive outcomes will exceed negative outcomes, and (ii) they expect to be able to obtain and manage the new information.

Depending on the results of evaluation, in the third stage of IM, decision, the individual chooses among three major options: to seek information, forgo or avoid information-seeking, or reappraise previous judgments (i.e. uncertainty discrepancy, outcome and/or efficacy assessments). In some writings, this decision is based on the direct effects of both OE and EE, as well as indirect effects of OE on EE (e.g. Afifi 2015; Afifi and Wiener 2004), whereas other writings posit only indirect effects of OE on decision via their effect on EE (e.g. Afifi and Weiner 2006; Fowler and Afifi 2011).

If the individual seeks information and approaches some potential source, the TMIM theorizes that the source, recognizing this intent, goes through similar processes of evaluation and decision. That is, the source appraises the likelihood and value of various outcomes of providing information to the seeker and perceived efficacy (i.e. whether the source has the information sought, can communicate it effectively, and can manage the consequences of sharing information with the seeker). The decision to provide or withhold information follows from these appraisals.

Applications

The TMIM has been tested in a number of health-related contexts. Two years after rolling out the model, Afifi and Weiner (2006) tested it in the context of seeking information from a partner about the partner's sexual health as a means of preventing the spread of sexually transmitted disease. Support for the model was mixed, and the findings of no or very small effects of outcome and efficacy expectancies on seeking information from partners about their sexual history and health were particularly noteworthy.

Afifi et al. (2006; also see Morse et al. 2009) studied information seeking and willingness to talk to one's family about their views on organ donation. Findings were generally consistent with the model, with perhaps the major exception that outcome expectancies had no direct effect on the main information management variable in this study (i.e. the directness of talk with family).

Fowler and Afifi (2011) tested the model in the context of adult children's conversations with elderly parents about care as parents age, including measures of two different affective reactions to uncertainty discrepancy. One, anxiety, was the sole affective reaction posited in the original model, as laid out by Afifi and Weiner (2004). However, drawing on the more extensive consideration of affective reactions posited in Afifi and Morse's refined model, Fowler and Afifi also included happiness as an emotional reaction to uncertainty discrepancy. Results were generally consistent with expectations. The model has also been used to study information management in domains such as family health history (Hovick 2014; Rauscher and Hesse 2014), illicit drug use (Morse et al. 2013), and spouse's preferences for end of life care (Rafferty et al. 2015).

Appraisal

The TMIM is among the most elaborate available descriptions of the cognitive and affective precursors of information seeking. Its foundation in the literature on rational behavior and cognitive processes provides both substantial conceptual grounding and solid methodological guidance. Not surprisingly, the model has been quite attractive to studies of information seeking across a growing range of contexts, and the empirical support has been generally congenial. Afifi (2015) concluded that evidence concerning the effect of OE on EE, and the influence of specific EE on decisions has been inconsistent. While this may be due to methodological variations, another possibility is simply that different contexts give rise to variations in the causal structure motivating information seeking.

In any case, the theory also has been used in interesting theory-building efforts, including Afifi and Morse's (2009) incorporation of appraisal theory to flesh out the emotional influences of uncertainty discrepancy, as well as its contribution to Kahlor's (2010) planned risk information seeking model, and syntheses with literatures on shared decision-making (Mikesell et al. 2016), religiosity (Morse et al. 2009), and social ties (Lewis and Martinez 2014).

Perhaps the most substantial empirical limitation is the paucity of efforts to test the model in the context of interaction, particularly its view of information source behavior and unfolding information-related behavior. Conceptually, Afifi (2015) has called for more attention to neurological and biological processes, but another approach to developing the model might be to pay closer attention to meanings. As it stands, writing about the model has uncritically accepted Brashers' (2001) gloss of various meanings of uncertainty. This issue becomes clearer in the context of problematic integration theory.

Problematic Integration Theory

Origins and Central Concepts

Problematic integration (PI) theory (Babrow 1992, 2001, 2016) grew out of interest in communication and uncertainty, which it shares with UMT and TMIM. It has, however, approached this relationship differently than do the latter perspectives. UMT and TMIM are both explicitly post-positivist perspectives, and both conceptualize uncertainty as a psychological state that sets in motion psychological processes, which in turn cause communication behavior in the form of either information seeking or avoidance. And, for both theories, these behaviors are intended to reduce, maintain, or increase uncertainty. By contrast, Babrow (2001, 2016) founded PI theory on a critique of strictly psychological perspectives, offering an alternative social constructionist conception of communication and uncertainty.

Babrow (1992, 2001, 2016) argued that people are continually constructing the meaning of their lives in the form of beliefs and evaluations. According to PI theory, communication is the constructive process that forms, maintains, and transforms these meanings. Communication and meaning-making are straightforward (non-problematic) when beliefs and evaluations are consistent: when what we want to be true is likely or certain, or when what we do not want to be so is unlikely or impossible. However, when beliefs (expectations) and evaluations (desires) are inconsistent, people struggle to construct meaning. These struggles take several forms: *Uncertainty* (i.e. when we are not sure what to believe or expect) about something quite valuable is one of four main forms of problematic meaning. In addition, meaning and understanding are troubled when we face substantial *ambivalence* (e.g. when what we want comes with considerable costs), *inconsistent or divergent expectations and desires* (i.e. when we believe that we are unlikely to realize significant desires or avoid substantial unpleasantness), or the *impossibility* of realizing desire (or what we dread is certain). Thus, in PI theory, uncertainty, ambivalence, divergent expectations and desires, and impossibility are the four major forms of troublesome or problematic meanings.

PI theory conceives of health communication as largely the construction and reconstruction of uncertainty, ambivalence, diverging expectation and desire, and impossibility. For example, health communication is essential to understanding health risks, illness diagnosis, treatment costs and benefits, and physical loss. Through communication, we work out bodily material understandings, as well as interweaving identity, relational, and other psychosocial meanings. Moreover, the theory focuses not on the meaning of any one message, but on the ongoing communicative construction of troubled, unsettling, unsettled understandings and lines of action.

PI theory is thus a more general perspective than UMT and TMIM, as it conceptualizes uncertainty as just one of several cardinal forms of troublesome meaning. In addition, PI research has excavated the nature of uncertainty, specifically, identified many of its distinctive forms, and studied the significance of these distinctions for the communicative construction of problematic meanings (e.g. Babrow 2001, 2016; Babrow, Kasch, and Ford 1998). Brashers (2001) used this research to formulate his own omnibus definition in explicating UMT: "uncertainty exists when details of situations are ambiguous, complex, unpredictable, or probabilistic; when information is unavailable or inconsistent; and when people feel insecure in their own state of knowledge or the state of knowledge in general" (Brashers 2001, p. 478). In turn, Afifi and Weiner (2004, p. 172) adopted this definition in their presentation of TMIM.

Beyond this definition, the distinctions in meanings of uncertainty play no explicit, systematic role in either UMT or TMIM. In contrast, PI researchers argue that, to understand the communicative construction of problematic meanings, we must attend carefully to the specific forms of uncertainty and other troublesome constellations of belief and desire, and particularly to the dynamics of their communicative formation and transformation through time. Focusing on these distinctions leads to claims that differ from those of the other theories. First, communication is not merely a source of information to be sought or avoided. Second, uncertainty is not merely "managed," or rationally controlled. Third, people do not deal with uncertainty only by maintaining it at its current level or ratcheting it up or down.

These ideas emerge when we explicitly and systematically disentangle the varied forms of troubled meanings and recognize that these meanings are worked out in unfolding communication processes. For instance, the meaning and aims of communication are quite different when we are ignorant of important information that we think others possess, in comparison to situations in which we believe that nobody knows what we wish to know (see Babrow 2020). As another example, communicative coping with ambivalence, such as when we accept that a given treatment is likely to be effective and to have unpleasant side-effects, is surely different than coping with suspicions about the motives or expertise of the care provider who delivers this information (see Gill and Morgan 2011, on ambivalence).

Further, as people communicate about problematic meanings, these meanings are likely to "chain" out or shift in their focus or configuration (see Babrow 2001). In other words, unlike the TMIM's static causal structure, PI researchers expect the focus or issue at the heart of troubled meanings at any one moment to shift to other issues as people work out the troubled/troubling meanings of their situation. For example, ambivalence about the therapeutic benefit of a treatment that comes with substantial unpleasant side-effects might chain into concerns about mixed messages about the likelihood of necessary support from the care provider, family, or friends. Meanings also chain as one form of PI shifts to another when people reflect on and communicate about a dilemma. For example, a person might seek information to reduce uncertainty (i.e. uncertainty as ignorance of available information) only to encounter inconsistent information (another form of uncertainty), an overwhelming avalanche of information (still another form of uncertainty), or learn that what one wants is simply impossible (not uncertainty at all, but another problematic meaning). PI theory holds that meanings are thus likely to change, and whatever they are at any one moment will be highly context dependent.

Applications

PI theory has been applied productively in a number of health and other contexts. For example, it has been used in studies of contraceptive choice (Sundstrom et al. 2017), genetic testing and counseling (Kirkscey 2017), the uncertainty of due dates (Vos et al. 2014), breast-feeding (Koerber, Brice, and Tombs 2012), the elimination of Asperger's syndrome as a diagnostic category in the DSM-V (Parsloe and Babrow 2016), the transition to assisted living (Gill and Morgan 2011), and end-of-life decision-making (Ohs, Trees, and Kurian 2017). As more specific examples, Matthias (2009) used the theory to illuminate the differences in pregnancy and childbirth care provided by midwives and OB/GYNs, and Parsloe (2017) used the theory (among others) to study activism among the disabled and chronically ill. In addition, PI theory, and particularly its analysis of uncertainty, has contributed to development of an alternative theory of uncertainty in medical care (see Han 2013; Han, Klein, and Arora 2011).

Appraisal

PI theory has been useful for both conceptual/theoretical development and empirical inquiry. It differs from UMT and the TMIM in that it (i) broadens understanding of problematic meanings beyond uncertainty, (ii) identifies varying forms of uncertainty and illuminates the importance of these varied meanings, (iii) broadens the conception of communication beyond the binary of information seeking and avoiding, (iv) offers a dynamic conception of communication as ongoing construction of (often problematic) meanings, and (v) broadens conceptions of communication outcomes beyond just decreasing, increasing, and maintaining uncertainty. In addition, unlike the TMIM post-positivist goals of explanation, prediction, and control of information management (UMT has also been characterized as a post-positivist; see Afifi and Matsunaga 2008), PI theory is intended to illuminate with greater subtlety the character of these troubled meanings and of the communication that constructs and reconstructs them. It is thus an interpretive perspective. Accordingly, in addition to enriching our understanding of particular forms of problematic meanings as they are communicatively constructed, PI theory also aims to "enhance communicator sophistication, . . . provide alternative ways of understanding and acting, and . . . foster empathy and compassion" (Babrow and Striley 2014, p. 105).

Conclusion

Uncertainty is a part of nearly every aspect of health and illness: beliefs about risk and risk factors, the utility of preventative measures of all sorts, screening options, symptoms and diagnosis, illness progression, treatments and side effects, remission and cure, and ongoing changes in medical knowledge and in the physical, social, and political-economic environments. Communication processes construct, maintain, and transform uncertainties in all of these phenomena. Not surprisingly, and as the literature reviewed here attests, uncertainty has been a fruitful focus for health communication theory development. However, attention to the interrelationships between communication and uncertainty is nowhere near as extensive as it could and should be.

A recent review of the literature illuminated the gap between potential and actual accomplishment in this area. In that work, Babrow (2020) studied publications on health and medicine as represented in PubMed, the 24 million-item database curated by the US National Library of Medicine, by searching for publications indexed with either "communication" or "uncertainty" as Medical Subject Headings. The search revealed that the number of publications focused on these terms has grown exponentially over the past 40 years. In each of the past 10 years, there were over 10 000 publications in which "communication" was a major topic and over 500 publications indexed with "uncertainty" as focal issue. However, the numbers of publications indexed with *both* "uncertainty" *and* "communication" as major topics ranged from just 41 to 71 per year. Clearly, there is enormous opportunity for research and theory development at the intersection of these important phenomena.

The theories reviewed here also demonstrate that this relationship can be studied productively from both post-positivist and interpretive perspectives. Although theorists may disagree over the reach and appropriateness of these approaches, such disagreements are best adjudicated by the accomplishments of research, rather than as debates about philosophy of science.

One other important open question is how to translate insights from this research and theory building into guidelines for practice. HR research has already been quite successful in this regard. Brashers et al.'s (2017) application of UMT in the domain of coping with a recent diagnosis of HIV is a promising demonstration project, as are practical implications drawn from applications of the TMIM (e.g. Afifi et al. 2006; Afifi and Weiner 2006). PI theory's emphasis on the importance of "form-specific adaptation" of messages (Babrow 2016, 2020), perhaps its single most practical implication, has not yet been applied, but such work is currently underway in the context of neonatal intensive care (Babrow and Sierra-Fernandez 2020). In short, the interdependence of uncertainty and health communication is an important focus for health communication theory-building. The most exciting developments are surely in what remains to be done.

Note

1. The authors used Lazarus's (1991) appraisal theory to flesh out their analysis of emotional reactions to uncertainty discrepancy, conceiving of anxiety as the result of a primary appraisal, and other more specific emotions as the result finer-grained secondary appraisals (Afifi & Morse, p. 90).

References

Abelman, D. D. (2017). Mitigating risks of students use of study drugs through understanding motivations for use and applying harm reduction theory: A literature review. *Harm Reduction Journal, 14*, 68. doi: 10.1186/s12954-017-0194-6.

Afifi, W. A. (2015). Theory of motivated information management. In C. R. Berger & M. E. Roloff (Eds.), *International encyclopedia of interpersonal communication* (pp. 1756–1765). New York, NY: Wiley Blackwell.

Afifi, W. A., & Matsunaga, M. (2008). Uncertainty management theories: Three approaches to a multifarious process. In L. A. Baxter & D. O. Braithwate (Eds.), *Engaging theories of interpersonal communication* (pp. 117–132). Thousand Oaks, CA: Sage.

Afifi, W. A., Morgan, S. E., Stephenson, M. T., Morse, C., Harrison, T., Reichert, T., & Long, S.D. (2006). Examining the decision to talk with family about organ donation: Applying the theory of motivated information management. *Communication Monographs, 73*(2), 188–215. doi:10.1080/03637750600690700

Afifi, W. A., & Morse, C. R. (2009). Expanding the role of emotion in the theory of motivated information management. In *Uncertainty, information management, and disclosure decisions: Theories and applications* (pp. 87–105). London: Routledge.

Afifi, W. A., & Weiner, J. L. (2004). Toward a theory of motivated information management. *Communication Theory, 14*(2), 167–190.

Afifi, W. A., & Weiner, J. L. (2006). Seeking information about sexual health: Applying the theory of motivated information management. *Human Communication Research, 32*(1), 35–57.

Albrecht, T. L., & Adelman, M. B. (1987). *Communicating social support.* Newbury Park, CA: Sage.

Babrow, A. S. (1992). Communication and problematic integration: Understanding diverging probability and value, ambiguity, ambivalence, and impossibility. *Communication Theory, 2*(2), 95–130. doi:10.1111/j.1468-2885.1992.tb00031.x

Babrow, A. S. (2001). Uncertainty, value, communication, and problematic integration. *Journal of Communication, 51,* 553–573.

Babrow, A. S. (2016). Problematic integration theory. In C. R. Berger & M. E. Roloff (Eds.), *International encyclopedia of interpersonal communication* (Vols. 1–3, pp. 1387–1395). Chichester, UK: John Wiley & Sons.

Babrow, A. S. (2020). Meeting the challenges of communication and uncertainty in medical care: Tradition, recent trends and their limits, and directions for further developments. In H. D. O'Hair & M. J. O'Hair (Eds.), *Handbook of applied communication research* (Vol. 2, pp. 827–846). Hoboken, NJ: Wiley.

Babrow, A. S., Kasch, C. R., & Ford, L. A. (1998). The many meanings of uncertainty in illness: Toward a systematic accounting. *Health Communication, 10*(1), 1–23. doi:10.1207/s15327027hc1001_1

Babrow, A.S., & Sierra-Fernandez, H. (2020). Surveying the topics and forms of uncertainty experienced by parents of children receiving neonatal and pediatric intensive care. (Unpublished manuscript).

Babrow, A. S., & Striley, K. M. (2014). Problematic integration theory and uncertainty management theory. In D. O. Braithwate & P. Schrodt (Eds.), *Engaging theories in interpersonal communication* (2nd ed., pp. 103–114). Los Angeles, CA: Sage.

Barbour, J. B., Rintamaki, L. S., Ramsey, J. A., & Brashers, D. E. (2012). Avoiding health information. *Journal of Health Communication, 17*(2), 212–229. doi:10.1080/10810730.2011.585691

Berger, C. R., & Calabrese, R. J. (1975). Some explorations in initial interaction and beyond: Toward a developmental theory of interpersonal communication. *Human Communication Research, 1*(2), 99–112. doi:10.1111/j.1468-2958.1975.tb00258.x

Brashers, D. E. (2001). Communication and uncertainty management. *Journal of Communication, 51*(3), 477–497.

Brashers, D. E. (2007). A theory of communication and uncertainty management. In B. Whaley & W. Samter (Eds.), *Explaining communication theory* (pp. 201–218). Mahwah, NJ: Erlbaum.

Brashers, D. E., Basinger, E. D., Rintamaki, L. S., Caughlin, J. P., Para, M. (2017). Taking control: The efficacy and durability of a peer-led uncertainty management intervention for people recently diagnosed with HIV. *Health Communication, 32,* 11–21. doi:10.1080/10410236.2015.1089469

Brashers, D. E., Goldsmith, D. J., & Hsieh, E. (2002). Information seeking and avoiding in health contexts. *Human Communication Research, 28,* 258–271.

Brashers, D. E., Neidig, J. L., Haas, S. M., Dobbs, L. K., Cardillo, L. W., & Russell, J. A. (2000). Communication in the management of uncertainty: The case of persons living with HIV or AIDS. *Communication Monographs, 67,* 63–84.

Carcioppolo, N., Yang, F., & Yang, Q. (2016). Reducing, maintaining, or escalating uncertainty? The development and validation of four uncertainty preference scales related to cancer information seeking and avoidance. *Journal of Health Communication, 21,* 979–988.

Donovan, E. E., Brown, L. E., LeFebvre, L., Tardif, S., & Love, B. (2015). "The uncertainty is what is driving me crazy": The tripartite model of uncertainty in the adolescent and young adult cancer context. *Health Communication, 30*, 702–713. doi:10.1080/10410236.2014.898193

Eversman, M. H. (2015) Harm reduction in U.S. tobacco control: Constructions in textual news media. *International Journal of Drug Policy, 26*(6), 575–582.

Ford, L. A., Babrow, A. S., & Stohl, C. (1996). Social support messages and the management of uncertainty in the experience of breast cancer: An application of problematic integration theory. *Communication Monographs, 63*, 189–207.

Fowler, C., & Afifi, W. A. (2011). Applying the theory of motivated information management to adult children's discussions of caregiving with aging parents. *Journal of Social & Personal Relationships, 28*(4), 507–535. doi:10.1177/0265407510384896

Geist-Martin, P., Ray, E. B., & Sharf, B. F. (2003). *Communicating health: Personal, cultural, and political complexities*. Belmont, CA: Wadsworth/ Thompson Learning.

Gill, E. A., & Morgan, M. (2011). Home sweet home: Conceptualizing and coping with the challenges of aging and the move to a care facility. *Health Communication, 26*(4), 332–342. doi:10.1080/10410236.2010.551579

Haas, E., & Mattson, M. (2014). Harm reduction theory. In T. Thompson (Ed.) *Encyclopedia of health communication* (Vol II, pp. 539–541). Los Angeles, CA: Sage.

Harm Reduction International. (2017). What is harm reduction? A position statement. https://www.hri.global/what-is-harm-reduction (accessed June 3, 2019).

Han, P. K. J. (2013). Conceptual, methodological, and ethical problems in communicating uncertainty in clinical evidence. *Medical Care Research and Review: MCRR, 70*(1 (Supplement)), 14S–36S. doi:10.1177/10775587 12459361

Han, P. K. J., Klein, W. M. P., & Arora, N. K. (2011). Varieties of uncertainty in health care: A conceptual taxonomy. *Medical Decision Making: An International Journal of the Society for Medical Decision Making, 31*(6), 828–838. doi:10.1177/0272989X11393976

Hathaway, A.D. (2001). Shortcomings of harm reduction: Toward a morally invested drug reform strategy. *International Journal of Drug Policy, 12*(2), 125–137.

Hilton, B. A., Thompson, R., Moore-Dempsey, L., & Janzen, R. G. (2001). Harm reduction theories and strategies for control of human immunodeficiency virus: A review of the literature. *Journal of Advanced Nursing, 33*(3), 357–370.

Hippocrates. (n.d.). *Aphorisms*. Internet Classics Archive. Retrieved June 29, 2019, from http://www.iupui.edu/~histwhs/h364.dir/hipp.aph.html

Hogan, T., & Brashers, D. (2009). The theory of communication and uncertainty management: Implications from the wider realm of information behavior. In T. Afifi & W. Afifi (Eds.), *Uncertainty, information management, and disclosure decisions: Theories and applications* (pp. 45–66). New York, NY: Routledge.

Hovick, S. R. (2014). Understanding family health information seeking: A test of the theory of motivated information management. *Journal of Health Communication, 19*(1), 6–23. doi:10.1080/10810730.2013.778369

Kahlor, L. (2010). PRISM: A planned risk information seeking model. *Health Communication, 25*(4), 345–356. doi:10.1080/10410231003775172

Katz, J. (1984). *The silent world of doctor and patient.* Baltimore, MD: Johns Hopkins Press.

Keane, H. (2003). Critiques of harm reduction, morality, and the promise of human rights. *International Journal of Drug Policy, 14*(3), 227–232.

Kirkscey, R. (2017). Patient decision aids for prenatal genetic testing: Probability, embodiment, and problematic integration. *Health Communication, 32*(5), 568–577. doi:10.1080/10410236.2016.1140500

Koerber, A., Brice, L., & Tombs, E. (2012). Breastfeeding and problematic integration: Results of a focus-group study. *Health Communication, 27*(2), 124–144. doi:10.1080/10410236.2011.571754

Lazarus, R. S. (1991). *Emotion and adaptation.* New York, NY: Oxford University Press.

Lewis, N., & Martinez, L. S. (2014). Does the number of cancer patients' close social ties affect cancer-related information seeking through communication efficacy? Testing a mediation model. *Journal of Health Communication, 19*(9), 1076–1097. doi:10.1080/10810730.2013.872724

Logan, D. E., & Marlatt, G. A. (2010). Harm reduction therapy: A practice-friendly review of research, *Journal of Clinical Psychology, 66*(2), 201–214. doi:10.1002/jclp.20669

Marlatt, G. A. (1998). Highlights of harm reduction: A personal report from the First National Harm Reduction Conference in the United States. In G.A. Marlatt (Ed.), *Harm reduction* (pp. 3–29). New York, NY: Guilford Press.

Martin, S. C., Stone, A. M., Scott, A. M., & Brashers, D. E. (2010). Medical, personal, and social forms of uncertainty across the transplantation trajectory. *Qualitative Health Research, 20*, 182–196.

Matthias, M. S. (2009). Problematic integration in pregnancy and childbirth: Contrasting approaches to uncertainty and desire in obstetric and midwifery care. *Health Communication, 24*, 60–70.

Matthias, M. S., & Babrow, A. S. (2007). Problematic integration of uncertainty and desire in pregnancy. *Qualitative Health Research, 17*(6), 786–798. doi:10.1177/1049732307303241

Mattson, M. (2000). Empowerment through agency-promoting dialogue: An explicit application of harm reduction theory to reframe HIV test counseling. *Journal of Health Communication, 5*(4), 333–349. doi:10.1080/10810730050199132

Mikesell, L., Bromley, E., Young, A. S., Vona, P., & Zima, B. (2016). Integrating client and clinician perspectives on psychotropic medication decisions: Developing a communication-centered epistemic model of shared decision making for mental health contexts. *Health Communication, 31*(6), 707–717. doi:10.1080/10410236.2014.993296

Miller, L. E. (2014). Uncertainty management and information seeking in cancer survivorship. *Health Communication, 29*, 233–243. doi:10.1080/10410236.2012.739949

Mishel, M. H. (1988). Uncertainty in illness. *Image–The Journal of Nursing Scholarship, 20*(4), 225–232.

Mishel, M. H. (1990). Reconceptualization of the uncertainty in illness theory. *Image – The Journal of Nursing Scholarship, 22*(4), 256–262.

Morse, C. R., Afifi, W. A., Morgan, S. E., Stephenson, M. T., Reichert, T., Harrison, T. R., & Long, S. D. (2009). Religiosity, anxiety, and discussions about organ donation: Understanding a complex system of associations. *Health Communication, 24*(2), 156–164. doi:10.1080/10410230802676755

Morse, C. R., Volkman, J. E., Samter, W., Trunzo, J., McClure, K., Kohn, C., & Logue, J. C. (2013). The influence of uncertainty and social support on information seeking concerning illicit stimulant use among young adults. *Health Communication, 28*(4), 366–377. doi:10.1080/10410236.2012. 689095

Ohs, J. E., Trees, A. R., & Kurian, N. (2017). Problematic integration and family communication about decisions at the end of life. *Journal of Family Communication, 17*(4), 356–371. doi:10.1080/15267431.2017.1348947

Parsloe, S. M. (2017). *"Real people. real stories.": Self-advocacy and collective connective action on the digital platform,* The Mighty (PhD dissertation). Ohio University. Retrieved from https://etd.ohiolink.edu/!etd.send_file? accession=ohiou1497536100831896&disposition=inline

Parsloe, S. M., & Babrow, A. S. (2016). Removal of Asperger's syndrome from the DSM V: Community response to uncertainty. *Health Communication, 31*(4), 485–494. doi:10.1080/10410236.2014.968828

Rafferty, K. A., Cramer, E., Priddis, D., & Allen, M. (2015). Talking about end-of-life preferences in marriage: Applying the theory of motivated information management. *Health Communication, 30*(4), 409–418. doi:10.1080/1041023 6.2014.889555

Rains, S. A. (2014). Health information seeking and the world wide web: An uncertainty management perspective. *Journal of Health Communication, 19*, 1296–1307.

Rauscher, E. A., & Hesse, C. (2014). Investigating uncertainty and emotions in conversations about family health history: A test of the theory of motivated information management. *Journal of Health Communication, 19*(8), 939–954. doi:10.1080/10810730.2013.837558

Sordo, L., Barrio, G., Bravo, M.J., Indave, B.I., Degenhardt, L., Wiessing, L., . . . Pastor-Barriuso, R. (2017). Mortality risk during and after opioid substitution treatment: Systematic review and meta-analysis of cohort studies, *BMJ, 357*, j1550. doi:10.1136/bmj.j1550

Stone, A. M., & Jones, C. L. (2009). Sources of uncertainty: Experiences of Alzheimer's disease. *Issues in Mental Health Nursing, 30*, 677–686.

Sundstrom, B., Ferrara, M., DeMaria, A. L., Baker-Whitcomb, A., & Payne, J. B. (2017). Integrating pregnancy ambivalence and effectiveness in contraceptive choice. *Health Communication, 32*(7), 820–827. doi:10.1080/10410236. 2016.1172294

Vos, S. C., Anthony, K. E., & O'Hair, H. D. (2014). Constructing the uncertainty of due dates. *Health Communication, 29*(9), 866–876. doi:10.1080/10410236.2 013.809501

14

Cultural Theories of Health Communication

Evelyn Y. Ho and Barbara F. Sharf

Health communication scholarship is quite varied in the ways it deals with culture. Theoretical approaches used to explain culture are equally variable, coming from different disciplines and not always easily compared. In this chapter we present one way of organizing and cataloging theories and approaches, recognizing that others may propose different categorizations. Because research that examines culture and communication in health settings is interdisciplinary and preexisted health communication, we begin with an historical review of interdisciplinary foundational research related to culture. We then follow with three sections focused on health communication theorizing about culture. In the first section, we examine research that focuses on the correlational study of one particular culture or cultural variable, such as race or ethnicity, as part of a broader health issue. In the second section, we cover ecological models of health that expand the concept of culture and take a contextual perspective, centralizing the study of culture. In the third section, we group together theoretical approaches that link the study of culture with critique of power imbalances, structures and institutions.

Health Communication Theory, First Edition. Edited by Teresa L. Thompson and Peter J. Schulz.
© 2021 John Wiley & Sons, Inc. Published 2021 by John Wiley & Sons, Inc.

Interdisciplinary Foundations

During the 1970s and 1980s as health communication was coalescing as a scholarly and organizational subdiscipline, simultaneously significant new ideas were emerging within medicine and public health, and from health-related social science and humanities. Of particular relevance are those concepts that realized the importance of culture as essential to health and medical care.

From the Biomedical to the Biopsychosocial Model

What has become known as scientific Western biomedicine dominates over other systems of healing in global influence. The biomedical model focuses on biological conceptions and explanations of disease affecting the human body with treatments that are evidenced-based, preferably from large-scale clinical trials. Health is conceived as the absence of disease. Symptoms of diseases are often referred to specialist practitioners, thus fragmenting the understanding and care of the disease. Internist and psychiatrist George L. Engel (1977) revolutionized medical thinking by proposing the biopsychosocial model that posits human illness is affected simultaneously by biological, psychological, and social factors.

A few years later, social psychologist and sociolinguist Elliot Mishler (1984) counterposed the discourse of clinicians, which he called the "voice of medicine" (heavily influenced by the biomedical model), with the "voice of the life world" – the way patients talk about their illness experiences. Using discourse analysis, he demonstrated how the differences between these two "voices" or discursive forms often lead to problems affecting clinical care. The voice of medicine reveals the practice of medicine to be a unique culture unto itself, while the voice of the life world implicitly includes ethnocultural influences. Like Mishler, psychiatrist-anthropologist Arthur Kleinman (1980, 1988) was one of the founders of the practice of narrative medicine, with its emphasis on stories as a basis for practice. He theorized that healthcare professionals are storytellers for one another who focus on narratives of *disease*, narrowly focused on the manifestations of pathophysiology, while patients tell stories of dis-ease, i.e. the subjective experiences suffered while living through *illness* or disability, including concepts rooted in patients' ethnocultural roots within their descriptions of illness. The natural dichotomy that emerges from the interaction of these two perspectives yields contrasting *explanatory models*, stories of what is wrong, why, and what should be done. These explanatory models are often recognized as the cultural difference between how groups of people understand illness.

The Biocultural Model

We often differentiate biomedicine from other modes of "alternative" types of healing, often originating in non-Western or non-"first world" cultures. However, journalist Lynn Payer (1988/1996) introduced the argument that modern scientific, Western-dominated medicine is not a global monolith of shared knowledge and modalities, but rather a collection of ideologies and practices shaped by local culture. Her assertion about the role of culture in shaping medical practice was soon followed by literary and medical humanities scholar David Morris, whose work has focused on the experience of pain, and introduced the idea of "postmodern illness," as "a mental, emotional, bodily event constructed at the crossroads of biology and culture" (Morris 1998, p. 19). The biocultural model, in contrast to the two previous models, seeks to explore how various biological states, from menopause to post-traumatic stress disorder, as well as how psychosocial epidemics of racism to gun violence, are shaped by historical and cultural forces.

Social Determinants of Health and Health Disparities

A great deal of research and public policy from medicine to public health has been focused on reducing recognized health disparities, often using a social determinants of health (SDH) approach. This approach considers that healthcare is complex, using many of the models already discussed. The World Health Organization (WHO) Commission on SDH states "the structural determinants and conditions of daily life constitute the social determinants of health and are responsible for a major part of health inequities between and within countries" (CSDH 2008, p. 1). An SDH perspective was important in institutionalizing a move away from individual level behavioral causes (and blame) for illness to one that recognized both an individual's behavior and their social, cultural, and material concerns.

Cultural Competency, Cultural Humility, and Structural Humility

An important shift in focus occurred in medical education from *cultural competency* to *cultural humility* and more recently to *structural humility*. Because of the increased racial and ethnic diversity of the US and the many racial/ethnic based health disparities (Smedley, Stith, and Nelson 2003), for the last 20–30 years, health and medicine have increasingly recognized the importance of race and ethnicity. More broadly, this has included the concept of culture in promoting health. To improve health disparities, the Liaison Committee on Medical Education (LCME), the accrediting body of US medical schools, has since 2000 stipulated that as part of their educational standards, universities offering medical degrees must "demonstrate an understanding of the manner in which people of diverse cultures and belief systems perceive health and illness and respond to various symptoms, diseases, and treatments" and "recognize and appropriately address gender and cultural biases in themselves and others, and in the process of health care delivery" (International Association of Medical Colleges, n.d.). Understood as the call for cultural competency, it is worth noting that even from the beginning, the LCME's stipulation included both a set of knowledge and a particular attitude towards culture. A commonly cited definition of cultural competence is:

> A set of congruent behaviors, attitudes, and policies that come together in a system, organization, or among professionals that enables effective work in cross-cultural situations. . ... Culture [is] . . . the integrated patterns of human behavior that include the language, thoughts, actions, customs, beliefs, and institutions of racial, ethnic, social, or religious groups. . .. Competence [is] . . . the capacity to function effectively. (Cross et al. 1989, p. 3)

Especially in situations where providers and patients are not racially or ethnic concordant (matching), research has found that cultural competence training leads to increased patient satisfaction and health promotion (Fortier and Bishop 2003), but not always improved health outcomes (Renzaho et al. 2013).

When providers learn more about the cultural beliefs, customs, and practices of patients, presumably, they should provide better care. However, scholars recognize that cultural competence should be more than trying to learn a finite set of knowledge, habits, and practices. Two health researchers who are women or color, Melanie Tervalon and Jann Murray-Garcia, introduced a now widely used alternative of *cultural humility*, where providers exercise self-reflection and recognize power inequalities, placing culture in a larger context and moving away from memorizing static facts about culture (Masters et al. 2019; Tervalon and Murray-Garcia 1998). In doing so, providers can respond flexibly to the patient in front of them. Cultural humility, however, has also been critiqued for not having measurable outcome variables (Ahmed et al. 2018).

While cultural humility adds complexity to cultural competency, both perspectives focus on the micro-level interpersonal communications between providers and patients. Health disparities scholars especially have brought attention to the institutional or macro-level factors by introducing a similarly named concept called *structural humility* or *structural competency* (Bourgois et al. 2017; Farmer et al. 2006; Metzl and Hansen 2014). Metzl and Hansen (2014) define structural competency as having four goals/concerns: (i) recognizing the social and professional structures that shape clinical interactions; (ii) developing an extra-clinical language of structure; (iii) rearticulating "cultural" presentations in structural terms; (iv) observing and imagining structural intervention; and (v) developing structural humility. Just as research in medicine covers an array of paradigmatic positions regarding the role of culture, as we present in the next three sections, health communication scholarship examining culture is wide-ranging and multilayered.

Culture as Variable: Correlational Studies of Culture in Health Communication

In this first category of theoretical approaches, culture is quite often undertheorized. Some have named this a "culture as variable" approach (Dutta 2007; Ho 2014) in which culture is an independent variable of interest affecting a host of dependent variables such as health status or behavior change. In addition, when culture is mentioned it is often used as a proxy for race or ethnicity (Ford and Harawa 2010) and often focused on non-White, or non-dominant ethnic groups. As a predictive variable, successful health communication is caused by meeting the needs, values, expectations, or practices of a particular "culture" of people. Because other health communication theories are typically developed in majority populations and treated as universal or culturally invisible, the cultural adjustments that scholars recognize as necessary in developing and measuring health communication are typically only recognized in non-dominant cultural groups. For example, a randomized control trial to increase mammography and fruit and vegetable intake in lower income African American women tailored health messages focused on religiosity, collectivism, racial pride, and time orientation (Kreuter and Haughton 2006).

Research of this type tends to be quantitative and often experimental, coming from a post-positivist and/or scientific perspective. In the following sections, we will review some theoretical approaches whose main goals are to craft and adjust health communication to match culture.

Targeting and Tailoring

Health communication and public health scholars interested in crafting health messages to affect behavior change in target populations often discuss the importance of cultural targeting and tailoring. Much of this early work was focused on cultural groups – meaning race and ethnic based groups – and was conducted with African Americans and Hispanic/Latinx populations (Resnicow et al. 1999). To design and implement behavior change in these populations, scholars needed to match materials to the *surface structure*, "observable social and behavioral characteristics of a target population" (Resnicow et al. 2000, p. 272) such as preferred languages or including pictures of target populations. However, health communication also needs to address how people understand illness, its causes and treatments, and core cultural values or *deep structures* (Resnicow et al. 2000, p. 272). As an example, a recent study found that Black audiences evaluated an entertainment education theatrical production of a White family's cancer journey more favorably than White or other people of color audiences (Beach et al. 2019). While on the surface, this could be seen as not culturally sensitive, from a deeper level, authors credit the oral storytelling aspects as deeply resonant with African American audiences perhaps more so than the race of the actors.

Kreuter et al. (2003) recognize the heterogeneity inherent in all cultural groups and takes this idea one step further in their definition of *cultural tailoring*. Differentiating from cultural targeting which focuses on meeting the cultural needs of a group, tailoring focuses on assessing an *individual* audience member, providing *individualized* information, and measuring change in individuals. Because much of what goes into the process of cultural targeting and tailoring overlaps the message design theories and behavior change theories, we suggest readers go to those sections of this book for more information.

Social Determinants of Health, Health Literacy, and Health Communication

There has been a wealth of research in the intersecting areas of medicine, public health, and health communication regarding the intersections of SDH including culture, and health literacy (HL) which we cannot cover thoroughly in this chapter. However, Dean Schillinger, an MD who does health communication research in vulnerable populations, has proposed a model bringing together these well-studied concepts (SDH, HL, and health communication) into an empirically testable correlational model (Schillinger 2020). The model begins from an SDH perspective, which incorporates culture-related intersecting components such as race/ethnicity, language, economic, social, and environmental factors. These SDH factors lead to health disparities through a public health pathway (that recognizes the unequal distribution of health-promoting resources and unhealthy life course exposures) and/or through a health-care pathway (that takes into account how health systems – such as hospitals and clinics – respond to the clinical needs of patients). Both of these pathways can be mediated by health literacy, which then affects health outcomes and can lead to health disparities. As a conceptual and empirically testable model, it posits that the combination of patient health literacy and provider communication skills leads to health and well-being via pathways including effective elicitation and explanation between provider and patient, concordance, the development of shared meaning, and a trusting therapeutic alliance, which should lead to appropriate decision-making and treatment adherence. While such a model may seem complex, it operates as a theoretically and empirically testable framework to measure the impact of health communication research, education, and interventions (Schillinger et al. 2017).

Concordance, Implicit Bias

Numerous studies find that racially discordant interactions (e.g. White physician and patient of color) result in a number of negative impacts such as lower patient satisfaction and less patient-centeredness (Bylund and Koenig 2015). One explanation for this is due to physician non-conscious or implicit bias, which may affect how physicians interact with patients. In studies of actual physician–patient interactions, physicians with higher levels of implicit bias were found to be less patient-centered and more verbally dominant (Cooper et al. 2012; Penner et al. 2016). Implicit bias is not just racially based but can also affect gender, age, and other social identities. However, research does show that education can reduce implicit bias (Girod et al. 2016).

Globalization and Development Communication

A final area of related research is global and development communication. A thorough review of this area goes beyond the scope of this chapter but readers interested may consult *The Handbook of Global Health Communication* (Obregon and Waisbord 2012).

Culture as Context: Ecological, Language, and Performance Perspectives in Health Communication

In contrast to studying culture as a specific trait, such as race, ethnicity, religion, or locality, as we have discussed in the previous section, other forms of scholarship define culture as a broad, anthropological understanding of taken-for-granted ways of living – language, implicit values, specified rules, rituals, celebrations, art forms, and so forth. The theories described in this section employ this perspective of culture as expansive and complex.

Ecological Theories

These theories share a common acknowledgment that health-related issues are embedded within broader, more general dynamics – social, political, cultural – that have bearing on the communication processes occurring in and about healthcare and promotion. Some of these theories come from an ecological perspective, taking into account the complex interrelationships among the communication phenomena being studied and circumstances, processes, and institutions within the surrounding environment, both material and discursive. However, other than sharing an intentionally ecological approach, the following examples are very different in terms of focus, methods, and definition or treatment of culture.

Though teaching communication skills in medical/health education had been ongoing since the 1970s, there were no curricular materials that addressed cross-cultural communication between clinicians and patients until 1990 (Sharf et al. 1990). A related theoretical model was developed to help physicians in training have greater awareness of how cultural differences may subtly contribute to misunderstandings in diagnosis and treatment. The *culturally sensitive model* (Sharf and Kahler 1996) depicts a broad conceptualization of culture that includes layers of meaning derived from (i) the deeply engrained *values and ideologies* developed through the history, laws, customs, and mores of communities of shared identities; (ii) *sociopolitical realities* that create the bases of power and resulting group differences based on demographics such as race, ethnicity, religion, gender, and sexuality; (iii) *institutional and professional influences* from organizations such as medical centers and hospitals, pharmaceutical companies, health insurance companies, legislation, health education and public health structures affecting access to and quality of healthcare; (iv) *ethnocultural/ familial influences*, which account for the traditional beliefs and practices of what constitutes good health and healing, causes of sickness, and effective treatments (what Kleinman [1980, 1988] referred to as explanatory models); and (v) *interpersonal dynamics* that stem from the uniqueness of individuals who interact with one another, such as in clinical encounters. This model posits that these levels of meaning are continuously present and in process, but that one or more may be more salient and influential at any particular stage of interaction. Furthermore, often the level of meaning emphasized by one participant differs from what is most meaningful to the other. Applying the model in guided discussion helps clinician-learners to understand interactions with patients in which aspects of culture may have come directly into conflict, or often were not engaging with one another at all. Such instances of disagreement or non-engagement, in turn, affect clinical rapport and partnership, accuracy in diagnosis, and efficacy of treatment recommendations.

The *ecological model of communication in medical encounters* (Street 2003) is a detailed attempt to account for the complex influences that shape medical provider–patient encounters. This model posits that each participant is subject to a variety of personal, individual factors including style of communication, self concept, personality, beliefs, perceptions of power, relationships, emotions, and communicative strategies. These elements constitute the "interpersonal context" which is the central core of the model. In turn, this central core is affected by at least four additional contexts including mediated (and technological), organizational, political-legal, and cultural. The latter is described as including "race, ethnicity, socioeconomic status, religion, etc." In sum, this model emphasizes that provider–patient dialogues are continuously subject to influences from a wide array of discourses, institutions, and regulations simultaneously.

Often, the model is not used in its entirety at once, but aspects of it may enrich in-depth understanding. For example, Street and colleagues made substantial contributions to how perceptions of race and ethnicity contribute to the quality of clinical consultations. In one of several studies using race as a key variable, he and colleagues discovered an important disparity in communication with lung cancer patients, comparing racially concordant patient–physician pairs (in which both identify as being of the same race) and racially discordant pairs (in which racial identification differs). The results showed that during consultations in the discordant pairs, black patients asked fewer questions and prompted less information from their doctors and, in turn, received less information.

This tendency may lead to very serious consequences in light of differences in treatments that have been evidenced among black patients with lung and other cancers (Gordon et al. 2006).

"Crossing borders in health communication research" (Ford, Crabtree, and Hubbell 2009), a study documenting public health education in the southwest US–Mexican borderlands, demonstrates an alternate way of theorizing from an ecological perspective. Based on their detailed description of a multi-year set of applied communication efforts to increase public understanding and change health behaviors, the authors show how a holistic ecology can work. Their explanation combines localized knowledge of geography, politics, culture, language, disease, and health beliefs with use of community networking and effective communication practices in order to prevent the spread of a viral pulmonary disease, instruct women on early detection and treatment of breast cancer, and cooperate with and advance community health educators (*promotoras*). All these activities took place within a high-risk, impoverished and underserved population and an understanding that state and national boundaries do not necessarily coincide with community identification.

Communication infrastructure theory (CIT; Kim and Ball-Rokeach 2006) is described as an ecological model of civic engagement that emerged from mass media studies of community engagement and recently health disparities in geographic and ethnic based communities (Wilkin 2013). Although not explicitly created as a cultural approach, we believe CIT offers a theoretical, community-based social change model to examine health narratives and storytellers (in a communicative network) as embedded within larger social, political, and cultural dynamics.

An asset-based model, the goal of CIT is to evaluate the strength of community networks through its local figures, ties, and information networks. Communication in CIT examines multiple levels of storytelling broadly across modes and media and pays close attention to meso-level storytelling agents, for example community organizations and local ethnic media and micro-level storytelling agents, such as the actual neighbors (Kim and Ball-Rokeach 2006). These agents form the storytelling networks (STNs; Wilkin et al. 2010) and the strength of the STN relies on the strength of integration of these agents (Kim and Ball-Rokeach 2006) which can be constrained or facilitated by the communication action context (CAC), or the cultural, social, economic, and physical components of a community environment. For example, the Metamorphosis Project in Los Angeles used CIT-based mapping to identify existing community communication resources, using this knowledge to later create a storytelling project where members discussed pressing community health issues (Wilkin et al. 2010). Studies have found STN to be related directly and indirectly to health outcomes, but strong STN does not always correlate with positive outcomes (Wilkin 2013). Studies using CIT have also engaged community members in health intervention research and expanded to examine how communication ecologies intersect with race/ethnicity and place, or what Wilkin (2013) calls geo-ethnicity.

Language, and Social Interaction

In 2001, the Office of Minority Health in the US Department of Health and Human Services (2001) introduced federal standards for culturally and linguistically appropriate care, also known as CLAS standards, to advance health equity among the diverse communities in the US, requiring language services for those with limited English proficiency. Health communication scholar, Elaine Hsieh (2006, 2007) has written extensively about the role of medical interpreters as not just an invisible conduit but as important co-diagnosticians in medical visits. This work recognizes that language and language translation always takes into account cultural norms, expectations, and meaning-making in the interaction.

The connection between language and culture is often studied within the subfield of language and social interaction (LSI; Fitch and Sanders 2005) which is interested in examining language as it is actually used in everyday contexts. LSI research focused on health and culture primarily comes from the subdisciplines of ethnography, discourse analysis, discursive psychology, and conversation analysis.

Originally an expansion of the way communication scholars studied culture and intercultural communication, speech codes theory (SCT; Philipsen 1997) has also been used to examine cultural ways of speaking in health contexts. A speech code is defined as a "system of socially constructed symbols and meanings, premises, and rules, pertaining to communicative conduct" (Philipsen 1997, p. 126). As such, what makes SCT different from other studies of culture is that culture is not the group one belongs to, but rather, the speech code(s) that one uses. SCT consists of six empirically testable propositions (Philipsen 1992, 1997; Philipsen, Coutu, and Covarrubias 2005).

As an example of SCT used to study health, Ho's (2006) ethnographic study of traditional Chinese medicine (TCM) explores the way TCM practitioners and students use the term "qi" (often translated as energy or vital force) in conversations at a student acupuncture clinic. Acknowledging that speaking about qi in a US/English-speaking context requires some explanation for patients unfamiliar with this word, the larger speech code requires not only the mention of qi but also the philosophical basis of acupuncture that comes from qi, as opposed to Western biomedical explanations. The qi-based speech code also operates to separate novice from experienced acupuncturists and to separate Chinese and Japanese style acupuncture. The speech code, therefore, is a way that people distinguish between culturally different subgroups. In other words, what is *cultural* about this research is as much about the communicative code as it is about Chinese vs. Western medicine. Ho and Bylund (2008) build on these findings, arguing for a different way to understand holistic medicine more broadly through examining the valued ways of speaking and codes in this same community. By separating how TCM providers and patients communicate (paternalistic, collaborative, consumerist) from the implied models of health (biological, biopsychosocial, holistic), they demonstrate that what is culturally "holistic" about TCM (e.g. a collaborative interpersonal dynamic) may actually be contested between providers and patients.

Ethnography and Analysis of Performance

Performance studies is an academic discipline unto itself, though it shares historical roots and contemporary connections with communication studies. In this section we present exemplary studies that used performance theory and analysis to investigate and explain cultural aspects of health and illness in creative and insightful ways.

Ethnography of performance is an investigative approach to studying aspects of everyday life, not as random acts or personal strategies, but as purposeful performances intended for public (as well as private) observation and meaning-making. As implied in the name, this is a research activity that is qualitative, interpretive, and often interactive in nature, wherein the researcher is frequently an active participant. Furthermore, theory and practice are intertwined and often inseparable in ethnographic research. Performance, as that term implies, encompasses not only discourse and dialogue, but also costume and decoration, gesture and movement, plot and character, scenery and props.

A highly acknowledged performance study scholar who significantly defined the field, Dwight Conquergood was both a theorist and ethnographer, known for sharing the lived experiences of his research participants in amazing depth and longevity. Those participants were disenfranchised social groups, including refugees and immigrants, gang members, and prisoners. In a landmark public health study (Conquergood 1988), he became a public health officer and the only WHO worker to live *with* the population of a Thai camp for Hmong refugees from Laos. Removed from their native environment and ways of living, sanitation and illness prevention conditions in the camp became perilous for the refugees. Working in conjunction with people living in the camp, Conquergood helped the refugees creatively adapt Hmong native folk stories and traditions to create a performative health campaign that addressed sanitation and health risk. Not only was this a successful case study of basing a health campaign on familiar native culture, it contributes to the theory of how ethnoculture, performance, and application may be employed for problem-solving in unexpected circumstances.

A similar, more recent community-based performance program, called The Bigger Picture, is a joint venture between a youth-focused poetry/ spoken word non-profit, Youth Speaks, and the University of California San Francisco's Center for Vulnerable Populations (Schillinger and Huey 2018). Through this program, young people of color who are disproportionately affected by type 2 diabetes participate in afterschool workshops to learn about diabetes, its connections to food insecurity, targeted food and sugary drinks advertising, and unequal access to recreation/ physical activity space. These workshops include Youth Speaks mentors, a UCSF primary care provider, and a health communication expert who help participants generate spoken word poetry that gives agency and voice to youth experiences and makes explicit links to the structural causes of diabetes. The program has generated numerous poems, over 1.5 million views on YouTube and is being adopted by numerous schools, demonstrating that performance is an effective way to "change the conversation about diabetes" (www.thebiggerpictureproject.org).

The final exemplar centers on a televised entertainment performance and social media response. In addition to somatic changes, Jill Yamasaki's (2014) astute analysis of a popular television scenario demonstrates how self-perceptions interact with cultural characterizations and social labeling to create the meanings of aging. In this study, a contestant on the reality TV show, *The Biggest Loser*, a 49-year-old woman chose to portray herself repeatedly as a "Southern grandmother of nine." She chose to emphasize that the show was her "last chance" since she had only "a good 20 years left." Audiences responded very negatively through social media to what was perceived as her unseemly, premature embrace of age as defeatism, in contrast to many examples of people who are older but more forward-thinking. This media ethnographic study demonstrates the power of performance in everyday life to affect thinking and public discussion about the ubiquitous process of human aging.

Culture as Critique: Political, Structural, and Ideological Considerations in Health Communication

In 1994, an essay by Australian sociologist Deborah Lupton published in *Health Communication* startled many readers (Lupton 1994). She characterized the then relatively new field of health communication as dominated by social-psychological behavioral research, while ignoring the actual discourse used in health contexts and "the ways in which the use of language in the medical settings acts to perpetuate the interests of some groups over others" (Lupton 1994, p. 55). She took the field to task for its alliances with practitioners, health policy-makers and funders, and for underestimating the intelligence and capabilities of patients and the public. Within the critical cultural approach she advocates, culture is not only conceptualized in terms of traditions, ideas, and conditions specific to particular communities, but also performances of everyday living and expression. Thus, "apart from their biomedical manifestations, health, medicine, and disease may be considered products of cultural practices" (Lupton 1994, p. 57), for example, understanding health and illness as "products of social systems and ideological processes" (Lupton 1994, p. 58) and approaching physician–patient communication as dynamics of symbolic and political power and control.

Finally, in addition to these emphases on language and sociopolitics, Lupton concludes that there is an obligation for health communication scholars to be advocates for those who are victimized or rendered without power by systematic and cultural imbalances. Rather than presenting a unified theory of culture or healthcare culture, Lupton opened the door within health communication to a new, underrepresented paradigm of how to understand culture and related implications for doing research.

In much the same way as Lupton discusses, physician and sociologist Howard Waitzkin (1991) combined critical theory and sociolinguistic analysis of physician–patient encounters to demonstrate how the practice of medicine at the micro-level of talk in the clinic constantly and subversively marginalizes the social aspects (e.g. finances, social support, gender roles, medical surveillance of work life) that significantly affect patients' illnesses and doctors' efforts to administer care. His analyses show how seamlessly these limitations are built into clinical encounters.

Collins O. Airhihenbuwa (1995) brought a critical perspective to public health theory and practice. He argued that an in-depth consideration of culture must be central and integral to any public health policy and interventions. In examining the mainstream health communication strategies based on social psychological theories of behavioral change used to curb the AIDS pandemic in the 1990s, Airhihenbuwa and Oregon (2000) found that culture was de-emphasized. When it was mentioned, culture was designated as artifacts from the past, exotified oddities of non-Western peoples, and considered a barrier to the recommendations of health authorities and researchers. As an alternative, he advocates the PEN-3 model that helps researchers and health strategists to delve deeply into aspects of culture from community members themselves to create interventions that will be adaptable, workable, and resonant with the designated communities. The PEN-3 model features three main domains: cultural identity, cultural empowerment, and relationships and expectations. Each domain, in turn, has three subcategories (each of these subcategory topics begin with the letters P, E, and N; Airhihenbuwa and Webster 2004).

Just a decade after Lupton's complaint, Heather Zoller and Kimberly Kline (Zoller and Kline 2008, p. 90) claimed that interpretive/critical perspectives had become "more mainstream" rather than "alternative" (p. 2) to what had been health communication's post-positivist dominance. Their painstakingly detailed and thorough analysis of the considerable body of works in this combined genre included studies that examine routine experiences related to health and illness, media constructions of health meanings, ideologies of identity and power embedded in health discourse, deconstruction of bias in policy, development of "context sensitive" health promotion campaigns, and possibilities for resistance to dominance and social change.

Iccha Basnyat (2017) draws from intersectionality theory (Crenshaw 1989), to examine the place of gender within a larger cultural and social context among female sex workers (FSWs) in Nepal. Intersectionality was originally developed by black feminist scholar activists to recognize the multiple forms of oppression that women of color face including not just race and gender, but also class, sexuality, and cultural ideologies and institutional arrangements (Davis 2008) such as (in Basnyat's research) mother and sex worker. By using an intersectional frame, FSWs' "health risk" is reconstructed as the particular gendered health context in which FSWs must negotiate multiple inequalities and lack of resources as mothers make the difficult choice between their own health and the health of the children.

What is likely the best known, widely used form of critical theory in health communication scholarship is the culture-centered approach (CCA; Dutta 2008). This theory is focused on understanding and improving the plight of subaltern communities which are disenfranchised and suffer consequences, health-related and otherwise, from sustained sociopolitical inequities. Within a critical theory perspective, subaltern refers to those of low status within the prevailing socioeconomic hierarchy or social structure. There are historical factors that have resulted in the origins and persistence of this low status that is often associated with oppression, inaccessibility of social and material resources, and conditions that result in ill-health. There are three basic and necessary components to a CCA analysis: culture, structure, and agency. *Culture*, of course, is at the center, continuously created within a community through the shared meanings, values, and practices, of its members, and, importantly, making possible "the creation of transformative spaces" (Dutta 2017, p. 336). The second component is *Structure*, defined as "those organizations, processes, and systems in society which determine how that society is organized, how it functions, and how individual members within it behave with respect to one another" (Dutta 2008, p. 62). These structures "enable and/or constrain access to resources of health" (Dutta 2017, p. 336). *Agency*, the third component, "reflects the active processes through which individuals, groups, and communities participate in a variety of actions which directly challenge the structures that constrain their lives, and simultaneously, work with the structures in finding healthful options" (Dutta 2008, p. 7). Agency may occur "in ordinary processes of sensemaking, in everyday acts of negotiation, in adapting to structures, and in collective participation in processes of structural transformation" (Dutta 2017, p. 337). All three elements of the CCA are continuously interacting with one another in ways that may continue, worsen, or improve the conditions and situations that constrain access to conditions conducive to better health. In line with Lupton's precept that critical theorist scholars should be advocates for subalterns who suffer from sociopolitical inequalities, the CCA constructs the role of scholars who use it to identify the aforementioned "transformative spaces" with participating community members in order to promote dialogue with the end goal of enacting helpful changes.

The CCA has been used in a wide variety of studies of and projects with communities in need throughout the world. In a systematic review of 47 empirical CCA articles, Sastry et al. (2019) distinguish between CCA projects that demonstrate use of the *ontological* axis of CCA for defining health problems (through attention to culture, structure and agency) and those that use the *epistemological* axis, or the dialogic co-construction with marginalized communities. In addition, Sastry et al. examine the use of the term reflexivity across CCA-named projects.

They differentiate between *methodological* reflexivity in which the researchers present and account for their own place and effect in the project, and *philosophical* reflexivity, or the political and emancipatory commitment (or axiology) of the CCA. In this way CCA scholars differentiate themselves from other community-based or development communication projects (Dutta 2015). While any one project that claims CCA may fall into any one or more of these three nested as opposed to completely separate "bowls," the stated goal of CCA is to encompass projects that do all three.

Conclusion

In writing this chapter, it was our goal to create a scheme to organize the expansive and often too-disciplinary-specific conceptualizations of culture used in health communication research in order to improve healthcare. Examining how culture in health communication has been defined and applied reveals a continuously interdisciplinary, paradigm-crossing endeavor by researchers from communication studies and other social sciences, humanities, medicine, allied health, and public health disciplines. Whether conceptualized as a specific variable that correlates with other factors, as a broad, encompassing context within which communication about health intersects with all facets of living, or as a conveyor of ideology and deep structures, theories of culture in health communication call forth a wide array of premises, methods, and emphases. These, in turn, enrich our understandings of how culture in its many forms influences and complexifies how illness is conceptualized, experienced, and treated, as well as how health may best be promoted. It is our hope that as this scholarship continues to grow and develop that it will be done with awareness of and striving toward both cultural and structural humility, as discussed earlier in this chapter.

References

Ahmed, S., Siad, F. M., Manalili, K., Lorenzetti, D. L., Barbosa, T., Lantion, V., . . . Santana, M. J. (2018). How to measure cultural competence when evaluating patient-centred care: A scoping review. *BMJ Open, 8*, e021525. doi:10.1136/bmjopen-2018-021525

Airhihenbuwa, C. O. (1995). *Health and culture: Beyond the western paradigm.* Thousand Oaks, CA: Sage.

Airhihenbuwa, C. O., & Obregon, R. (2000). A critical assessment of theories/ models used in health communication for HIV/AIDS. *Journal of Health Communication, 5*(Supp.1), 5–15. doi:10.1080/10810730050019528

Airhihenbuwa, C. O., & Webster, J. D. (2004). Culture and African contexts of HIV/AIDS prevention, care and support. *SAHARA-J: Journal of Social Aspects of HIV/AIDS, 1*(1), 4–13. doi:10.1080/17290376.2004.9724822

Basnyat, I. (2017). Theorizing the relationship between gender and health through a case study of Nepalese street-based female sex workers. *Communication Theory, 27*(4), 388–406. doi:10.1111/comt.12114

Beach, W. A., Dozier, D. M., Allen, B. J., Chapman, C., & Gutzmer, K. (2019). A White family's oral storytelling about cancer generates more favorable evaluations from Black American audiences. *Health Communication, 35*(12), 1520–1530. doi:10.1080/10410236.2019.1652387

Bourgois, P., Holmes, S. M., Sue, K., & Quesada, J. (2017). Structural vulnerability: Operationalizing the concept to address health disparities in clinical care. *Academic Medicine, 92*, 299–307. doi:10.1097/acm.0000000000001294

Bylund, C. L., & Koenig, C. J. (2015). Approaches to studying provider-patient communication. In N. G. Harrington (Ed.), *Health communication: An introduction to theory, method and application* (pp. 116–146). New York, NY: Routledge.

Conquergood, D. (1988). Heath theatre in a Hmong refugee camp. *TDR, 32*, 174–208.

Cooper, L. A., Roter, D. L., Carson, K. A., Beach, M. C., Sabin, J. A., Greenwald, A. G., & Inui, T. S. (2012). The associations of clinicians' implicit attitudes about race with medical visit communication and patient ratings of interpersonal care. *American Journal of Public Health, 102*, 979–987. doi:10.2105/ajph.2011.300558

Crenshaw, K. (1989). Demarginalizing the intersection of race and sex: A Black feminist critique of antidiscrimination doctrine, feminist theory and antiracist politics. *The University of Chicago Legal Forum, 140*, 139–167.

Cross, T. L., Bazron, B. J., Dennis, K. W., & Isaacs, M. R. (1989). *Towards a culturally competent system of care*. Child Development Center, Georgetown University, Washington DC. Retrieved from https://files.eric.ed.gov/fulltext/ED330171.pdf

CSDH. (2008). *Closing the gap in a generation: Health equity through action on the social determinants of health. Final report of the Commission on social determinants of health*. Geneva, Swizerland: World Health Organization. Retrieved from: https://www.who.int/social_determinants/thecommission/finalreport/en/

Davis, K. (2008). Intersectionality as buzzword: A sociology of science perspective on what makes a feminist theory successful. *Feminist Theory, 9*(1), 67–85. doi:10.1177/1464700108086364

Dutta, M. J. (2007). Communicating about culture and health: Theorizing culture-centered and cultural sensitivity approaches. *Communication Theory, 17*(3), 304–328. doi:10.1111/j.1468-2885.2007.00297.x

Dutta, M. J. (2008). *Communicating health*. Cambridge, England: Polity Press.

Dutta, M. J. (2015). Decolonizing communication for social change: A culture-centered approach. *Communication Theory, 25*(2), 123–143. doi:10.1111/comt.12067

Dutta, M. J. (2017). Communicating the culture-centered approach to health disparities. In J. Yamasaki, P. Geist-Martin, & B. F. Sharf (Eds.), *Storied health and illness: Communication personal, cultural, & political complexities* (pp. 333–356). Long Grove, IL: Waveland Press.

Engel, G. L. (1977). The need for a new medical model: A challenge for biomedicine. *Science, 196*, 129–196. doi:10.1126/science.847460

Farmer, P. E., Nizeye, B., Stulac, S., & Keshavjee, S. (2006). Structural violence and clinical medicine. *PLoS Med, 3*. doi:10.1371/journal.pmed.0030449

Fitch, K., & Sanders, R. E. (Eds.). (2005). *Handbook of language and social interaction* Mahwah, NJ: Erlbaum.

Ford, C. L., & Harawa, N. T. (2010). A new conceptualization of ethnicity for social epidemiologic and health equity research. *Social Science & Medicine, 71*, 251–258. doi:10.1016/j.socscimed.2010.04.008

Ford, L. A., Crabtree, R. D., & Hubbell, A. (2009). Crossing borders in health communication research: Toward an ecological understanding of context, complexity, and consequences in community-based health education in the U.S.–Mexico borderlands. *Health Communication, 24*(7), 608–618. doi:10.1080/10410230903242218

Fortier, J. P., & Bishop, D. (2003). *Setting the agenda for research on cultural competence in health care: Final report.* Rockville, MD: U.S. Department of Health and Human Services Office of Minority Health and Agency for Healthcare Research and Quality.

Girod, S., Fassiotto, M., Grewal, D., Ku, M. C., Sriram, N., Nosek, B. A., & Valantine, H. (2016). Reducing implicit gender leadership bias in academic medicine with an educational intervention. *Academic Medicine, 91*, 1143–1150. doi:10.1097/acm.0000000000001099

Gordon, H. S., Street, R. L., Jr., Sharf, B. F., & Souchek, J. (2006). Racial differences in doctors' information-giving and patients' participation. *Cancer, 107*(6), 1313–1320. doi:10.1002/cncr.22122

Ho, E. Y. (2006). Behold the power of Qi: The importance of Qi in the discourse of acupuncture. *Research on Language and Social Interaction, 39*, 411–440. doi:10.1207/s15327973rlsi3904_3

Ho, E. Y. (2014). Socio-cultural factors in health communication. In N. G. Harrington (Ed.), *Health communication: Theory, method, and application* (pp. 212–239). New York and London: Routledge.

Ho, E. Y., & Bylund, C. L. (2008). Models of health and models of interaction in the practitioner-client relationship in acupuncture. *Health Communication, 23*, 506–515. doi:10.1080/10410230802460234

Hsieh, E. (2006). Understanding medical interpreters: Reconceptualizing bilingual health communication. *Health Communication, 20*, 177–186. doi:10.1207/s15327027hc2002_9

Hsieh, E. (2007). Interpreters as co-diagnosticians: Overlapping roles and services between providers and interpreters. *Social Science and Medicine, 64*, 924–937.

International Association of Medical Colleges. (n.d.) LCME Accreditation Standards. Retrieved from http://www.iaomc.org/lcme.htm

Kim, Y.-C., & Ball-Rokeach, S. J. (2006). Civic engagement from a communication infrastructure perspective. *Communication Theory, 16*, 173–197. doi:10.1111/j.1468-2885.2006.00267.x

Kleinman, A. (1980). *Patients and healers in the context of culture* (Vol. 3). Berkeley, CA: University of California.

Kleinman, A. (1988). *The illness narratives*. New York, NY: Basic Books.

Kreuter, M. W., & Haughton, L. T. (2006). Integrating culture into health information for African American women. *American Behavioral Scientist, 49*, 794–811. doi:10.1177/0002764205283801

Kreuter, M. W., Lukwago, S. N., Bucholtz, R. D., Clark, E. M., & Sanders-Thompson, V. (2003). Achieving cultural appropriateness in health promotion programs: Targeted and tailored approaches. *Health Education & Behavior, 30*, 133–146. doi.org/10.1177/1090198102251021

Lupton, D. (1994). Toward the development of critical health communication praxis. *Health Communication, 6*, 55–67. doi:10.1207/s15327027hc0601_4

Masters, C., Robinson, D., Faulkner, S., Patterson, E., McIlraith, T., & Ansari, A. (2019). Addressing biases in patient care with The 5Rs of cultural humility, a clinician coaching tool. *Journal of General Internal Medicine, 34*, 627–630. doi:10.1007/s11606-018-4814-y

Metzl, J. M., & Hansen, H. (2014). Structural competency: Theorizing a new medical engagement with stigma and inequality. *Social Science & Medicine, 103*, 126–133. doi:10.1016/j.socscimed.2013.06.032

Mishler, E. G. (1984). *The discourse of medicine: Dialectics of medical interviews*. Norwood, NJ: Ablex.

Morris, D. B. (1998). *Illness and culture in the postmodern age*. Berkeley, CA: University of California.

Obregon, R., & Waisbord, S. (Eds.). (2012). *The handbook of global health communication*. Malden, MA: John Wiley & Sons.

Payer, L. (1988/1996). *Medicine & culture*. New York, NY: Henry Holt.

Penner, L. A., Dovidio, J. F., Gonzalez, R., Albrecht, T. L., Chapman, R., Foster, T., . . . Eggly, S. (2016). The effects of oncologist implicit racial bias in racially discordant oncology interactions. *Journal of Clinical Oncology, 34*, 2874–2880. doi:10.1200/jco.2015.66.3658

Philipsen, G. (1992). *Speaking culturally: Explorations in social communication*. Albany, NY: SUNY Press.

Philipsen, G. (1997). A theory of speech codes. In G. Philipsen & T. L. Albrecht (Eds.), *Developing communication theories* (pp. 119–156). Albany, NY: SUNY Press.

Philipsen, G., Coutu, L. M., & Covarrubias, P. (2005). Speech codes theory: Revision, restatement, and response to criticisms. In W. Gudykunst (Ed.), *Theorizing about intercultural communication* (pp. 55–68). Thousand Oaks, CA: Sage.

Renzaho, A. M., Romios, P., Crock, C., & Sønderlund, A. L. (2013). The effectiveness of cultural competence programs in ethnic minority patient-centered health care – a systematic review of the literature. *International Journal for Quality in Health Care, 25*(3), 261–269. doi:10.1093/intqhc/mzt006

Resnicow, K., Baranowski, T., Ahluwalia, J. S., & Braithwaite, R. L. (1999). Cultural sensitivity in public health: Defined and demystified. *Ethnicity & Disease, 9*, 10–21.

Resnicow, K., Soler, R., Braithwaite, R. L., Ahluwalia, J. S., & Butler, J. (2000). Cultural sensitivity in substance use prevention. *Journal of Community Psychology, 28*, 271–290. doi:10.1002/(SICI)1520-6629(200005)28:3<271::AID-JCOP4>3.0.CO;2-I

Sastry, S., Stephenson, M., Dillon, P. D., & Carter, A. L. (2019). A meta-theoretical systematic review of the culture-centered approach to health comunication: Toward a refined, "nested" model. *Communication Theory*. doi:10.1093/ct/qtz024

Schillinger, D. (2020). The intersections between social determinants of health, health literacy, and health disparities. In R. A. Logan & E. R. Siegel (Eds.), *Health literacy in clinical practice and public health: New initiatives and lessons learned at the intersection with other disciplines* (pp. 22–41). IOS Press.

Schillinger, D., & Huey, N. (2018). Messengers of truth and health – Young artists of color raise their voices to prevent diabetes. *JAMA, 319*(11), 1076–1078. doi:10.1001/jama.2018.0986

Schillinger, D., McNamara, D., Crossley, S., Lyles, C., Moffet, H. H., Sarkar, U., . . . Karter, A. J. (2017). The next frontier in communication and the ECLIPPSE study: Bridging the linguistic divide in secure messaging. *Journal of Diabetes Research, 2017*, 9. doi:10.1155/2017/1348242

Sharf, B. F., & Kahler, J. (1996). Victims of the franchise: A culturally sensitive model of teaching patient-doctor communication in the inner city. In E. B. Ray (Ed.), *Communication and disenfranchisement: Social health issues and implications* (pp. 95–115). Mahwah, NJ: Erlbaum.

Sharf, B. F., Kahler, J., Foley, R., Bomgaars, M., Grant, D., & Harper, S. (1990). A shared understanding: Bridging racial and class differences in patient-doctor communication (video and instructors' manual). Chapel Hill, NC: Health Sciences Consortium.

Smedley, B. D., Stith, A. Y., & Nelson, A. R. (Eds.). (2003). *Unequal treatment: Confronting racial and ethnic disparities in health care.* Washington, DC: The National Academies Press.

Street Jr, R. L. (2003). Communication in medical encounters: An ecological perspective. In T. L. Thompson, A. M. Dorsey, K. I. Miller, & R. Parrott (Eds.), *Handbook of health communication* (pp. 63–89). Mahwah, NJ: Erlbaum.

Tervalon, M., & Murray-Garcia, J. (1998). Cultural humility versus cultural competence: A critical distinction in defining physician training outcomes in multicultural education. *Journal of Health Care for the Poor and Underserved, 9*, 117–125.

US Department of Health & Human Services, Office of Minority Health (2001). *National Standards for Culturally and Linguistically Appropriate Services in Health Care.* Rockville, MD.

Waitzkin, H. (1991). *The politics of medical encounters: How patients and doctors deal wtih social problems.* New Haven, CT: Yale University Press.

Wilkin, H. A. (2013). Exploring the potential of communication infrastructure theory for informing efforts to reduce health disparities. *Journal of Communication, 63*, 181–200. doi:10.1111/jcom.12006

Wilkin, H. A., Moran, M. B., Ball-Rokeach, S. J., Gonzalez, C., & Kim, Y.-C. (2010). Applications of Communication Infrastructure Theory. *Health Communication, 25*, 611–612. doi:10.1080/10410236.2010.496839

Yamasaki, J. (2014). Age accomplished, performed, and failed: Liz Young as old on The Biggest Loser. *Text and Performance Quarterly, 34*, 354–371. doi:1 0.1080/10462937.2014.942871

Zoller, H. M., & Kline, K. N. (2008). Theoretical contributions of interpretive and critical research in health communication. In C. S. Beck (Ed.), *Communication Yearbook 32* (pp. 89–35). New York: Routledge.

15

Effects of Digital Media Technology on Health Communication

Maria D. Molina and S. Shyam Sundar

Traditionally, media and communication technology have been viewed as channels for the transmission of information between sender and receiver (Shannon and Weaver 1949). Following this premise, research has often centered on investigating the development of messages for distribution in online platforms with the goal of persuading users into engaging in better health behaviors. However, features of the medium can also have powerful persuasive effects. This is because affordances, or action possibilities, offered by different features of media technology, have psychological correlates that can persuade users in two distinct ways: (i) by providing visual representations or cues that guide perceptions and (ii) by motivating action (Sundar et al. 2015). These are referred to by the theory of interactive media effects (TIME) as the cue route and the action route. This dual-process framework can be used to understand several theories pertaining to the effects of technology in health communication.

Health Communication Theory, First Edition. Edited by Teresa L. Thompson and Peter J. Schulz.
© 2021 John Wiley & Sons, Inc. Published 2021 by John Wiley & Sons, Inc.

Cue route

Technological affordances are a bundle of cues that are often visible on the media interface. To begin with, the sheer presence of certain affordances in the form of features (e.g. interactive tools, Like button) can be a psychologically salient cue with potential to persuade individuals. Furthermore, the outcomes resulting from the use of such features by other individuals (in the form of visible metrics such as the number of comments and number of likes) can also serve as cues that can affect one's perceptions of the underlying health message and/or source.

MAIN Model

The modality-agency-interactivity-navigability (MAIN) model (Sundar 2008b) epitomizes the cue route. It posits that technological affordances can cue cognitive heuristics, or "rules of thumb," that guide user perceptions about the quality and credibility of the content they are reading. For example, in Lin and Spence (2018), users perceived a Twitter post warning about food safety as more trustworthy when it had received a high number of retweets, compared to a low number of retweets. This occurred because the number of retweets serves as a visual cue that triggers the *bandwagon heuristic* or the perception that "if others like or share this post then it must be true." Likewise, there are other cues on the interfaces of contemporary media that guide users' perceptions of content. The MAIN model identifies four broad categories of affordances that serve as repositories of interface cues: modality, agency, interactivity, and navigability.

Modality affordances refer to the "the means through which information is conveyed" (Sundar et al. 2015, p.72) and they can cue heuristics individually (i.e. text, audio, video) or in combination. For example, when exposed to a false news article through video compared to audio or text, users perceived the article as more credible and were also more likely to share it with their family (Sundar, Molina, and Cho 2020). This is because video modality cues the *realism heuristic* (i.e. the rule of thumb: "seeing is believing") due to its higher similarity to the real world (Sundar 2008b). Similarly, in Perrault and Silk (2014), users who were exposed to a website including a video promoting practices to reduce environmental breast cancer risk performed more risk prevention behaviors after 15 days of exposure, compared to those who were exposed to the explanatory website alone, but without the associated video. Another heuristic related with modality is the *being there heuristic*. This heuristic can be triggered by new media technologies, such as virtual and augmented reality (VR/AR). The ability of VR and AR in promoting immersion has been linked with several health benefits, particularly reducing anxiety disorders. This is because "mental health problems are inseparable from the environment," and VR can help recreate those difficult environments and experiences lived by individuals by triggering the being-there heuristic (Freeman et al. 2017, p. 2392).

Agency affordances refer to the multiple ways in which content can be sourced in new media. While in traditional media the sources of information were largely media organizations who served as the gatekeepers of content, this is not the case in online environments where we receive information from a variety of sources, ranging from news organization to friends and family. Likewise, we ourselves can act as sources of information by creating or curating content and sharing it with our network. This ability to serve as a source oneself, as well as the identity of other sources, can both be conveyed via cues on the interface, triggering a number of heuristics. An example is the *bandwagon heuristic* explained previously, where other users indirectly serve as sources in the form of social endorsement cues that provide users a sense of what others think about a particular topic. Such bandwagon cues not only alter our perceptions but can also alter our behaviors. For instance, in Molina (2019), when participants were provided meal options on a tracking device, they were more likely to select the highly rated meals for their next dinner, compared to meals that had a low star rating. Another relevant agency heuristic is the *authority heuristic* or the rule of thumb "if the source of information is an authority, then the information is likely true." For example, Lee and Sundar (2013) found that health tweets are perceived as more credible when they come from a doctor with many followers, compared to one with just a few followers.

Interactivity affordances pertain to features that enable individuals to interact with the media interface and other users (Sundar 2008b). One interactivity heuristic relevant to the health context is the *contingency heuristic*, or the "way that messages are threaded to reflect a sequence of interactions" (Sundar 2008b, p.87). A message is said to be contingent when it is related to not only the message immediately before it, but the one before that (Rafaeli 1988). Research reveals the mere presence of message interactivity in a site can cue the contingency heuristic, en route to persuasive outcomes. For instance, in Wise, Hamman, and Thorson (2006), participants were more likely to participate in an online community with slow response rate when messages were interactive and contingent upon each other (vs. not interactive). Message interactivity also has powerful effects on behavioral intentions. In Bellur and Sundar (2017), users assigned to an online health risk assessment tool with high message interactivity (chat service with threaded conversations) reported more likelihood to perform preventive health behaviors such as diet and exercising, as well as safer sex and alcohol consumption, compared to participants in the low interactivity condition (assigned to a chat that was simple Q&A). These effects were mediated by perceived contingency.

Finally, *navigability affordances* are those that give users the ability to explore the mediated environment (Sundar et al. 2015). For example, search engines provide relevance rankings based on several aspects such as previous browsing behavior. These rankings can trigger the *prominence heuristic*, or the rule of thumb that results that appear first on a search are the best (Sundar 2008b). Research reveals that the prominence of the link influences users' selection of the link even more than the associated abstract (Pan et al. 2007). Considering that more than 80 percent of patients go online for a health diagnosis (Wong and Cheung 2019), this heuristic can have a profound influence on health-related decisions by a large number of individuals, with important implications for public health. This is especially concerning in an online environment that is full of health misinformation. For example, a recent study found that 77% of YouTube videos about prostate cancer contained biased information and/or misinformation (Loeb et al. 2019).

Aside from search engines, a key source of health information is social media, where exposure tends to be incidental rather than planned. Importantly as well, this information often comes from a variety of sources, most of which are of unknown credibility in this content domain. The sheer variety of sources and volume of information found online can lead to information overload, forcing users to make their decisions and credibility assessments by relying on heuristic cues (Metzger, Flanagin, and Medders 2010).

Network Influence and Social Contagion

Another distinguishing element of social media is the network of direct and indirect ties surrounding each user. While other users can influence our decision-making online through agency affordances such as the bandwagon cue or the identity cue, they can also influence our behaviors online through *social contagion*. Social contagion is a theory posed by Christakis and Fowler (2007, 2013) which posits that social networks typically exhibit "three degrees of influence," meaning that our social connections have influence on our behavior, and this influence does not end with a direct friend. In other words, people influence their direct friends (one degree), who then influence their friends (second degree), who in turn influence their friends (third degree). For example, Christakis and Fowler (2007) analyzed the Framingham Heart Study, a longitudinal database of cohorts including information about the types of connections (friends, relatives, or neighbors) of each participant for 30 years. The researchers found that obesity in social networks was clustered into discernable ties and that the risk of obesity among people connected with someone with obesity was about 45% higher in the observed versus random network (one degree of separation). Similarly, the risk of obesity for a friend's friend was 20% higher (two degrees of separation), and that of a friend's friend's friend was 10% higher (three degrees of separation). However, the researchers did not find evidence of contagion effects by the fourth degree, suggesting that the reach of contagion was three degrees.

Social contagion effects are also evident in social media. For instance, Coviello et al. (2014) found that on Facebook, rainfall influenced the emotional tone of users' status and it also affected the status of users' friends who were in cities where there was no precipitation. This means that emotions "ripple through social networks to generate large-scale synchrony that gives rise to clusters of happy and unhappy individuals" (Coviello et al. 2014, p.5). With new media technologies, users have unique opportunities to express their thoughts and opinions to a wide range of users. This means that we could see "spikes in global emotion that could generate increased volatility" (Coviello et al. 2014, p.5). For instance, posts revealing suicidal ideation are increasingly common in social media. A recent study revealed that exposure to self-harm posts on Instagram was associated with emotional disturbance and suicidal ideation (Arendt, Scherr, and Romer 2019).

But why does contagion occur? As Christakis and Fowler (2013) explain, "not everything spreads by the same mechanisms" (p. 563). For instance, while it is possible that weight gain/loss spreads due to social learning or imitation of eating or workout behaviors, it is also possible that it occurs due to a transmitted social norm. Likewise, it is also possible that contagion occurs due to the operation of a particular cue or heuristic, such as the similarity heuristic, where one imitates the behavior of another person who is evaluated as similar to oneself. Centola (2011) demonstrates the influence of homophily in an experimental study where participants were randomly assigned to a structured or unstructured network. In the structured network, participants were clustered by health characteristics within a social network neighborhood, whereas the nonstructured networks were composed of integrated neighborhoods despite such characteristics. Findings of the study reveal that structured networks adapted an internet-based diet diary significantly more than the unstructured network. Importantly as well, this difference held true not only for fit participants, but also obese members of the population. In fact, "homophilous networks promoted greater uptake of the behavior among obese individuals than among nonobese individuals" (Centola 2011, p.1270). Findings of this study also reveal the effect of homophily on adoption of a behavior occurs regardless of how homophily is generated. In other words, people do not necessarily have to make a choice on forming homophilous relationships. Homophilous relationships based on individual characteristics alone, regardless of the shared history that people might have, can lead to social influence. This is consistent with Christakis and Fowler's (2013) work revealing that social distance is of greater importance than geographical distance in the spread of obesity. Furthermore, despite homophily being an important variable to explain diffusion in social networks, Christakis and Fowler (2007) found that the influence of friends is directional, revealing that the "covariance in traits between friends is unlikely to be the result of unobserved contemporaneous exposures experienced by the two persons in a friendship" because if this were the case, then there should not be a difference in directionality (Christakis and Fowler 2013, p. 570). In other words, influence within a network has a social nature, regardless of people's tendencies to select friends based on similarities.

Proteus Effect

Another theory pertinent to the cue route is the Proteus effect, which seeks to explain the relationship between avatar representation during an online interaction and user behavior (Yee and Bailenson 2007). According to the Proteus effect, users infer their expected action during an interaction based on the avatar image, and conform to that behavior during the interaction or game. This is possible due to the anonymity afforded by online environments where a loss of self-awareness or individuality might occur. In these instances, users "are free to take over or essentially possess other objects in the world, which grants them unique abilities" (Yee 2014, p. 206). The avatar, thus, is not simply used as a tool during the online experience, but it becomes part of the user's self-representation, influencing how the user behaves (Yee and Bailenson 2007). For example, in Li, Lwin, and Jung's (2014) analysis of body size and workout motivation in overweight children, children assigned to conditions where their avatar had a normal body size performed significantly better in a running game than those assigned to conditions where the avatar had a larger body size. Furthermore, children in the normal body size condition also had more positive attitudes and motivation toward working out after the activity.

The inferring of expected action in the Proteus effect occurs because of self-perception, where users "conform to the expectations and stereotypes of the identity of their avatars" (Yee and Bailenson 2007, p.274). In other words, people examine an avatar's appearance from a third-person perspective and behave in accordance with the stereotypical expectation associated with that appearance. In this regard, virtual worlds are similar to the real world in that we interpret our own attitudes based not only on how we act, but also on how we look (Yee and Bailenson 2007). This explains why in the Li et al. (2014) study participants in the large body size conditions performed worse than those in the normal body size condition. As the authors explain, being stereotyped, whether positively (normal body size) or negatively (large body size), transcends the "real" world into virtual environments. Thus, designing avatars that suggest the behavior that we would like to see enacted (i.e. fit avatars to encourage workout behavior) would increase attitudinal and behavioral changes.

Action Route

While the aforementioned theories are premised on the subtle influence of contextual cues on relatively passive consumers of information, the next set of theories focuses on the interactivity afforded by contemporary media technologies. As new technologies provide newer and more varied opportunities for the user to interact with the system, they call for motivated users to engage with the information in more effortful ways and process it more systematically rather than heuristically. This can have a range of psychological effects that go well beyond the perceptual effects of cognitive heuristics and nudges described thus far.

Agency Model

The agency model of customization discusses the psychological outcomes of the user becoming, in effect, the source of communication with the help of interactivity, modality, and navigability affordances in the medium. The "self as source" perception is theorized to increase user involvement in the content of the system, project their identity onto the interface and help provide control over the system, leading to powerful psychological outcomes pertaining to cognition, affect, and behavior, respectively (Sundar 2008a). When the user can customize the online environment or generate his/her own content, it allows them to assert identity, which can be both ego-gratifying and can instill a sense of importance of their own agency. Furthermore, the degree to which a user can generate new content is the degree of choice the user perceives s/he has over the information environment.

For example, in Kalyanaraman and Sundar (2006), users who received articles through websites tailored to their own interests had better attitudes toward the sites, compared to conditions with low and medium customization. This relationship was mediated by perceived involvement and perceived interactivity. Likewise, in Kang and Sundar (2016), when users read a health-related message from a site that allowed them to customize by selecting themes or gadgets of their choice, they were more likely to engage in the health-related messages in the article. This occurred because users who were allowed to customize perceived the site as being a reflection of their own identity. Importantly as well, customization or user-initiated tailoring is typically more effective than personalization or system-initiated tailoring because it provides higher levels of choice. In a study exploring personalization versus customization as strategies to promote preventive health information delivered via smart watches, users who were allowed to select from a category of topics expressed better attitudes toward the health message, compared to those who were provided with a topic based on their previous browsing behavior (Kim, Shin, and Yoon 2017).

The effects of personalization and customization on health attitudes and behaviors have also been explored in the context of new technologies such as conversational agents and avatars. For example, Fulmer et al. (2018) utilized a conversational agent (Tess) to relieve depression and anxiety. The system was programmed to follow-up with users daily on previously discussed topics and personalized responses by "adjusting their style to accommodate a client's therapeutic preference over time" and "gathering feedback to deliver interventions that best meet a user's needs" (p. 4). Results reveal that depression symptoms of participants who interacted with Tess decreased over the course of the study. Conversely, symptoms increased for those assigned to a control group who received general information through an electronic link about depression without any form of customization.

Similar health interventions for treatment of mental health have been conducted utilizing avatar customization. In Birk and Mandryk's (2019) study, customizing an avatar (vs. receiving a predetermined avatar) improved the efficacy of a cognitive training program designed for mental health intervention. Participants in the customized avatar condition were more likely to feel identified with the avatar. Notably, avatar identification was correlated with reduction of anxiety for participants on the training. Similarly, in Fox and Bailenson's study (2009), when the avatar resembled the user, users were more motivated to exercise than when the avatar represented another model, even when this possessed the same sex and gender as the participant. More than resemblance, the extent to which participants are able to visualize their ideal body through their avatar is positively related to the level of motivation they have to engage in preventive health behaviors like quitting smoking or drinking (Kim and Sundar 2012).

Although providing users with customization tools is associated with positive attitudes toward the system and behavioral intentions to follow advocated health behaviors, it is important to consider its potential drawbacks. For instance, allowing users to choose what content to consume can lead to selective exposure or a systematic bias in the kind of media content that is consumed (Knobloch-Westerwick 2015a), with problematic consequences, as explained in the next section.

Selective Exposure Self- and Affect-Management Model

The selective exposure self- and affect-management (SESAM) model (Knobloch-Westerwick 2015b) explains that when selecting messages for consumption users do so to regulate their self-concept, as well as their affective and cognitive states. An important concept for understanding the SESAM model is the dynamic self-concept, which postulates that a person's self-concept is not stable, but is composed of many self-representations (Knobloch-Westerwick 2015b; Markus and Wurf 1987). While some self-representation can be activated automatically as a result of situational stimuli, others are sought out by people. Markus and Wurf (1987) describe three motives for the activation of self-representations: self-enhancement, self-consistency, and self-actualization. These motives determine what self-concept will be activated at any given time and in turn that "working self-concept regulates ongoing responses and behaviors" (Knobloch-Westerwick 2015b, p. 967). While there are many individual characteristics that influence users' selection of content, these will not influence responses to a media message at a given time unless they are activated and salient. For instance, Knobloch-Westerwick

(2015b) found that weight management salience measured at time 1 influenced user's tracking of food intake (time 3). This relationship was mediated by selective exposure to weight loss messages at time 2.

Studies exploring selective exposure in online environments caution that some affordances of technology such as customization can exacerbate selective exposure and lead to negative consequences. This is because when users are allowed to select what topics and articles to read through customization, they will likely encounter pro-attitudinal messages, while reducing engagement with counter-attitudinal information (Dylko et al. 2017). Scholars warn about the possible creation of echo-chambers or filter bubbles where users mainly encounter information that aligns with their own beliefs and attitudes (Sunstein 2002). This is especially important in social media where we receive information from an array of sources ranging from news organizations, to unreliable sources, to our network of friends and family. Del Vicario et al. (2016) analyzed the spread of information online, specifically rumors, and found that "users mostly tend to select and share content related to a specific narrative and ignore the rest" (p. 558) and that social homogeneity was the primary predictor of content diffusion, meaning users who take information from others belong to the same echo chamber.

Such an online ecosystem can be a dangerous breeding ground for misinformation. As Southwell, Thorson, and Sheble (2017) explain, misinformation can lead people to have misperceptions about particular events or phenomena. When these misperceptions occur among large groups of people, these can have "downstream consequences for health, social harmony, and political life" (p. 368). For instance, Broniatowski et al. (2018) found that Russian trolls and bots spread misinformation about vaccines, intensifying the division between supporters and those against vaccination. The easiness through which such rumors diffuse online and their effects has led many to recognize misinformation as a threat to public health and a pandemic risk (Larson 2018).

Motivational Technology Model

While the agency model of customization predicts that features of technology can persuade users by imbuing a sense of agency, the motivational technology model (MoTech; Sundar, Bellur, and Jia 2012) predicts affordances can do so by enhancing self-determination (see chapter 11 in this volume). The model explains that technological affordances of modern media can help satisfy the basic psychological needs outlined by self-determination theory (SDT). For example, the presence of interactivity on an interface can afford users the ability to relate to others with similar health issues and thereby fulfill the need for relatedness. Customization, or the ability to tailor content in the medium, can fulfill human need for autonomy. Good navigability features on a media interface can render it more usable and serve to enhance the feeling of competence among users. Satisfying users' needs of relatedness, autonomy, and competence through these technological affordances can, in turn, increase users' intrinsic motivation to use health systems and applications, as predicted by SDT. The repeated use of the health applications will translate into positive preventive health attitudes and behaviors.

Empirical research using this model has shown a systematic association between the provision of interface features and the key predictors and outcomes of intrinsic motivation. For example, Bellur and DeVoss (2018) found that perceived interactivity afforded by mHealth apps was a predictor of attitudes toward the health app and users' intention to continue using the app. Similarly, Jung and Sundar (2016) showed that the number of comments and replies in a user's Facebook profile was associated with higher feelings of relatedness and enjoyment of Facebook among senior citizens.

Furthermore, affording interactivity provides a venue to receive informational and emotional support to help patients cope with their situation (e.g. Leimeister et al. 2008; Nimrod 2013). Although online social support shares several of the characteristics of face-to-face social support, the ability to communicate both synchronously and asynchronously, and the anonymity associated with these spaces make online social support unique (Lacoursiere 2001). As Lacoursiere (2001) explains, the absence of social context cues in online environments allows for more egalitarian participation across users because social differences get eliminated. In turn, users of online communities are brought together by common interests rather than background or offline networks (Ferreday 2009), thus enhancing the relatability among members of those communities.

Just as interactivity affordances can increase users' sense of relatedness, agency affordances are known to imbue the sense of control necessary to satisfy users' need for autonomy (Sundar et al. 2012). One such feature of technology provided by tracking applications is allowing users to choose among different workouts or exercises. A recent study found that users who chose workouts from a series of options on a fitness app reported more engagement in physical activity, more cardio hours, and more total weight lifted (Molina and Sundar 2020). In fact, a unit increase in the number of workouts a user followed increased the amount of weight lifted at a rate of 3.2% and cardio hours by 3.9%.

Finally, MoTech predicts that navigability affordances can build competence by allowing users to explore the interface or application. This is because easy navigation allows users to achieve their goals more efficiently (Sundar et al. 2012). For example, providing navigational features such as steering control in VR environments is associated with increased spatial presence (Balakrishnan and Sundar 2011). Evidence suggests spatial presence is correlated with increased likelihood of enacting protective health behaviors (Westerman, Spence, and Lin, 2015). Aside from navigability, modality affordances related to posting pictures can also promote user competence. For example, in Jung and Sundar's (2016) study exploring older adults' Facebook interactions, the number of photos participants posted over the year was associated with feelings of competence. This is because posting pictures requires a higher level of skill than a text entry. Similarly, in Molina and Sundar (2020) the number of pictures a user posted was positively associated with more weight lifted in a tracking application. This pattern was especially prominent for male users of the platform.

Gamification

Self-determination theory has also been applied to the gaming context, specifically studying how different features of games can increase or thwart the needs of relatedness, competence, and autonomy (e.g. Peng et al. 2012; Tamborini et al. 2011). "The intentional use of game elements for a gameful experience of non-game tasks and contexts" (Seaborn and Fels 2015, p. 17) – a strategy known as gamification – has been shown to increase engagement with health applications and important health outcomes. Game elements include leaderboards, achievement ranks, competition and challenges, and rewards, among others.

The purpose behind the use of gamification in different contexts is to engage users with a brand or application, motivate users, and promote behavioral change. The latter objective is particularly important in the health context. A systematic review assessing the effectiveness of gamification in promoting health and well-being revealed that 59% of studies included in the review found positive results (Johnson et al. 2016). For example, Shameli et al. (2017) analyzed the use of competition in promoting physical activity. In their study, participants engaged in a walking challenge using a mobile tracking application. On average, participants increased physical activity by 23% during these competitions. Notwithstanding, participants who were last in the competition did not increase their activity after the competition. For these participants, their physical activity actually dropped below baseline levels. This finding reveals that for competition to be successful, participants should be equal in their physical activity pre-competition. Other studies have analyzed gamification elements for treating anxiety. For example, in Pramana et al.'s (2018) study, gamification was used to improve the delivery of cognitive behavioral therapy treatment to children. Findings reveal that children who used the gamified therapy used the app more frequently and longer compared to children who used the previous non-gamified version.

All these findings support a general theory of gamification which argues that game elements are intrinsically motivating for users and therefore increase the likelihood of uptake of health message, leading to desired consequences. The sheer attractiveness of gameplay ensures that individuals use the interactive tools offered by the interface, which translates to greater engagement with advocated health content embedded in the interface. There are several mechanisms underlying the effects of gamification, many of which derive from specific elements of technology. For instance, Frost and Eden (2014) analyzed the effects of private versus shared feedback on motivation to play brain games. They found that when feedback such as leaderboards is shared on social networks, participants are more motivated and enjoyed the game more. The authors explain that this could have occurred because shared feedback satisfies users' needs of relatedness and competence. On the other hand, Carissoli and Villani (2019) found that video games can help foster emotional intelligence because students are guided to "pay attention to their emotions" (p. 411) increasing their awareness of their own emotional states and functioning. Despite several mechanisms guiding the success of gamification, Ushaw, Eyre, and Morgan,(2017) argue that the main reason for the success of games designed for serious contexts such as health is the interactivity through which the benefit is being delivered.

Interactivity Effects Model

The action route of TIME is best epitomized by the interactivity effects model (Sundar 2007) which identifies three different species of interactive tools offered by media interfaces – modality interactivity, message interactivity, and source interactivity. *Modality interactivity* refers to the different modalities we use when interacting with our media, ranging from text, audio and video to newer forms of interaction such as swiping and gesturing. These modalities differ in the degree to which they afford sensory experience of the mediated environment because they differ in the degree to which they map our natural actions in real life, and the extent to which they are intuitive and ease to use. Certain modalities like sliding (i.e. using a slider to move across an interface) are known to increase the "perceptual bandwidth" of users, allowing them to take in more of the mediated content and leading to greater engagement with messages embedded in that content. In a series of studies, Oh and colleagues have shown that modality interactivity in the form of a slider can be quite instrumental in increasing the effectiveness of preventive health messages on websites. This is because modality interactivity increases cognitive absorption, leading to better attitudes toward the interface and its message (Oh and Sundar 2015). A recent study found that the number of clicks and drags that users perform on sliders on an anti-smoking website is positively associated with their attitudes toward anti-smoking messages and smoking outcome beliefs among non-smoking power users. The increase in "perceptual bandwidth" caused by the use of sliders can be a double-edged sword, however, with non-smokers becoming more engaged with the health advocacy message but smokers becoming more defensive in their processing of the message (Oh and Sundar 2019).

Message interactivity is quite different from modality interactivity in that it refers to the exchange of messages with the system or with others, often in textual form. The widespread popularity of instant messaging via a variety of platforms such as SMS, WhatsApp, and chatbots signifies the appeal of this form of interactivity. Message interactivity engages users by offering contingent messages, i.e. subsequent messages are contingent upon the content of the preceding messages leading to a threaded conversation. Contingency can also be achieved by explicitly acknowledging interaction history. Oh and Sundar (2015) found that when they embedded an anti-smoking website with message interactivity (by branching its content based on user actions and using visual indicators of interaction history to show the path they traversed through the site), users were more cognitively engaged with content, elaborating on the prevention message embedded in the site. Aside from building interaction, message interactivity can also be used to create a dialogue quite akin to interpersonal communication, as often happens in doctor–patient communications. Bellur and Sundar (2017) operationalized it in the form of an online health risk assessment tool that asked pointed questions and provided health advice by taking into account not only user responses to those questions but also their responses to earlier questions, thus mimicking a threaded conversation. They found that high levels of such contingency in message exchange were associated with higher levels of perceived contingency and dialogue, which in turn was associated with more positive attitudes toward the online tool and its contents, but more importantly higher intentions for future preventive health behaviors.

Source interactivity refers to affordances that enable users to serve as sources of content, either by way of gatekeeping for oneself (customization) and others (curation) or by creating one's own messages (e.g. blogs). The model argues that opportunities for self-expression can boost user engagement with the interface and its contents. This is quite evident from research on online social support wherein laypersons act as important sources of informational and social support to others. For instance, frequency of blogging is associated with greater levels of perceived support from readers, and perceived reader support is a positive predictor of health self-efficacy (Rains and Keating 2011). The model of digital coping with illness (Rains 2018) further outlines how affordances of communication technology can be systematically used for coping with illness. The model explains two initial steps. First, people assess the event or illness and its relevance. Five forms of distress are identified: emotional upset, inadequate information, insufficient support, physical pain, and existential concerns. Then, users evaluate affordances of communication technology for its use in that particular distress. For instance, if distress stems from insufficient support, then the person would likely benefit from utilizing visibility affordances of communication in order to identify themselves to others who might provide that support. Other situational or individual differences will also play a role in users' selection and evaluation of technological affordances. The form of distress, affordances of technology, and individual difference together will contribute to the digital coping activity that a person will utilize (e.g. acquiring and sharing information, managing upset, sensemaking). For instance, in the above example, a person whose distress is due to inadequate information might use visibility affordances of technology to acquire information and expand connections.

Source interactivity can also be manifest in terms of user comments and ratings of helpfulness. Such feedback received from others who exercise their source interactivity in a support forum by way of site metrics (e.g. number of people who found your post helpful) and system-generated status markers (e.g. the label of frequent contributor) are shown by research to motivate individuals to post more in online health forums (Kim and Sundar 2011).

Captology

There are two possible interactions that can occur with technology: interacting with others through technology (computer-mediated communication) or interacting *with* computers (human–computer interaction). Captology studies the latter, specifically "how people are motivated or persuaded when interacting with computing products" (Fogg 2003, p.16). Thus, the goal of captology is to motivate attitude and behavioral change through interactions with technology. Importantly, these interactions should be planned or intentional, meaning that they must be designed with a particular persuasive goal in mind. Persuasion through technology can occur through two levels – macrosuasion and microsuasion. The first is when the overall goal of a designed product is to persuade. For instance, in Miloff et al. (2016), the authors tested a VR exposure therapy for treating spider phobia. This VR experience was specifically created with this goal in mind. On the other hand, microsuasion occurs when elements of the designed technology include persuasive components (e.g. dialogue boxes, interaction patterns). For instance, to persuade about a product's effectiveness, sites often use testimonials from other users. Testimonials have been associated with greater trust toward a site, and have a greater impact on users with less online shopping experience (Spillinger and Parush 2012).

According to captology, there are three strategies through which technology persuades depending on the role that is played by computers. Fogg (2003) refers to these roles as the functional triad. On one hand, technology can serve as a tool, making behavior easier to accomplish or leading users through a particular process. For instance, digital technologies can allow users with an illness to document and maintain diaries, helping in the sensemaking process of coping with that illness (Rains 2018). Secondly, technology can serve as a medium. In this sense, technology can be persuasive by providing users with vicarious experiences and helping people practice a behavior (Fogg 2003). A representation of the self through virtual environments, for instance, has been associated with exercise motivation (Fox and Bailenson 2009). Finally, technology can persuade by being a social actor, or creating relationships with the user (Fogg 2003). For example, conversational agents can be utilized for treatment of depression and anxiety by providing therapy to users in need (Fulmer et al. 2018).

Conclusion

In sum, a range of emergent theories and associated research delineates how affordances of digital media technologies can play a critical role in shaping the presentation, uses, and effects of a variety of health communications, ranging from preventive campaigns by public health advocates to doctor's advice about healthy behaviors to informational and emotional support from laypersons in online forums. As such, the theories covered in this chapter signal a departure from the earlier generation of "technology theories" (e.g. diffusion of innovation, technology acceptance model) that tended to treat technologies as boxes, often black boxes, without considering their constituent properties, instead focusing on user perceptions of existing technologies. The new breed of technology theories drills down to specific features of digital media technologies (e.g. modality, interactivity, customization) and attempts to articulate the processes (e.g. heuristics, contagion, gamification) by which they shape user perceptions and actions in the health domain. While the first set of theories in this chapter focused on the "cue effect" of technological affordances in promoting persuasion, the latter set emphasized the "action effect" wherein users need to engage with the medium in order to co-create a reality that is personally relevant to individual users' health status and aspirations. Together, both serve to advance our knowledge about social cognition, motivation, and a whole host of social psychological factors that underlie the effects of modern media technologies on individual health.

References

Arendt, F., Scherr, S., & Romer, D. (2019). Effects of exposure to self-harm on social media: Evidence from a two-wave panel study among young adults. *New Media & Society, 21*(11–12), 2422–2442. doi:10.1177/1461444819850106

Balakrishnan, B., & Sundar, S. S. (2011). Where am I? How can I get there? Impact of navigability and narrative transportation on spatial presence. *Human–Computer Interaction, 26*(3), 161–204. doi:10.1080/07370024.2011.601689

Bellur, S., & DeVoss, C. (2018). Apps and autonomy: Perceived interactivity and autonomous regulation in mHealth applications. *Communication Research Reports, 35*(4), 314–324. doi:10.1080/08824096.2018.1501672

Bellur, S., & Sundar, S. S. (2017). Talking health with a machine: How does message interactivity affect attitudes and cognitions? *Human Communication Research, 43*(1), 25–53. doi:10.1111/hcre.12094

Birk, M. V., & Mandryk, R. L. (2019). Improving the efficacy of cognitive training for digital mental health interventions through avatar customization: Crowdsourced quasi-experimental study. *Journal of Medical Internet Research, 21*(1). doi:10.2196/10133

Broniatowski, D. A., Jamison, A. M., Qi, S., AlKulaib, L., Chen, T., Benton, A., . . . Dredze, M. (2018). Weaponized health communication: Twitter bots and Russian trolls amplify the vaccine debate. *American Journal of Public Health, 108*(10), 1378–1384. doi:10.2105/AJPH.2018.304567

Carissoli, C., & Villani, D. (2019). Can videogames be used to promote emotional intelligence in teenagers? Results from EmotivaMente, a school program. *Games for Health Journal, 8*(6), 407–413. doi:10.1089/g4h.2018.0148

Centola, D. (2011). An experimental study of homophily in the adoption of health behavior. *Science, 334*(6060), 1269–1272. doi:10.1126/science.1207055

Christakis, N. A., & Fowler, J. H. (2007). The spread of obesity in a large social network over 32 years. *The New England Journal of Medicine, 357*(4), 370–379. doi:10.1056/NEJMsa066082

Christakis, N. A., & Fowler, J. H. (2013). Social contagion theory: Examining dynamic social networks and human behavior. *Statistics in Medicine, 32*(4), 556–577. doi:10.1002/sim.5408

Coviello, L., Sohn, Y., Kramer, A. D. I., Marlow, C., Franceschetti, M., Christakis, N. A., & Fowler, J. H. (2014). Detecting emotional contagion in massive social networks. *PLOS ONE, 9*(3), e90315. doi:10.1371/journal.pone.0090315

Del Vicario, M., Bessi, A., Zollo, F., Petroni, F., Scala, A., Caldarelli, G., . . . Quattrociocchi, W. (2016). The spreading of misinformation online. *Proceedings of the National Academy of Sciences, 113*(3), 554. doi:10.1073/pnas.1517441113

Dylko, I., Dolgov, I., Hoffman, W., Eckhart, N., Molina, M., & Aaziz, O. (2017). The dark side of technology: An experimental investigation of the influence of customizability technology on online political selective exposure. *Computers in Human Behavior, 73*, 181–190. doi:10.1016/j.chb.2017.03.031

Ferreday, D. (2009). *Online belongings: Fantasy, affect and web communities.* New York, NY: Peter Lang.

Fogg, B. J. (2003). *Persuasive technology: Using computers to change what we think and do.* San Francisco, CA: Morgan Kaufmann.

Fox, J., & Bailenson, J. N. (2009). Virtual self-modeling: The effects of vicarious reinforcement and identification on exercise behaviors. *Media Psychology, 12*(1), 1–25. doi:10.1080/15213260802669474

Freeman, D., Reeve, S., Robinson, A., Ehlers, A., Clark, D., Spanlang, B., & Slater, M. (2017). Virtual reality in the assessment, understanding, and treatment of mental health disorders. *Psychological Medicine, 47*(14), 2393–2400. doi:10.1017/S003329171700040X

Frost, J., & Eden, A. (2014). The effect of social sharing games and game performance on motivation to play brain games. In B. Schouten, S. Fedtke, M. Schijven, M. Vosmeer, & A. Gekker (Eds.), *Games for health 2014* (pp. 48–55). Wiesbaden: Springer Vieweg.

Fulmer, R., Joerin, A., Gentile, B., Lakerink, L., & Rauws, M. (2018). Using psychological artificial intelligence (Tess) to relieve symptoms of depression and anxiety: Randomized controlled trial. *JMIR Mental Health, 5*(4), e64. doi:10.2196/mental.9782

Johnson, D., Deterding, S., Kuhn, K.-A., Staneva, A., Stoyanov, S., & Hides, L. (2016). Gamification for health and wellbeing: A systematic review of the literature. *Internet Interventions, 6*, 89–106. doi:10.1016/j.invent.2016.10.002

Jung, E. H., & Sundar, S. S. (2016). Senior citizens on Facebook: How do they interact and why? *Computers in Human Behavior, 61*, 27–35. doi:10.1016/j.chb.2016.02.080

Kalyanaraman, S., & Sundar, S. S. (2006). The psychological appeal of personalized content in web portals: Does customization affect attitudes and behavior? *Journal of Communication, 56*(1), 110–132. doi:10.1111/j.1460-2466.2006.00006.x

Kang, H., & Sundar, S. S. (2016). When self is the source: Effects of media customization on message processing. *Media Psychology, 19*(4), 561–588. doi:10.1080/15213269.2015.1121829

Kim, H.-S., & Sundar, S. (2011). Using interface cues in online health community boards to change impressions and encourage user contribution. *Proceedings of the SIGCHI Conference on Human Factors in Computing Systems*, 599–608. doi:10.1145/1978942.1979028

Kim, K. J., Shin, D.-H., & Yoon, H. (2017). Information tailoring and framing in wearable health communication. *Information Processing and Management, 53*(2), 351–358. doi:10.1016/j.ipm.2016.11.005

Kim, Y., & Sundar, S. S. (2012). Visualizing ideal self vs. actual self through avatars: Impact on preventive health outcomes. *Computers in Human Behavior, 28*(4), 1356–1364. doi:10.1016/j.chb.2012.02.021

Knobloch-Westerwick, S. (2015a). *Choice and preference in media use: Advances in selective exposure theory and research*. Routledge.

Knobloch-Westerwick, S. (2015b). The selective exposure self- and affect-management (SESAM) model: Applications in the realms of race, politics, and health. *Communication Research, 42*(7), 959–985. doi:10.1177/0093650214539173

Lacoursiere, S. P. (2001). A theory of online social support. *Advances in Nursing Science, 24*(1), 60–77. doi:10.1097/00012272-200109000-00008

Larson, H. J. (2018). The biggest pandemic risk? Viral misinformation. *Nature, 562*, 309. doi:10.1038/d41586-018-07034-4

Lee, J. Y., & Sundar, S. S. (2013). To tweet or to retweet? That is the question for health professionals on twitter. *Health Communication, 28*(5), 509–524. doi:10.1080/10410236.2012.700391

Leimeister, J. M., Schweizer, K., Leimeister, S., & Krcmar, H. (2008). Do virtual communities matter for the social support of patients? Antecedents and effects of virtual relationships in online communities. *Information Technology & People, 21*(4), 350–374. doi:10.1108/09593840810919671

Li, B. J., Lwin, M. O., & Jung, Y. (2014). Wii, myself, and size: The influence of proteus effect and stereotype threat on overweight children's exercise motivation and behavior in exergames. *Games for Health, 3*(1), 40–48.

Lin, X., & Spence, P. R. (2018). Identity on social networks as a cue: Identity, retweets, and credibility. *Communication Studies, 69*(5), 461–482. doi:10.1 080/10510974.2018.1489295

Loeb, S., Sengupta, S., Butaney, M., Macaluso, J. N., Czarniecki, S. W., Robbins, R.,. . . Langford, A. (2019). Dissemination of misinformative and biased information about prostate cancer on YouTube. *European Urology, 75*(4), 564–567. doi:10.1016/j.eururo.2018.10.056

Markus, H., & Wurf, E. (1987). The dynamic self-concept: A social psychological perspective. *Annual Review of Psychology, 38*(1), 299–337. doi:10.1146/ annurev.ps.38.020187.001503

Metzger, M. J., Flanagin, A. J., & Medders, R. B. (2010). Social and heuristic approaches to credibility evaluation online. *Journal of Communication, 60*(3), 413–439. doi:10.1111/j.1460-2466.2010.01488.x

Miloff, A., Lindner, P., Hamilton, W., Reuterskiöld, L., Andersson, G., & Carlbring, P. (2016). Single-session gamified virtual reality exposure therapy for spider phobia vs. traditional exposure therapy: Study protocol for a randomized controlled non-inferiority trial. *Trials, 17*, 1–8. doi:10.1186/ s13063-016-1171-1

Molina, M. D. (2019). I am what you eat: Effects of social influence on meal selection online. *Proceedings of CHI'19 Extended Abstracts of Human Factors in Computing Systems*, SRC09:1–6. doi:10.1145/3290607.3308451

Molina, M. D., & Sundar, S. S. (2020). Can mobile apps motivate fitness tracking? A study of technological affordances and workout behaviors. *Health Communication, 35*(1), 65–74. doi:10.1080/10410236.2018.1536961

Nimrod, G. (2013). Online depression communities: Members' interests and perceived benefits. *Health Communication, 28*(5), 425–434. doi:10.1080/10410 236.2012.691068

Oh, J., & Sundar, S. S. (2015). How does interactivity persuade? An experimental test of interactivity on cognitive absorption, elaboration, and attitudes. *Journal of Communication, 65*(2), 213–236. doi:10.1111/jcom.12147

Oh, J., & Sundar, S. S. (2019). What happens when you click and drag: Unpacking the relationship between on-screen interaction and user engagement with an anti-smoking website. *Health Communication*, 1–12. doi:10.1080/10410 236.2018.1560578

Pan, B., Hembrooke, H., Joachims, T., Lorigo, L., Gay, G., & Granka, L. (2007). In Google we trust: Users' decisions on rank, position, and relevance. *Journal of Computer-Mediated Communication, 12*(3), 801–823. doi:10.1111/ j.1083-6101.2007.00351.x

Peng, W., Lin, J.-H., Pfeiffer, K. A., & Winn, B. (2012). Need satisfaction supportive game features as motivational determinants: An experimental study of a self-determination theory guided exergame. *Media Psychology, 15*(2), 175–196. doi:10.1080/15213269.2012.673850

Perrault, E. K., & Silk, K. J. (2014). Testing the effects of the addition of videos to a website promoting environmental breast cancer risk reduction practices: Are videos worth it? *Journal of Applied Communication Research, 42*(1), 20–40. doi:10.1080/00909882.2013.854400

Pramana, G., Parmanto, B., Lomas, J., Lindhiem, O., Kendall, P. C., & Silk, J. (2018). Using mobile health gamification to facilitate cognitive behavioral therapy skills practice in child anxiety treatment: Open clinical trial. *Journal of Medical Internet Research, 20*(5), e9. doi:10.2196/games.8902

Rafaeli, S. (1988). From new media to communication. *Sage Annual Review of Communication Research: Advancing Communication Science, 16,* 110–134.

Rains, S. A. (2018). *Coping with illness digitally.* Cambridge, MA: The MIT Press.

Rains, S. A., & Keating, D. M. (2011). The social dimension of blogging about health: Health blogging, social support, and well-being. *Communication Monographs, 78*(4), 511–534. doi:10.1080/03637751.2011.618142

Seaborn, K., & Fels, D. I. (2015). Gamification in theory and action: A survey. *International Journal of Human-Computer Studies, 74,* 14–31.

Shameli, A., Althoff, T., Saberi, A., & Leskovec, J. (2017). How gamification affects physical activity: Large-scale analysis of walking challenges in a mobile application. *Proceedings of the 26th International Conference on World Wide Web Companion (WWW '17 Companion),* 455–463. doi:10.1145/3041021.3054172

Shannon, C. E., & Weaver, W. (1949). *The mathematical theory of communication.* Urbana, IL: University of Illinois Press.

Southwell, B. G., Thorson, E. A., & Sheble, L. (2017). The persistence and peril of misinformation. *American Scientist, 105*(6), 372–375.

Spillinger, A., & Parush, A. (2012). The impact of testimonials on purchase intentions in a mock e-commerce web site. *Journal of Theoretical and Applied Electronic Commerce Research, 7*(1), 9–10. doi:10.4067/S0718-18762012000100005

Sundar, S. S (2007). Social psychology of interactivity in human-website interaction. In A. N. Joinson, K. Y. A. McKenna, T. Postmes, & U.-D. Reips (Eds.), *The Oxford handbook of internet psychology* (pp. 89–104). Oxford University Press. doi:10.1093/oxfordhb/9780199561803.013.0007

Sundar, S. S. (2008a). Self as source: Agency and customization in interactive media. In E. Konijn, S. Utz, M. Tanis, & S. Barnes (Eds.), *Mediated interpersonal communication* (pp. 58–74). New York, NY: Routledge. doi:10.4324/9780203926864

Sundar, S.S. (2008b). The MAIN model: A heuristic approach to understanding technology effects on credibility. In M. J. Metzger & A. J. Flanagin (Eds.), *Digital media, youth, and credibility* (pp. 72–100). Cambridge, MA: The MIT Press.

Sundar, S. S, Bellur, S., & Jia, H. (2012). Motivational technologies: A theoretical framework for designing preventive health applications. In M. Bang & E. L. Ragnemalm (Eds.), *Proceedings of the 7th International Conference on Persuasive Technology (PERSUASIVE 2012), Lecture notes in Computer Science* (pp. 112–122). Berlin/Heidelberg: Springer. doi:10.1007/978-3-642-31037-9_10

Sundar, S.S, Jia, H., Waddell, T. F., & Huang, Y. (2015). Toward a theory of interactive media effects (TIME): Four models for explaining how interface features affect user psychology. In S.S. Sundar (Ed.), *The handbook of the psychology of communication technology* (pp. 47–86). Malden, MA: Wiley Blackwell.

Sundar, S.S., Molina, M.D., & Cho, E. (2020). *Seeing is believing: Is video modality more powerful in spreading fake news via online messaging apps?* Unpublished manuscript.

Sunstein, C. R. (2002). The law of group polarization. *Journal of Political Philosophy, 10*(2), 175–195. doi:10.1111/1467-9760.00148

Tamborini, R., Grizzard, M., David Bowman, N., Reinecke, L., Lewis, R. J., & Eden, A. (2011). Media enjoyment as need satisfaction: The contribution of hedonic and nonhedonic needs. *Journal of Communication, 61*(6), 1025–1042. doi:10.1111/j.1460-2466.2011.01593.x

Ushaw, G., Eyre, J., & Morgan, G. (2017, April). A paradigm for the development of serious games for health as benefit delivery systems. *2017 IEEE 5th International Conference on Serious Games and Applications for Health (SeGAH)*, 1–8. doi:10.1109/SeGAH.2017.7939264

Westerman, D., Spence, P. R., & Lin, X. (2015). Telepresence and exemplification in health messages: The relationships among spatial and social presence and exemplars and exemplification effects. *Communication Reports, 28*(2), 92–102. doi:10.1080/08934215.2014.971838

Wise, K., Hamman, B., & Thorson, K. (2006). Moderation, response rate, and message interactivity: Features of online communities and their effects on intent to participate. *Journal of Computer-Mediated Communication, 12*(1), 24–41. doi:10.1111/j.1083-6101.2006.00313.x

Wong, D. K.-K., & Cheung, M.-K. (2019). Online health information seeking and eHealth literacy among patients attending a primary care clinic in Hong Kong: A cross-sectional survey. *Journal of Medical Internet Research, 21*(3), e10831. doi:10.2196/10831

Yee, N. (2014). *The Proteus paradox: How online games and virtual worlds change us – and how they don't*. New Haven, CT: Yale University Press.

Yee, N., & Bailenson, J. (2007). The Proteus effect: The effect of transformed self-representation on behavior. *Human Communication Research, 33*(3), 271–290. doi:10.1111/j.1468-2958.2007.00299.x

PART V

Perspectives on the Future

16

Directions in Health Communication Theory

Dannielle E. Kelley and Brian G. Southwell

Health communication researchers have engaged a wide range of human experiences in recent decades. The chapters in this volume demonstrate that diversity. Despite that exploration, our theorizing is incomplete. As we look ahead, there are important specific questions about methods and hypotheses within each of the lines of inquiry outlined in the chapters in this volume that we should address. At the same time, we also can point to a series of general considerations about insufficiently explored theoretical dimensions of the intersection of human communication and health that could guide future health communication research.

In this chapter, we outline ways to expand health communication theorizing to reflect the dynamic communication environment we have faced and will continue to face. We also highlight ways we can better contribute to the conduct of applied health research and generate actionable insights through health communication inquiry. At least five needs, outlined below, highlight historically underdeveloped dimensions in health communication theory.

Health Communication Theory, First Edition. Edited by Teresa L. Thompson and Peter J. Schulz.
© 2021 John Wiley & Sons, Inc. Published 2021 by John Wiley & Sons, Inc.

1. The need for multilevel, systems-oriented thinking about health
2. The need for longitudinal theorizing
3. The need to consider translation, implementation, and dissemination
4. The need for integration with regulatory science
5. The need to theorize about misinformation

The Need for Multilevel, Systems-Oriented Thinking about Health

As an entity for social science, communication poses subtle challenges. Where exactly does communication reside? What is the substance to be studied? As we attempt to understand communication related to health, we not only face a process that occurs through time, but we also have various levels of human organization to consider. Some health communication researchers ask questions about interactions between patients and physicians, others ask questions about mass media systems, and yet others ask questions about message effects that involve both individuals and messages. Communication research generally faces a challenge as a body of inquiry that sits at many intersections between macro-level theorizing and available micro-level measurement, a situation that calls for multilevel theorizing and analysis in many cases (Price, Ritchie, and Eulau 1991; Southwell 2005).

What future moves could we make to acknowledge a multilevel perspective in health communication research? On an organizational level, we should find ways to encourage more multidisciplinary training among graduate students and early career researchers. Analysis methods for multilevel modeling that are now used in various social sciences, for example, highlight an interdisciplinary diffusion success story: multilevel modeling arose in part from the needs of educational researchers who attempted to study students who were growing over time as they were nested within classrooms that were nested within schools and geographic areas. Those techniques are equally relevant to patients to be screened for cancer who are nested in neighborhoods and social networks or parents making vaccination decisions as they are nested in communities and health systems. We can learn and adapt multilevel methods from various areas of inquiry that have needed such analytical tools and can articulate multilevel theories to account for key outcomes.

Health communication scholars may benefit from theoretical engagement with areas of work such as social epidemiology, in which theorizing is often done with multiple levels of influence and various actors in mind.

For example, the social contextual framework (Sorensen et al. 2003), defines a set of factors and conditions across multiple levels of influence on the pathway to behavior change. There are sociodemographic factors (e.g. social class, race, gender, age) that influence modifying conditions such as social context interpersonal factors (e.g. material circumstances, daily hassles), interpersonal factors (e.g. social ties, diversity of friendship patterns), organizational factors (e.g. social capital, job strain), neighborhood and community factors (e.g. safety, access to resources, transportation), and society factors (e.g. discrimination or stigma). These factors in turn can influence mediating mechanisms such as social norms, self-efficacy, attitudes, intentions, as well as intervention effects on variables. The sociodemographic characteristics, modifying conditions, and mediating mechanisms all sit within a set of cultural norms, standards, and expectations that also are relevant when designing interventions. From this perspective, an intervention operates either directly on a desired behavior or outcome or through mediating processes to achieve a desired change. Either way, the approach sensitizes us to the importance of considering multiple levels of variables at once.

Sorensen and colleagues (2004) demonstrate the value of using this framework in the context of smoking disparities. While individual-level behavioral theories, such as the reasoned action approach to behavior (Fishbein and Ajzen 2010) have informed smoking interventions in the United States, social inequalities in smoking prevalence persist. Using the social contextual framework, Sorensen et al. demonstrate the importance of identifying a multilevel set of potential modifying factors that can influence the success of intervention on smoking cessation among blue-collar workers (such as income-related stress, smoking prevalence within one's social network, job stress, exposure to tobacco advertising, tobacco industry targeting, and relevant policies on advertising in the communities frequented by blue-collar populations. With this multilevel framework in mind, formative research for this intervention led researchers to focus on smoking cessation interventions that also address nutrition and the need to reduce hazardous occupational exposures. Results showed that among hourly employees (who are most often exposed to hazardous occupational exposures), interventions that addressed tobacco, nutrition, and hazardous occupational exposures together were most effective in reducing the smoking prevalence, whereas the interventions that just addressed tobacco and nutrition were most effective among salaried employees who have minimal hazardous occupational exposures. By using a multilevel theoretical framework, researchers were able to address smoking prevalence among blue-collar workers with interventions implemented in the workplace.

By identifying a population and key modifying factors using a multi-level lens, message designers may design effective and salient messages to be implemented in appropriate contexts to achieve a desired health-related behavioral outcome. A multilevel framework also allows us to theorize the various ways in which factors interact within and between levels, providing the researcher with a clear map of potential influences to guide research questions and methods beyond what individual-level considerations alone might provide. Consider the effect of available social network ties on individual sharing of health information, such as in Southwell et al. (2010).

Another benefit of considering multiple levels of context is that, by doing so, key actors are more readily identified and may be intervened upon where they are physically situated, allowing for a more comprehensive solution to any health issue of concern. An example of the importance of meeting people where they are and understanding multiple facets of an issue can be found in Jeffrey Kelly's work on HIV-related behavior. Recognizing the issue of HIV stigma and risk behaviors, Kelly and colleagues sought to understand attitudes about AIDS and patients with AIDS among physicians (Kelly et al. 1987a), medical students (Kelly et al. 1987b), nurses (Kelly et al. 1988), and students (St. Lawrence et al. 1990). The researchers then went on to assess predictors of risky behavior among populations of men who have sex with men (e.g. Kelly et al. 1990) and heterosexual at-risk women (e.g. Kalichman, Hunter, and Kelly 1992). With an understanding of the cultural sensitivity and prevalence of stigma around the topic and the risk factors for key populations, researchers identified community-specific interventions that included community members as key components of the intervention as effective means in populations such as men who have sex with men (e.g. Kelly et al. 1992), and African American women (e.g. Kalichman et al. 1993). Researchers have used this perspective to find multiple influences on risk behaviors and treatment adherence (e.g. Quinn et al. 2018; Broaddus et al. 2015). In this literature, researchers have explored perceptions and behaviors relevant to HIV and AIDS through the exploration of individual, interpersonal, organizational, and cultural factors, ultimately enabling theorizing about this issue in multiple dimensions as opposed to more conventional cross-sectional approaches that focus only on individual-level factors.

Importantly, multilevel modeling techniques offer new and useful ways to empirically study questions that are familiar to many health communication researchers already. Paek, Hove, and Jeon (2013), for example, used multilevel modeling to simultaneously study the effects of message characteristics, content producer characteristics, and viewer factors on viewer response to social media content. Such empirical ability to appropriately combine data describing various entities, such as messages, people, and groups, will continue to be useful for health communication analysis and should inform theorizing for the foreseeable future.

The Need for Longitudinal Theorizing

Communication is a process that unfolds across time, a reality that complicates theorizing about health communication. Scholars of music face a similar challenge: music essentially does not exist in any one cross-sectional moment, per se, but rather resides across or through time. A longitudinal perspective, in other words, is helpful to understand music, and it is helpful to understand health-related communication. There are many instances in which health communication experts are called upon to address an immediate or precise issue for a population without adequate consideration of history or longitudinal perspective.

Here we present an example, in hindsight, of a public health problem, response, and related consequences through a 100-year case study as a starting point of discussion about ways in which longitudinal theorizing in health communication could be useful. In the early 1900s, an Argentinian doctor and chemist named Angel Honorio Roffo presented his first findings linking malignant tumors in animals to tobacco tars (Robert 2006). Between 1920 and 1940, Dr. Roffo published a series of papers linking tobacco, with and without nicotine, to cancer, spurring a series of seminal papers promoting the association that were published in top medical journals during the early 1950s (e.g. Auerbach et al. 1957; Hammond and Horn 1954; Levin, Goldstein, and Gerhardt 1953; Schrek et al. 1950; Wynder and Graham 1950). In 1954, the tobacco companies jointly published a statement of rebuttal that reached over 43 million US Americans titled, "A Frank Statement to Cigarette Smokers," in which the industry questioned the scientific evidence linking smoking to cancer, ensured consumers that cigarettes were safe (even though the same companies behind this statement often made comparative health claims to market their products), and even announced the founding of their own research council, the Tobacco Industry Research Council (TIRC), promising that they would conduct their own research to investigate the allegations against smoking and work closely with those tasked with protecting the public health (TIRC 1954). To lend credibility to the research institution, they recruited prominent and respected public health figures, such as Clarence Cook Little, director of what is now the American Cancer Society before leaving for TIRC. Despite official Surgeon General warnings of the harmful effects of smoking and health in a televised press conference in 1957, and again in the 1964 Surgeon General's Report on Smoking and Health, the tobacco industry continued to deny any harmful effects of their products. This they did by discrediting the evidence, rejecting the addictive nature of smoking and claiming smokers could quit at any time, and publishing appealing advertisements claiming the safety and health benefits of smoking through appeals to credibility with images of doctors and scientists, and through the use of attractive models and lifestyle appeals, even targeting children through the use of cartoons and strategic media placement. Right up to their testimony before Congress in 1994, US tobacco companies maintained that the evidence on smoking-related diseases was inconclusive, cigarettes were not addictive, and they did not market to children. Years later industry documents revealed the tobacco industry was aware of the link between smoking and diseases such as cancer, the addictive nature of their product, and advertising tactics that targeted vulnerable populations (Cummings, Brown, and O'Connor 2006).

Eventually, the US tobacco industries would be charged with racketeering under the RICO (Racketeer Influenced and Corrupt Organizations) Act in a 1999 ruling declaring the industry had committed unlawful deceit of the American public about the health effects of smoking for over 50 years. The industry appealed this ruling, but it was upheld and finalized in 2006, at which time the industry was mandated to release statements called the "tobacco corrective statements," to correct their deceit, These statements were not released until 2017, due to 11 years of ongoing negotiations prompted by the tobacco industry's legal team.

Why does this history matter? False and misleading communication from the industry evolved over decades. Looking only cross-sectionally at current campaign message effects elides this cultural history and could miss past missteps that also continue to affect consumer perceptions.

In 1967, the Federal Communications Commission (FCC) decided to implement a balance of cigarette advertisements and anti-smoking advertisements under the Fairness Doctrine. The initial public health campaigns often focused on the smoker as a negative role model (e.g. an advertisement depicting a son copying his father's actions, from painting the outside of the house, watering the lawn, to picking up a cigarette and to negative health effects). As time progressed, anti-smoking campaigns began to depict smokers as making an individual choice to harm themselves and those around them (prompting the Bill for Nonsmoker's Rights 1976), as stupid, unattractive, and gross, and dangerous to others through secondhand smoke. Only later did the focus began to shift to industry manipulation and the devastating consequences and loss of control from nicotine addiction (Farrelly, Niederdeppe, and Yarsevich 2003). Although campaigns proved effective in contributing to the reduction of smoking prevalence in conjunction with state and federal policy initiatives (e.g. increased cigarette tax), decades of communication focused on the smoker as an unappealing prototype to reduce smoking initiation. At the time of this focus on the smoker, many were already hooked on nicotine and smoking was a socially normative behavior in many communities. The consequence of this combined effect of industry lies and industry's stigmatizing of public health campaigns portraying a negative smoking persona – effects that likely accumulated over time – theoretically has been detrimental to current short-term efforts to help smokers quit. Stigma among social peers and the medical community, self-stigma, nihilism, and reluctance to seek help for cessation and screening service could make quitting even more difficult than it already is due to nicotine addiction. A longitudinal or historical lens could help sensitize theories of campaign effects to the potential for ingrained beliefs or preexisting communication patterns that could condition current circumstances.

The Need to Consider Translation, Implementation, and Dissemination

Another dimension for future health communication theory involves the logistical details of how messages are presented and spread through society. Glib pronouncements about the general utility of health communication campaigns to affect behavior – punditry as to whether health communication campaigns work or do not work – often do not sufficiently acknowledge that all campaigns are not equal in terms of implementation. In other words, we may not yet have sufficient information to judge the efficacy of certain campaigns because we do not know whether they actually were implemented as planned. Not only do we need to monitor campaign implementation but we also need to theorize regarding dimensions of implementation that matter most.

For example, we know that campaign exposure matters in generating viewer attention and memory for content (Southwell et al. 2002). Such exposure can be a precursor to behavior change in many instances and despite that we often do not track indicators of the extent to which a campaign has ensured adequate exposure. That measurement oversight suggests that health communication researchers could benefit from better alignment with the emerging body of work on dissemination and implementation sciences, a literature in which researchers theorize about the details of how interventions are operationalized and how that affects outcomes.

Implementation science focuses on organizational processes such as service delivery and clinical interaction. Practitioners involved in the delivery of care or the diffusion of policies often point to a range of situational factors that can affect whether organizations achieve the outcomes intended when new innovations are introduced. Those factors include, among others, considerations of innovation acceptability among staff, feasibility of implementation, fidelity of implementation, and even sustainability of adoption over time (Weiner et al. 2017). Measurement of such factors is still not settled practice in all cases, but an active body of research has regularly moved us closer to widely available tools for assessing such considerations.

By adopting practices from the implementation science arena in our future research on public health communication, particularly with regard to campaigns, we will not only gain new empirical evidence to inform theory, e.g. suggesting weight loss or weight maintenance campaigns work best not only with certain message strategies but under certain conditions of implementation, but we also might set the stage for more productive learning across campaign and intervention experiences. Rather than highlighting evidence for success or failure of interventions that are somewhat inscrutable as to their logistical details, we might contribute to a collective learning environment by finding ways to inquire about and publicize the details of various project experiences.

Consider two examples to publicize implementation details that could inform future theorizing about campaigns: the VERB and The Real Cost campaigns, both widely considered to be successful in achieving purported goals. The VERB campaign was released in 2003 and was based on a social marketing approach that relied on theories of message design, information processing, and behavior change to promote physical activity among adolescents aged 9 to 13 years old (Huhman, Hetzler, and Wong 2004). Evidence suggests the campaign encouraged positive changes in physical activity among the target population that persisted as children grew outside of the target age range (Huhman et al. 2005; Huhman et al. 2007; Huhman et al. 2010). The Real Cost campaign was released in 2014 and has sought to make youth (12–17) aware of the real cost of each cigarette with novel portrayals of the health effects and addiction associated with smoking; after two years, this campaign was credited with preventing over 300 000 youth from starting smoking (Crosby 2019).

Both campaigns were implemented based on a priori development of behavior change logic models, a best practice in social marketing that provides campaign planners with an illustration of how the proposed campaign is hypothesized to work to achieve desired outcomes through campaign activities and theoretical mechanisms. However, these campaigns developed logic models in different ways and used a variety of methods for message development and testing; we know about these different experiences through descriptions of implementation.

The VERB campaign incorporated theories of message design and behavior and information processing along with branding theory (Huhman, Hetzler, and Wong 2004). The Real Cost campaign uses a media market approach that emphasizes iterative audience research and allows them to adapt to changes in the communication environment and compete with companies asking for much simpler exchange – money for a product promising immediate satisfaction (Crosby 2019) – while The Real Cost is trying to prevent adolescents from making that exchange when it comes to cigarettes (Farrelly et al. 2017). The VERB campaign relied on stated theories of message design, information processing, behavior change, and branding to develop and test messages using extensive formative research; the exact tools and findings appear as a supplement in an article published in the *American Journal of Preventive Medicine* (Berkowitz et al. 2008).

The Real Cost campaign took a different approach by analyzing quantitative data and developing a set of 151 beliefs representing different potential messaging themes (Brennan et al. 2017). These beliefs were subsequently tested in additional quantitative and qualitative testing before the most promising beliefs were taken to production and concept tested. Details of the development, formative research, and initial five years of campaign evaluation also can be found in a special issue of the *American Journal of Preventive Medicine* (see Brubach 2019).

When health communication scholars publish formative research and the details of how campaign efforts were implemented, rather than just focusing on reporting whether an effort worked, this provides future generations of health communication researchers with data that could inform theory. Theorizing about health communication effects could and should include accounts of exactly how messages are presented in addition to accounts of what types of messages will have desired effects.

Moreover, theorizing about implementation and dissemination can allow us to connect health communication scholarship to health services research, media sociology, and a variety of other relevant areas of inquiry.

The Need for Integration with Regulatory Science

A crucial observation among twentieth-century health communication scholars was the notion that mass media content can affect health-related behavior regardless of the impact of any specific public health campaign or educational intervention (Hornik 2000). To rightly conceptualize the effect of media content on health-related perceptions and behavior linked to health, we need to understand the information environment in which people operate every day and not just focus on materials developed by health professionals. That information environment can include the fruits of outreach by public health professionals, but it also can include television shows and movies and advertisements for commercial goods. At least some of those advertised goods fall under the jurisdiction of regulatory agencies, suggesting a role for communication researchers in supporting regulation and another avenue for future health communication theory. In the United States, for example, the US Food and Drug Administration (FDA) reviews direct-to-consumer advertising and marketing related to prescription drugs, tobacco, and other products. Social science research by communication scholars has begun to inform that regulation in recent years and future years will likely offer numerous opportunities for health communication researchers to support decision-making about shaping the information environments with which patients and consumers interact.

Noar, Cappella, and Price (2019) have written about opportunities for communication researchers to provide empirical evidence of consumer interaction with information about tobacco and nicotine, for example. Under the 2009 Family Smoking Prevention and Tobacco Control Act, the FDA received authority to regulate tobacco products in the United States. Under the act, the FDA must use scientific evidence to inform its actions. Regarding the marketing of tobacco, communication research that documents and explains consumer understanding of the language used to promote tobacco offers a vital resource. Noar and colleagues note the example of FDA action to ask cigarette manufacturers to cease using the words "natural" and "additive-free" in advertising. Such a decision reflects evidence that such terms can mislead consumers by suggesting cigarettes advertised with those labels are somehow less harmful than others to consumer health.

To be useful to regulatory considerations, the kinds of questions health communication researchers can ask about advertised products need to resonate with regulatory decision-making. To this end, communication research in recent years has begun to focus on specific elements of advertisements that are subject to regulatory input. One example of this is a price comparison claim in a prescription drug advertisement that compares the price of drug products from different companies. Researchers have investigated physician and patient response to such claims in a prescription drug and specifically have investigated whether contextualizing such information, e.g. by noting that price equivalence does not necessarily indicate drug efficacy equivalence, can usefully affect viewer response to an advertisements' claims (Betts et al. 2017).

One aspect of regulatory science that offers nuance and complexity for communication researchers to consider is the reactive nature of some regulatory responses to the unfolding information environment. The FDA can identify and respond to problematic advertising claims, for example, by requesting corrective advertising efforts by the advertisers responsible for the original problematic claims. Here again, communication research can be relevant for consideration, e.g. Aikin et al. (2015).

What exactly the most relevant and appropriate outcomes to investigate are is not always a straightforward consideration in the case of correction. Whereas a conventional campaign evaluation might investigate whether population-level behavior simply has increased, research on the effects of corrective advertising should consider whether exposure to a corrective advertisement eliminates the effect of originally problematic claims, a claim effect itself which likely does not occur in a vacuum. Ensuring that corrective information counteracts a problematic claim in an essentially surgical fashion, only affecting perceptions encouraged by the problematic claims, can be challenging work requiring careful experimental designs that nonetheless also reflect the realities of the consumer marketplace.

Communication researchers can contribute to regulatory science in numerous ways, including support through innovative study methods and development of reliable and valid measures of perceptions. Kelly et al. (2017) report on the validation of a bank of measures of viewer perceptions of direct-to-consumer prescription drugs and direct-to-consumer prescription drug advertisements, for example. The range of potentially relevant patient perceptions is considerable, as it needs to reflect various ways that patients understand drugs to work. Not only do we need to know the extent to which patients believe a drug will have its purported effects generally, for example, but we also need to understand for whom patients think those effects are most likely to occur. We need to know what patients think the benefits of a prescription drug to be, but we also need to know what patients think the risks of drugs will be. We also need to know when and how often patients are physically exposed to direct-to-consumer advertisements and the extent to which they accurately learn information from them.

Importantly, the consumer marketplace also tends to evolve over time, sometimes offering new, previously unavailable products. That suggests another role for communication research. Consider the example of dissolvable tobacco products that arrived in US consumer markets in the early part of the twenty-first century. In 2009 and 2010, advertising for dissolvable tobacco products increased substantially, which meant consumers faced more information about this new type of product than previously (RTI International 2011). Understanding how current smokers respond to various descriptions of dissolvable products and how such new products tend to be used, e.g. as supplements to, rather than replacements for, smoked products, became relevant questions for the FDA. Social scientists, in turn, could help to answer such questions, e.g. O'Connor et al. (2011).

Regulatory science needs communication research insofar as regulation involves oversight of communication between various entities. In order to most helpfully contribute in the future, however, communication researchers nonetheless will need to be cognizant of the needs of regulatory decision-makers, which sometimes differ from those of the clients for evaluations of public health media campaigns.

The Need to Theorize about Misinformation

Misinformation has been a topic of concern for social scientists in recent years given the speed and frequency with which information may be composed, disseminated, and shared across networks through a variety of platforms, and yet deception and inaccuracy in communication is deeply rooted in the human experience. How might health communication theory address and accommodate misinformation?

A first step will be continued refinement in the definition of what we mean by misinformation. The term misinformation is sometimes conflated with disinformation, which we can think of as deliberately false information created with the intent to cause harm; for our discussion here, we can use the broader umbrella notion of misinformation, which focuses on factual inaccuracy regardless of authorial intention (Southwell, Thorson, and Sheble 2017; Stahl 2006). Both misinformation and disinformation theoretically are relevant to health communication theorizing insofar as inaccurate information could lead people to behave (or not behave) in ways that are at odds with what they might do in circumstances of fully accurate information.

As a consideration for future health communication theorizing, there also are numerous caveats about the concept of misinformation we should raise. We can consider misinformation not as a monolithic force, for example, but as theoretically variable content that can range in harm (from inconsequential to acute threat), can stem from a multitude of actors or circumstances, can appear in numerous communication channels, and is potentially dependent upon context and time for meaning (Southwell et al. 2019). Rather than seeking to wrangle the multifaceted notion of misinformation into a concise and consistent source of harm, we can take a broader approach that considers misinformation as a set of different types of inaccuracies occurring in different situations that sometimes could be relevant for health communication theory. We need to develop a set of comprehensive theories and frameworks around misinformation relevant across a continuum of harms, stages (development, dissemination, processing, sharing), modes of communication, regulatory environments, and individual and cultural differences.

Although misinformation could be the consequence of a simple misunderstanding or misremembering, in some cases dissemination of misinformation also sometimes may signal a wealth of valuable information about cultural values, fears, desires, discrimination, or desperation as people try to make sense of health threats, all of which are worth considering when searching for effective ways to communicate about health with various populations. The mere presence of misinformation does not always constitute a problem among people, per se, as many pieces of misinformation fail to gain traction or agreement among others, and yet some types of misinformation spread rapidly and may call for remedy. Scholars have acknowledged that not all misinformation is necessarily bad and, in fact, may serve some social purpose sometimes (e.g. endorsing something known to be false but nonetheless topically resonate with a group's values can be a way to assimilate into a social group). We must also consider the unintended consequences of correcting misinformation, from wasted resources chasing down facts in order to combat a trivial piece of misinformation likely to dissipate on its own to overlooking a community's cultural and social values related to an instance of misinformation.

Various new projects and commentary from researchers about misinformation have highlighted different aspects of misinformation-related processes (e.g. message construction, reception, or dissemination). From this work, a variety of concepts have emerged that could inform future health communication theorizing involving misinformation. For example, a partnership between the social media platform Twitter and the nonprofit organization Cortico – see https://www.cortico.ai – has focused on what researchers at those organizations call the "health of a conversation" that can be described in terms of four indicators: shared attention, shared reality, variety of opinion, and receptivity (civility and the ability to listen to different opinions). Such indicators may be relevant in judging the diffusion and response to misinformation over time.

Some researchers such as Hastak and Mazis (2011) have developed ideas about types of misleading communication in advertising that are relevant to future theory. They highlight five main categories of problems: (i) omission of facts; (ii) semantic confusion (unclear language, symbols, imagery); (iii) intra-attribute misleadingness (e.g. "No cholesterol" claims on food packaging implying other brands contain cholesterol without an explicit statement of such); (iv) inter-attribute misleadingness (e.g. "low cholesterol" leading people to believe the product is low in fat, even though that's not necessarily true), and (v) source-based misleadingness (e.g. a doctor's endorsement for a product leading consumers to believe the product is safe and healthy). Such efforts at problem categorization are important, but we also now need theory to account for the interaction of the many actors, contexts, and subsequent psychological and behavioral mechanisms that we are identifying.

What can we say about visual misinformation or other forms of misinformation beyond written text? Many varieties of communication media have been insufficiently considered to date in the case of misinformation. How do visuals act on their own or in tandem with text to convey and persuade the spread of misinformation, for example? What about videos? Popular music lyrics? How do these challenges interact with information disparities? Ultimately, misinformation is a systems-level challenge that requires an orientation towards systems-level and future-oriented remedies that acknowledges the complexity of our current information environment (Southwell et al. 2019). Invoking misinformation in future health communication theories similarly should acknowledge these complexities.

Summary

We have identified five dimensions of theory that current and future generations of health communication scholars should pursue. This set of ideas may inspire programs of research that move health communication toward actionable insights to address current public health issues. Scholars can reenvision existing demographic variables, community descriptors, message characteristics, and behavioral outcomes in multilevel models. They should consider health communication processes and consequences over time and should consider the historical context of interventions. We can develop theoretical accounts of why and how intervention logistics matter. We also can connect our work to the work of regulatory agencies and watchdogs. We can theorize about the roles of misinformation as well as of information. By doing so, health communication scholars will improve the chances of their work being leveraged to achieve positive change. In an age in which technologies create opportunities to advance public health and introduce detriments to public health, health communication scholars are positioned to ask new questions about how and why communication using new and old technologies might affect (and be affected by) health. Optimizing real-life application of our work will require interdisciplinary and multidisciplinary efforts in addition to identifying ways in which health communication theory may complement and contribute to public health and medicine.

References

Aikin, K. J., Betts, K. R., O'Donoghue, A. C., Rupert, D. J., Lee, P. K., Amoozegar, J. B., & Southwell, B. G. (2015). Correction of overstatement and omission in direct-to-consumer prescription drug advertising. *Journal of Communication, 65*(4), 596–618.

Auerbach, O., Gere, J. B., Forman, J. B., Petrick, T. G., Smolin, H. J., Muehsam, G. E., . . . Stout, A. P. (1957). Changes in the bronchial epithelium in relation to smoking and cancer of the lung: A report of progress. *New England Journal of Medicine, 256*(3), 97–104.

Betts, K., Aikin, K., Boudewyns, V., Johnson, M., Stine, A., & Southwell, B. (2017). Physician response to contextualized price-comparison claims in prescription drug advertising. *Journal of Communication in Healthcare, 10*(3), 195–204.

Berkowitz, J. M., Huhman, M., Heitzler, C. D., Potter, L. D., Nolin, M. J., & Banspach, S. W. (2008). Overview of formative, process, and outcome evaluation methods used in the VERB™ campaign. *American Journal of Preventive Medicine, 34*(6), S222–S229.

Brennan, E., Gibson, L. A., Kybert-Momjian, A., Liu, J., & Hornik, R. C. (2017). Promising themes for antismoking campaigns targeting youth and young adults. *Tobacco Regulatory Science, 3*(1), 29–46.

Broaddus, M. R., DiFranceisco, W. J., Kelly, J. A., Lawrence, J. S. S., Amirkhanian, Y. A., & Dickson-Gomez, J. D. (2015). Social media use and high-risk sexual behavior among black men who have sex with men: A three-city study. *AIDS and Behavior, 19*(2), 90–97.

Brubach, A. L. (2019). The case and context for "The Real Cost" campaign. *American Journal of Preventive Medicine, 56*(2, Suppl. 1), s5–s8.

Crosby, K. (2019). How the Food and Drug Administration convinced teens to rethink their relationship with cigarettes. *American Journal of Preventive Medicine, 56*(2), s1–s4.

Cummings, K. M., Brown, A., & O'Connor, R. (2007). The cigarette controversy. *Cancer Epidemiology and Prevention Biomarkers, 16*(6), 1070–1076.

Farrelly, M. C., Duke, J. C., Nonnemaker, J., MacMonegle, A. J., Alexander, T. N., Zhao, X., . . . Allen, J. A. (2017). Association between the real cost media campaign and smoking initiation among youths – United States, 2014–2016. *MMWR. Morbidity and Mortality Weekly Report, 66*(2), 47.

Farrelly, M. C., Niederdeppe, J., & Yarsevich, J. (2003). Youth tobacco prevention mass media campaigns: Past, present, and future directions. *Tobacco Control, 12*(suppl. 1), i35–i47.

Fishbein, M., & Ajzen, I. (2010). *Predicting and changing behavior: The reasoned action approach.* New York, NY: Psychology Press.

Hammond, E. C., & Horn, D. (1954). The relationship between human smoking habits and death rates: A follow-up study of 187,766 men. *JAMA, 155*, 1316–1328.

Hastak, M., & Mazis, M. B. (2011). Deception by implication: A typology of truthful but misleading advertising and labeling claims. *Journal of Public Policy & Marketing, 30*(2), 157–167.

Hornik, R.C. (Ed.). (2000). *Public health communication: Evidence for behavior change.* Mahwah, NJ: Erlbaum.

Huhman, M., Heitzler, C., & Wong, F. (2004). The VERB™ campaign logic model: A tool for planning and evaluation. *Preventing Chronic Disease, 1*(3).

Huhman, M., Potter, L. D., Wong, F. L., Banspach, S. W., Duke, J. C., & Heitzler, C. D. (2005). Effects of a mass media campaign to increase physical activity among children: Year-1 results of the VERB campaign. *Pediatrics, 116*(2), e277.

Huhman, M. E., Potter, L. D., Duke, J. C., Judkins, D. R., Heitzler, C. D., & Wong, F. L. (2007). Evaluation of a national physical activity intervention for children: VERB™ campaign, 2002–2004. *American Journal of Preventive Medicine, 32*(1), 38–43.

Huhman, M. E., Potter, L. D., Nolin, M. J., Piesse, A., Judkins, D. R., Banspach, S. W., & Wong, F. L. (2010). The influence of the VERB campaign on children's physical activity in 2002 to 2006. *American Journal of Public Health, 100*(4), 638–645.

Kalichman, S. C., Hunter, T. L., & Kelly, J. A. (1992). Perceptions of AIDS susceptibility among minority and nonminority women at risk for HIV infection. *Journal of Consulting and Clinical Psychology, 60*(5), 725.

Kalichman, S. C., Kelly, J. A., Hunter, T. L., Murphy, D. A., & Tyler, R. (1993). Culturally tailored HIV-AIDS risk-reduction messages targeted to African-American urban women: Impact on risk sensitization and risk reduction. *Journal of Consulting and Clinical Psychology, 61*(2), 291.

Kelly, B. J., Rupert, D., Aikin, K., Sullivan, H., Johnson, M., West, S., . . . Rabre, A. (2017). Development and validation of patient-reported risk, efficacy and benefit measures in the context of DTC prescription drug advertising. *Pharmacoepidemiology and Drug Safety, 26*, 447–448.

Kelly, J. A., St. Lawrence, J. S., Smith Jr, S., Hood, H. V., & Cook, D. J. (1987a). Stigmatization of AIDS patients by physicians. *American Journal of Public Health, 77*(7), 789–791.

Kelly, J. A., St. Lawrence, J. S., Smith, S., Hood, H. V., & Cook, D. J. (1987b). Medical students' attitudes toward AIDS and homosexual patients. *Journal of Medical Education, 62*(7), 549–556.

Kelly, J. A., St. Lawrence, J. S., Hood, H. V., Smith, S., & Cook, D. J. (1988). Nurses' attitudes toward AIDS. *Journal of Continuing Education in Nursing, 19*(2), 78–83.

Kelly, J. A., St. Lawrence, J. S., Brasfield, T. L., Lemke, A., Amidei, T., Roffman, R. E., . . . McNeill Jr, C. (1990). Psychological factors that predict AIDS high-risk versus AIDS precautionary behavior. *Journal of Consulting and Clinical Psychology, 58*(1), 117.

Kelly, J. A., St Lawrence, J. S., Stevenson, L. Y., Hauth, A. C., Kalichman, S. C., Diaz, Y. E., . . . Morgan, M. G. (1992). Community AIDS/HIV risk reduction: The effects of endorsements by popular people in three cities. *American Journal of Public Health, 82*(11), 1483–1489.

Levin, M. L., Goldstein, H., & Gerhardt, P. R. (1950). Cancer and tobacco smoking: A preliminary report. *Journal of the American Medical Association, 143*(4), 336–338.

Noar, S. M., Cappella, J. N., & Price, S. (2019). Communication regulatory science: Mapping a new field. *Health Communication, 34*(3), 273–279.

O'Connor, R. J., Norton, K. J., Bansal-Travers, M., Mahoney, M. C., Cummings, M., Borland, R. (2011). US smokers' reactions to a brief trial of oral nicotine products. *Harm Reduction Journal, 8*(1). doi:10.1186/1477-7517-8-1

Paek, H. J., Hove, T., & Jeon, J. (2013). Social media for message testing: A multilevel approach to linking favorable viewer responses with message, producer, and viewer influence on YouTube. *Health Communication, 28*(3), 226–236.

Price, V., Ritchie, L. D., & Eulau, H. (1991). Cross-level challenges for communication research: Epilogue. *Communication Research, 18*(2), 262–271.

Quinn, K. G., Reed, S. J., Dickson-Gomez, J., & Kelly, J. A. (2018). An exploration of syndemic factors that influence engagement in HIV care among Black men. *Qualitative Health Research, 28*(7), 1077–1087.

RTI International. (2011). *Tobacco industry monitoring monthly report: April 2011* (Report prepared for the Florida Bureau of Tobacco Prevention Program). Research Triangle Park, NC: RTI International.

Robert, P. N., (2006). The forgotten father of experimental tobacco carcinogenesis. *Bulletin of the World Health Organization, 84*: 494–496.

Schrek, R., Baker, L.A., Ballard, G.P., & Dolgoff, S. (1950). Tobacco smoking as an etiologic factor in disease. *Cancer Research, 10,* 49–58.

Sorensen, G., Barbeau, E., Hunt, M. K., & Emmons, K. (2004). Reducing social disparities in tobacco use: A social-contextual model for reducing tobacco use among blue-collar workers. *American Journal of Public Health, 94*(2), 230–239.

Sorensen, G., Emmons, K., Hunt, M. K., Barbeau, E., Goldman, R., Peterson, K., . . . Berkman, L. (2003). Model for incorporating social context in health behavior interventions: Applications for cancer prevention for working-class, multiethnic populations. *Preventive Medicine, 37*(3), 188–197.

Southwell, B. G. (2005). Between messages and people: A multilevel model of memory for television content. *Communication Research, 32*(1), 112–140.

Southwell, B. G., Barmada, C. H., Hornik, R. C., & Maklan, D. M. (2002). Can we measure encoded exposure? Validation evidence from a national campaign. *Journal of Health Communication, 7*(5), 445–453.

Southwell, B. G., Kim, A. E., Tessman, G. K., MacMonegle, A. J., Choiniere, C. J., Evans, S. E., & Johnson, R. D. (2012). The marketing of dissolvable tobacco: Social science and public policy research needs. *American Journal of Health Promotion, 26*(6), 331–332.

Southwell, B. G., Slater, J. S., Rothman, A. J., Friedenberg, L. M., Allison, T. R., & Nelson, C. L. (2010). The availability of community ties predicts likelihood of peer referral for mammography: Geographic constraints on viral marketing. *Social Science & Medicine, 71*(9), 1627–1635.

Southwell, B. G., Thorson, E. A., & Sheble, L. (2017). The persistence and peril of misinformation. *American Scientist, 105*(6), 372–375.

St. Lawrence, J. S., Husfeldt, B. A., Kelly, J. A., Hood, H. V., & Smith, Jr, S. (1990). The stigma of AIDS: Fear of disease and prejudice toward gay men. *Journal of Homosexuality, 19*(3), 85–102.

Stahl, B. C. (2006). On the difference or equality of information, misinformation, and disinformation: A critical research perspective. *Informing Science, 9.*

Tobacco Industry Research Committee. (1954, Jan 4). *A frank statement to cigarette smokers.* (Bates Number: 980014685).

Weiner, B. J., Lewis, C. C., Stanick, C., Powell, B. J., Dorsey, C. N., Clary, A. S., . . . Halko, H. (2017). Psychometric assessment of three newly developed implementation outcome measures. *Implementation Science, 12*: 108. doi:10.1186/s13012-017-0635-3

Wynder, E. L., & Graham, E. A., (1950). Tobacco smoking as a possible etiologic factor in bronchogenic carcinoma. *JAMA, 143,* 329–336.

Index

Health Communication Theory, First Edition. Edited by Teresa L. Thompson
and Peter J. Schulz.
© 2021 John Wiley & Sons, Inc. Published 2021 by John Wiley & Sons, Inc.